NATIONAL COLLEGE OF EXERCISE PROFESSIONALS

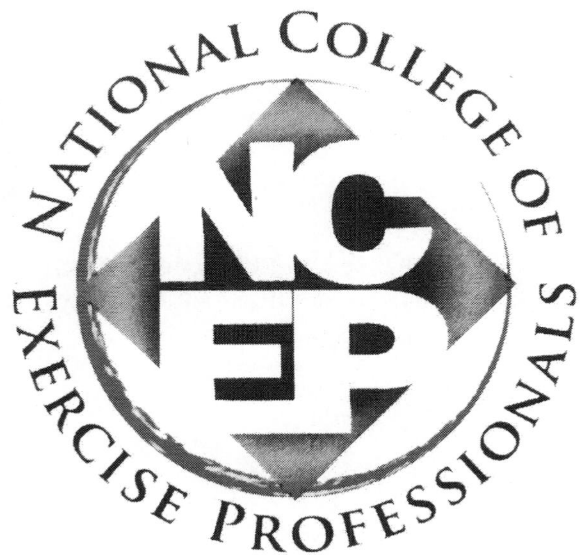

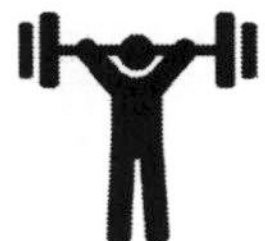 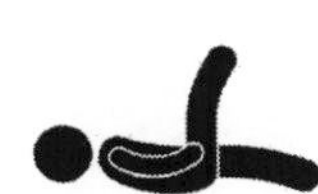 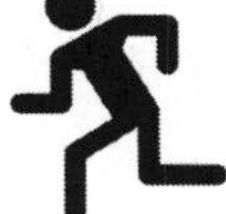 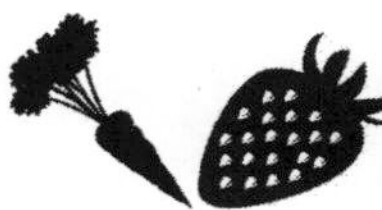 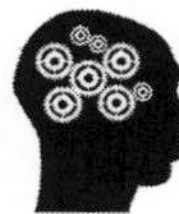

Standard Certification Manual

and

Study Guide

NCEPFITNESS.COM

Published by Critical Minds Press in Los Angeles, CA

THIRD EDITION published in December 2017.

Manual written by Michael DeMora and Barry M. Goldenberg
Chapter Eight written by Adam James, Michael DeMora, and Barry M. Goldenberg
Chapter Nine written by Michele Bond

Cover Design and Interior Layout by Barry M. Goldenberg

Cover photo courtesy of K.C. Ushijima at www.kcworkout.com

All photographs used in this manual are part of the 'public domain', under a Creative Commons license (in which attributions are provided), used with permission, or owned by NCEP.

ISBN-13: 978-0692512708
ISBN-10: 0692512705

Printed in the United States of America

A WELCOME LETTER

First and foremost, thank you for choosing NCEP. We sincerely appreciate your business, and so will all your future clients. Admittedly, that probably sounds a little odd coming from a personal training organization. The fact is, however, is that we are much, much more than an organization that teaches personal training—we are an organization dedicated to creating knowledgeable exercise professionals whom are passionate about changing lives. One major aspect that sets us apart is that our pedagogy focuses more on personal coaching than just personal training alone. In connection, our philosophy is that the coach works together with the client to help him/her co-create a new healthier lifestyle through a holistic approach.

A *Holistic* Personal Trainer Certification

Yet, what do we mean by the commonly repeated phrase, a 'healthy lifestyle'? To us, a healthy lifestyle consists of more than just running on a treadmill or lifting some weights, and it is far more extensive than just what we do in the gym. For decades, we at the NCEP have recognized that a healthy lifestyle is all-encompassing, and have designed a certification around this underlying fact. Thus, we believe that this manual and our accompanying Standard Certification course is one of the first ***holistic personal training certifications.*** The goal of this course is, in part, to provide you both the tools to design personalized and cutting-edge training sessions for clients—generally made up of resistance training—as well as fill in the gaps between these sessions in ways that can vastly improve your clients' (and your own) quality of life. Far too many trainers fail to become knowledgeable about the latter and it is this holistic approach, we believe, that can separate you from other trainers. Knowing more practical threads of knowledge, quite simply, means you can offer more life-changing information and instruction to your clientele—and we strive to only present material that is practical and directly applicable for clients of all ages and abilities.

To be sure, holistic is certainly another popular "buzz" word common in our industry, one that is often misunderstood and frequently diluted by slick marketing. (Our industry has a whole list of these "buzz" words, such as "functional training" and "core," both of which we discuss throughout this manual.) To avoid any such confusion with the term holistic, here is a dictionary definition:

Holistic: *relating to or concerned with wholes or with complete systems rather than with the analysis of, treatment of, or dissection into parts*

Jargon aside, that definition really makes sense to us, and we hope it will eventually make sense to you, too. This idea that we, as humans, should be concerned with "wholes or complete systems" rather than separate parts is profound (even if this concept itself is as old as civilization). Now, think about this definition with regards to personal training on both micro and macro levels. On a micro level, for example, kinesiology (the science of how the body moves) tells us that the body is not just a hodgepodge of muscles working in isolation, but a collection of muscles working together to perform complex movements. On a macro level, to be healthy, people need more than resistance training alone (i.e., to increase bone density and muscle mass), but also need to have a high level of cardiovascular health (i.e., a healthy heart) and proper nutritional intake (i.e., to receive life-sustaining nutrients). Thinking holistically about how the body moves as well as what the body needs overall is, in our minds, extremely important to helping yourself and others live a healthy lifestyle. This concept of holistic practices, while not always explicit throughout the manual and the course, is the foundation for which our Five Components of Fitness and entire our curricular model is premised on.

Ultimately, we believe that understanding this important principle will not only make you a better trainer, but a more successful one, too. The information, tools, and guidelines in this manual and emphasized throughout the course will help you create true and lasting lifestyle changes for your clients by getting them healthy. In turn, others will notice that what you do is different and that it works, as being a holistic personal trainer will set you apart within the health and fitness world.

An Overview of the NCEP Manual and Standard Certification Course

Returning to our mantra around the importance of a holistic approach, we at the NCEP have put together this course in which you will learn far more than a series of exercises and simple charts. For example, this manual and course teaches **resistance training** by focusing on movements, not muscles, because that is a more holistic (not to mention a more scientifically sound) view. You will learn that **nutritional guidance** is more than simply calories in and calories out because if that were true, then cookies would be just as healthy as organic carrots. **Cardiovascular training** is understood as more than a means of fat loss, but how to train for a healthy heart and circulatory system. **Flexibility training** becomes more than just stretching, but the maintenance of healthy joints and their range of motion. And finally, we introduce the notion of **attitude training** by explaining that a person's mental capacity can significantly influence his/her physical state. Each of these topics make up what we believe to be the **Five Components of Fitness.** Learning about all of these components alone would be well worth your time and efforts, and you would already be one of the more knowledgeable trainers within the industry. Of course, our course is much more than just these five components, as we also cover additional standard topics such as anatomy, metabolic pathways, postural assessments, physiology, health history, etc.

However, what will truly make you stand out as a trainer and, most importantly, what will make you so well equipped to change the lives of your clients is an understanding of the relationship that each one of these components has with the other. You will understand the amazing and intricate woven web of a healthy lifestyle. To refer back to the aforementioned holistic definition, you can only view the body correctly as a series of interacting systems. Remember, your health and the health of your clients is a by-product of many healthy systems interacting. Again, although it is necessary to understand resistance training on its own, you also need to know that resistance training affects cardiovascular training and vice versa. As we have already stated, we wholeheartedly believe that you will learn how to change lifestyles and lives, but we continue to re-iterate it because it is the heart of who we are as an organization and what we believe should be your mission as an exercise professional. This manual and our course reflect this core belief.

Yet, to achieve these goals, you need the proper tools and information presented in a digestible and accessible way—a way that is heavily based on science but can be easily understood and applied by the everyday person. Thus, this manual and our course also reflect our attempt to satisfy the dire need for a practical handbook for beginning personal trainers (or, as we hope, trainers seeking to learn a holistic approach or simply seeking more education). Everything in this manual is carefully selected to provide you with all the baseline information we believe is needed to be a highly knowledgeable trainer while also making sure to provide additional reference information and training advice that can be used throughout your career as a valuable resource.

The Role of Motivation and the Difficulty of Adopting a Healthy Lifestyle

Although we will discuss this more in our first chapter on the definition of personal training, it is crucial to initially understand that the concept of motivation connects to every aspect of the profession. We believe that one of the most important pieces of advice that every trainer should internalize revolves around being acutely aware, at all times, of the trainer-client relationship; your job as a trainer is to keep your client from getting de-motivated and to inspire him/her to live a healthy lifestyle. Unsurprisingly, this is one of the biggest challenges of personal coaching—trying to keep a person motivated long enough to create a lasting lifestyle change (plus not to mention continue his/her training sessions with you). All of your clients will have been motivated to some degree to schedule an appointment with you, but maintaining that motivation can be quite challenging. Too often, trainers forget that keeping clients motivated—if not inspired and energized—is the key to their success in this industry. For this reason, we believe that you should always keep this notion of motivation front and center, as every exercise you suggest and program you design should be predicated on this notion of keeping a client motivated.

Yet, why is it so difficult to get people to adopt and maintain a healthy lifestyle? Everyone knows that there are endless benefits to being healthy that we all want to receive. For us to understand why people lack motivation, we need to look at why people want to be healthy in the first place.
Part of this can be understood by realizing that our clients' health and nutrition objectives are multi-fold, as knowing the client's individual needs allows you to develop a variety of motivational strategies. Getting people started on a healthy program and maintaining him/her as a client should be as important to you as it to them.

More specifically, it is common to divide the motivation factors into intrinsic and extrinsic rewards. Intrinsic means that you are motivated internally and you want it for yourself whereas extrinsic means there is an outside force that is motivating you to do something. Although both types of motivation can help your clients begin, it is more likely for clients to continue with a healthy lifestyle over time if they are intrinsically motivated. Remember, your job, if you are willing to accept it, is to get your client to enjoy being healthy and all that it entails. Internalize that you are more than just a personal trainer, but a coach and a true exercise professional dedicated helping people live healthy lives. It all starts with motivation, and we begin the manual with this note because no matter how knowledgeable a trainer might be or how great his/her program is, it matters little if the client is no longer motivated to reach his/her goals. Always remember this important principle as you progress both through this manual and throughout your career.

Responsibilities as an NCEP Trainer

Whether you are entering the world of personal training for the first time or only continuing your education after many years of experience, know that we are proud to be your certification of choice and/or your choice for continuing education. All we ask of you is to keep an open mind and again, always stay committed to helping people adopt a healthy lifestyle. We are committed to staying on the cutting edge of exercise science and personal training, and we hope you are too. We welcome you as NCEP alumni and congratulate your professionalism, which, we believe, will be second to none. By taking this course with us, we always welcome your input and suggestions for improving, so do no not hesitate to drop us note and stay connected. With your help, we can make a difference in people's lives now and in the future.

Also understand, however, that as a certified exercise professional from NCEP, you are asked to follow the guidelines outlined in this manual. We hope you live by the professional responsibilities discussed therein, and that you take your profession as a personal trainer very seriously. Thus, it is important to first understand the scope of your responsibility, particularly since clients often ask for a variety of services. Even though we believe your NCEP certification will provide you both the necessary science and practical skills to become a successful trainer in the industry, there are inherent limitations to your position. You are not a physician, physical therapist, chiropractor, registered dietician, massage therapist, or social worker. Practicing these disciplines is not within the scope of your responsibilities or professional training. This applies to assessing clients, too; we believe in assessing the client only to determine how they are functioning and never to diagnose or treat conditions. The purpose of the assessment process is to make better exercise choices for our clients witih specific regards to program design and general health.

In connection, understand that trainers provide exercise programs—*not* exercise prescriptions. Even the word prescription has the connotation that it has been given by a doctor. We produce exercise programs that we suggest our clients follow, not mandate. The NCEP has very high standards of professionalism and we would like our coaches to hold themselves to this same standard. For example, and as we discuss throughout this course, we think it is important to document client information that is pertinent to the his/her well being and always put the client's health first. As a general guideline, we suggest that all coaches follow not only our NCEP guidelines but established guidelines by the American College of Sports Medicine (ACSM) and the World Health Organization (WHO) that are referred to throughout. Also, we suggest you follow your given common sense—when it comes to your health, no one knows better than you what is right.

Conclusion: Changing the World, One Trainer at a Time

In conclusion, always internalize that you have a tremendous impact on how your clients feel about the profession of personal training. By creating a very positive and motivating experience for your clients, they will enjoy your coaching so much—all the while becoming healthier—that they will suggest both your services and lifestyle changes to their peers. Our mission is to change people's lives by co-creating a healthy lifestyle and at the same time redefine the personal training industry that is more holistic in scope. Our mission depends on you. You must never forget that coaching an individual to better health is both a tremendous opportunity *and* responsibility. There is an old saying that people do not care what you know until they know that you care. Please care, find your passion in fitness, and go share it with the world—we will all be better for it.

In good health,
National College of Exercise Professionals

TABLE OF CONTENTS

STANDARD CERTIFICATION
STUDY GUIDE

Chapter One – *WHAT IS PERSONAL TRAINING?*

1. Name at least 5 benefits of exercise.

Chapter Two – *FIVE COMPONENTS OF FITNESS*

1. What are the five components of fitness?
2. What is a calorie?
3. Define active stretching. Give an example.
4. Define passive stretching. Give an example.
5. Define static stretching. Give an example.
6. Define ballistic stretching. Give an example.
7. What is the blood pressure?
8. What is the formula for training heart rate?
9. Define endurance.
10. Define strength.
11. Define power.
12. What is your core?

Chapter Three – *HEALTH HISTORY*

1. List at least 5 cardiac risk factors.
2. List at least 3 signs and symptoms of cardiopulmonary disease.
3. What are the 3 risk stratifications?

Chapter Four – *ASSESSMENTS*

1. Why do we start any program with assessments?
2. What is the purpose of the overhead squat?
3. What is the purpose of the push-up hold?
4. Why do we assess leg lowering?
5. What does the term multi-planar mean in the multi-planar step and hold?
6. What are the bio-motor abilities?

Chapter Five – *NUTRITION*

1. What are the 5 components to a healthy eating strategy?
2. What are the 6 essential nutrients?
3. How many calories are given off from 1 gram of Protein? Carbs? Fat?
4. How do you measure body fat?

Chapter Six – *PROGRAM DESIGN*

1. What is the heart rate intensity for a beginner in the testing phase?
2. What are the 3 tests given in the cardiovascular testing phase?
3. Why do we test anyone?
4. What is the goal of Level 1 resistance training? Level 2? Level 3? Level 4? Level 5?
5. How many reps do you perform for hypertrophy (to get "bigger")? Strength? Endurance?
6. What do we mean by the term neuro pathways? Why is it important?

Chapter Seven – *ENHANCING MOBILITY*

1. What are some benefits of increasing a person's range of movement/motion (ROM)?

2. Name one Stick Mobility™ stretch, fix, or solution, and describe it.

Chapter Eight – *ATTITUDE TRAINING*

1. Why is it important to keep clients from getting de-motivated?

2. Name one "tool" or strategy that can be used to build attitude training.

Chapter Nine – *PHYSIOLOGY*

1. What is a motor unit?

2. What is the all or none principle?

3. What is a slow twitch muscle? Fast twitch muscle? What types are they each?

4. What is the function of a muscle spindle?

5. What is a golgi tendon organ?

6. List 4 components of the sliding filament theory.

7. What are the 3 types of contractions? Describe how they work with force.

Chapter Ten – *ENERGY SYSTEMS*

1. What is another name for energy system?

2. What are the 3 energy systems?

3. What is the time and intensity associated with each energy system? (HINT: Look on the chart of energy systems.)

Chapter Eleven – *ANATOMY*
(NOTE: This is one of the most extensive chapters to study.)

1. What is the force around a joint called?

2. How can you increase the force around a joint without increasing load?

3. What are the curves of the spine called and where are they located?

4. What are the bones of the spine?
5. What is in between the bones of the spine? (except the sacrum and coccyx)
6. Where is the sacroiliac joint? What 2 bones make up the SI joint?
7. What bones make up the shoulder complex?
8. Name 2 joints of the shoulder complex?
9. What muscles act as ligaments and hold the gleno-humeral joint together?
10. What bones make up the elbow?
11. What muscles abduct the hip?
12. What muscles extend the knee?
13. What muscle extends the knee *and* flexes the hip?

Chapter Twelve – *MECHANICS OF EXERCISE*

1. What should you do before you move (create mobility)?
2. What muscle is integral in posture?
3. What are the joint actions of the hip, knee and ankle during the CONCENTRIC phase of the squat? (i.e., coming up)
4. What are the joint actions of the shoulder, elbow and scapula during the CONCENTRIC phase of the bench press?
5. What are the joint actions of the shoulder, elbow, and scapula during the CONCENTRIC phase of a seated row?

Chapter Thirteen – *POSTURAL DYSFUNCTIONS*

1. What are the possible tight muscles of someone who has rounded shoulder pattern?
2. What are the possible tight muscles of someone who has pelvic tilt pattern?
3. What are the possible tight muscles of someone who has pronation pattern?

NOTE: *The anatomy portion of your test will be the most challenging for most people. We have designed this portion of the study guide to help you prepare for the exam. Please do not take this lightly, it will have a huge impact on whether or not you pass the exam.*

I. VOCABULARY

- *Joint* – where two bones articulate or come together
- *Ligament* – attaches bone to bone, does not stretch
- *Tendon* – attaches muscle to bone, does not stretch
- *Disc* – cushion between each vertebra
- *Meniscus* – cushion between the tibia and femur
- *Fossa* – hole or depression in bone
- *Process* – protrusion on a bone
- *Kyphotic curve* – concave curve of upper back, thoracic region
- *Lordotic curve* – convex curve of lower back, lumbar region

II. TERMS OF MOVEMENT

- *Flexion* – decreasing the angle between two bones
- *Extension* – increasing the angle between two bones
- *Hyperextension* – movement beyond normal extension
- *Abduction* – moving away from midline
- *Adduction* – moving towards midline
- *Horizontal abduction* – moving upper arm away from midline in horizontal plane
- *Horizontal adduction* – moving upper arms towards midline in horizontal plane
- *Pronation* – rotating palms up to palms down
- *Supination* – rotating palms down to palms up

III. MUSCLES AND ACTIONS DIAGRAMS

➢ For each of the movements below, a diagram will illustrate the resulting action. Please learn each of the *JOINT ACTIONS, MUSCLES* AND *ATTACHMENTS* that are shown on the following pages. Example format:

JOINT ACTION
<u>Muscles that create the joint action</u>
Attachments of that muscle

WARNING: The anatomy portion of the test will be the most challenging for a majority of people. We have designed this portion of the study guide to help you prepare for the exam. Again, please do not take this section lightly, as it will have a huge impact on whether or not you pass the exam.

Part of what will separate you as an NCEP trainer will be your ability to recognize the movement patterns—specifically, the joint actions—of your clients. Remember, muscles do not "move" (they contract or "flex"), joints do.

MUSCLES/ACTIONS

(A) Spinal Flexion and (B) Spinal Extension

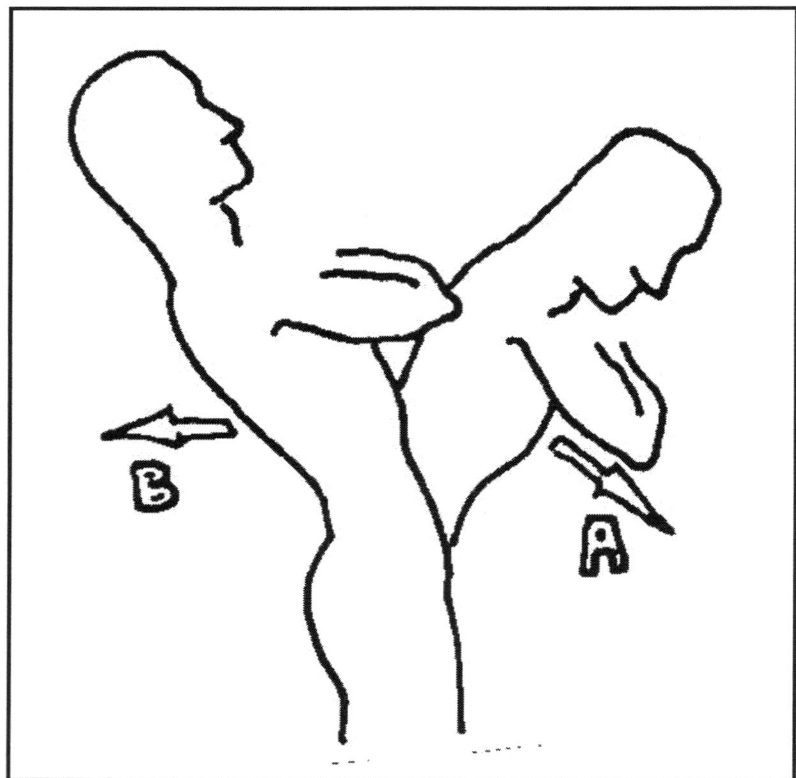

BONES
1. Vertebrae

JOINT
1. Spine

ACTIONS
1. Flexion
2. Extension
3. Stabilization

Exam

FLEXION
Rectus Abdominus -muscle
Rib cage to Pelvis - Action

EXTENSION
Erector Spinae
Sacrum to Vertebrae

STABILIZATION
Transverse Abdominus (TVA)
Ribs to Pelvis to Vertebrae

MUSCLES/ACTIONS

(A) Shoulder Flexion and (B) Shoulder Extension

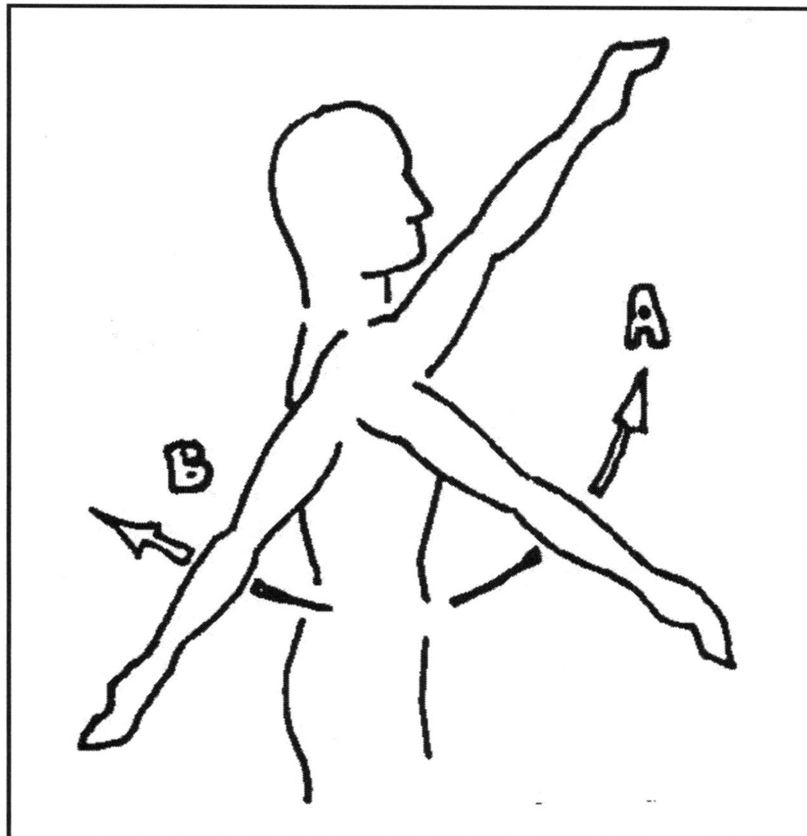

BONES
1. Scapula
2. Humerus
3. Clavicle

JOINT
1. Gleno-humeral

ACTIONS
1. Flexion
2. Extension
3. Stabilization

FLEXION

Anterior Deltoid
Scapula to Humerus

Pectorals
Sternum to Humerus

EXTENSION

Latissimus Dorsi
Humerus to Vertebrae

Posterior Deltoid
Scapula to Humors

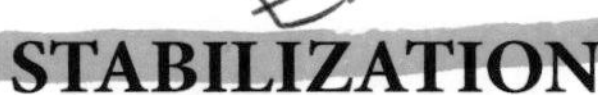

STABILIZATION

"Rotator Cuff" (Teres Minor, Supraspinatus, Infraspinatus, Subscapularis)
Scapula to Humerus

MUSCLES/ACTIONS

Shoulder Adduction(A) and Shoulder Abduction (B)

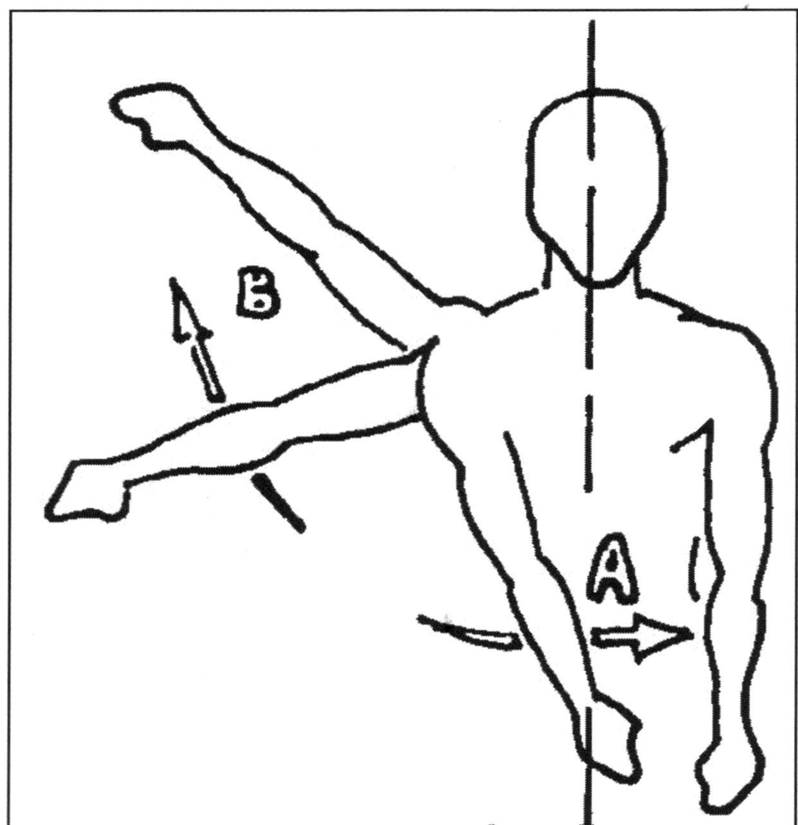

BONES
1. Clavicle
2. Humerus
3. Scapula

JOINT
1. Gleno-humeral

ACTIONS
1. Abduction
2. Adduction

SHOULDER ADDUCTION

Latissimus Dorsi
Humerus to Vertebrae

Posterior Deltoids
Scapula to Humerus

SHOULDER ABDUCTION

Deltoids
Scapula to Humerus

MUSCLES/ACTIONS

Horizontal: Shoulder Adduction(A) and Shoulder Abduction (B)

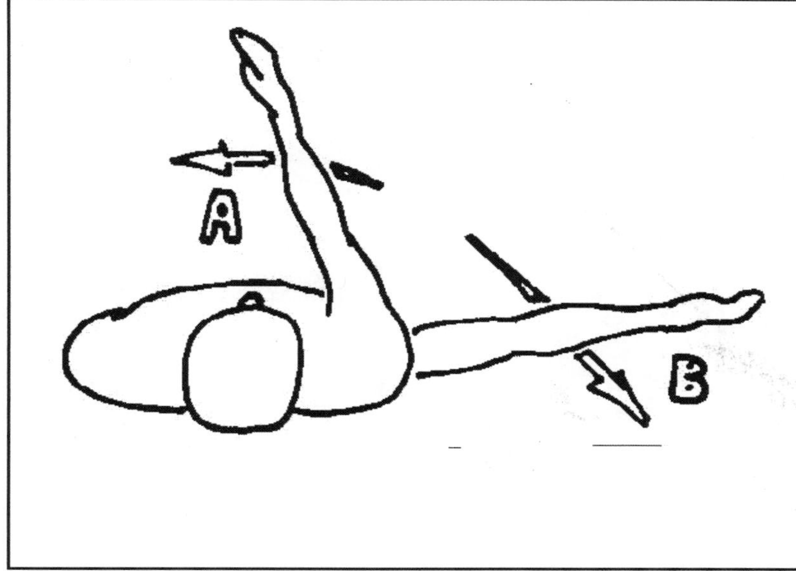

BONES
1. Clavicle
2. Humerus
3. Scapula

JOINT
1. Gleno-humeral

ACTIONS
1. Horiz. Abduction
2. Horiz. Adduction

HORIZONTAL SHOULDER ADDUCTION

Anterior Deltoids
Scapula to Humerus

Pectorals
Sternum to Humerus

HORIZONTAL SHOULDER ABDUCTION

Latissimus Dorsi
Humerus to Vertebrae

Posterior Deltoids
Scapula to Humerus

MUSCLES/ACTIONS

(A) Scapula Adduction and (B) Scapula Abduction

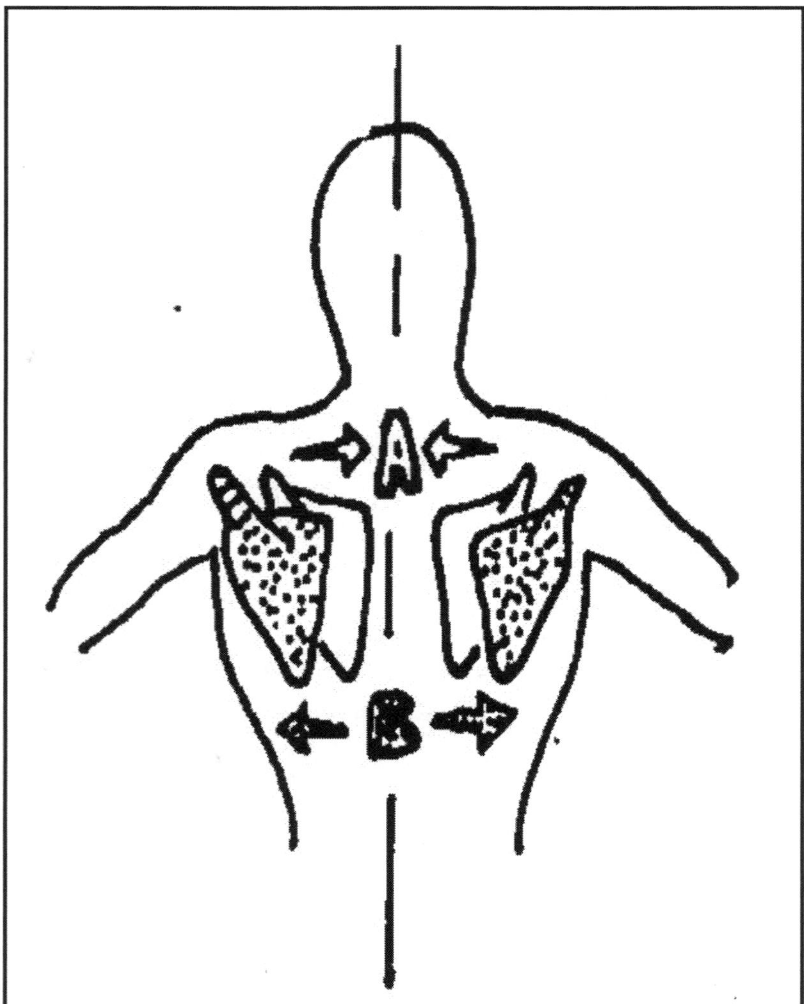

BONES
1. Scapula
2. Thoracic Vertebrae

JOINT
1. Scapulo-Thoracic

ACTIONS
1. Scapular Abduction
2. Scapular Adduction

Exam

SCAPULAR ADDUCTION
Rhomboids
Scapula to Vertebrae

SCAPULAR ABDUCTION
Serratus Anterior
Ribs to Scapula

Exam

Exam

Lats
Rhomboids
biceps
? pushups

MUSCLES/ACTIONS

(A) Scapula Elevation and (B) Scapula Depression

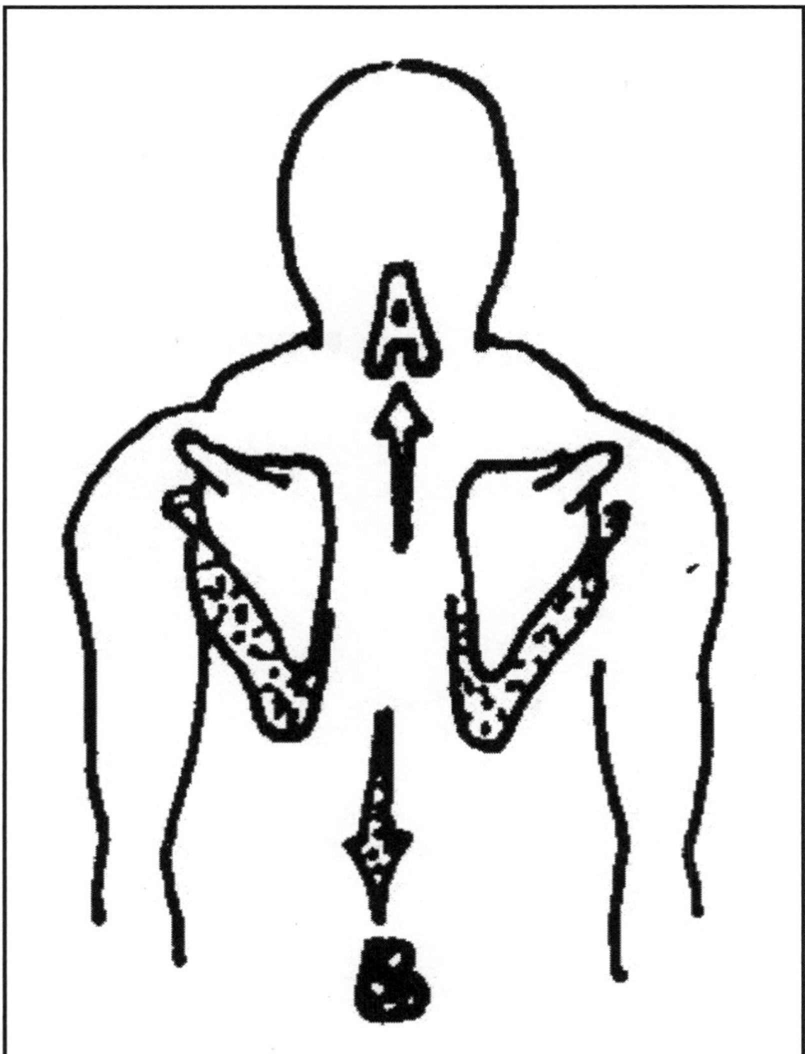

BONES

1. Scapula
2. Thoracic Vertebrae

JOINT

1. Scapulo-Thoracic

ACTIONS

1. Scapular Elevation
2. Scapular Depression

SCAPULAR ELEVATION

(Upper) Trapezius

Back of head (Cranium) to Scapula

SCAPULAR DEPRESSION

Latissimus Dorsi (+ gravity)

Humerus to Vertebrae

MUSCLES/ACTIONS

(A) Elbow Flexion and (B) Elbow Extension

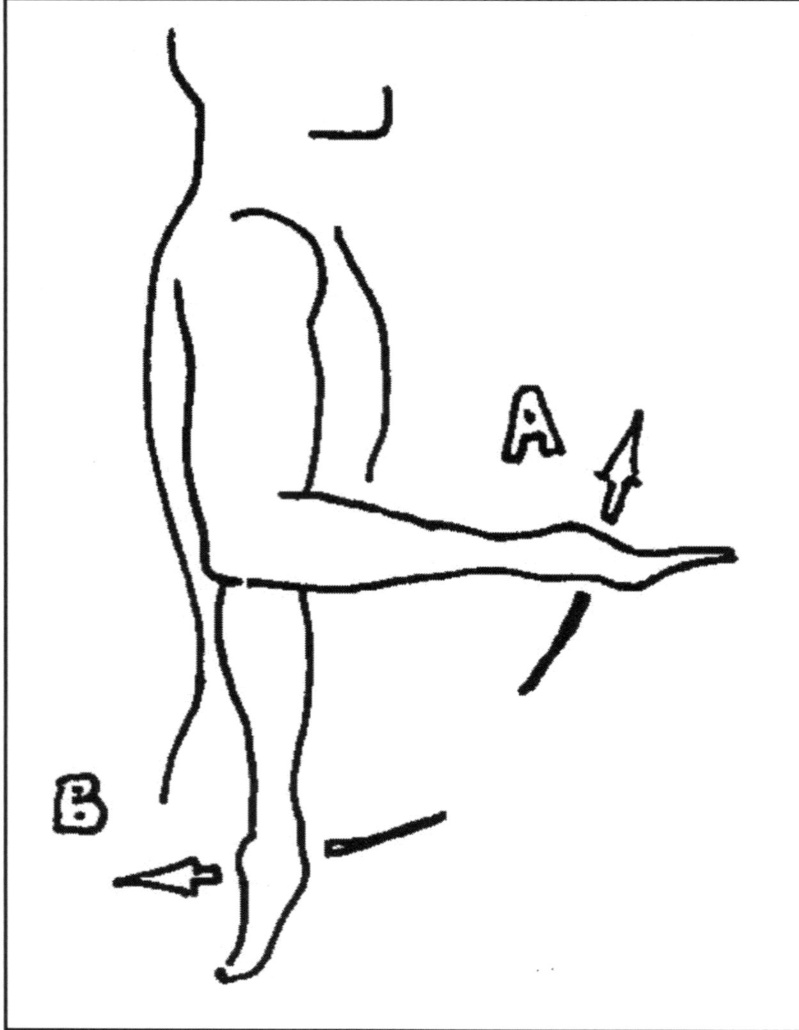

BONES
1. Humerus
2. Radius
3. Ulna

JOINT
1. Elbow

ACTIONS
1. Elbow Flexion
2. Elbow Flexion

ELBOW FLEXION
Biceps
Scapula to Radius

ELBOW EXTENSION
Triceps
Scapula to Ulna

MUSCLES/ACTIONS

(A) Hip Flexion and (B) Hip Extension

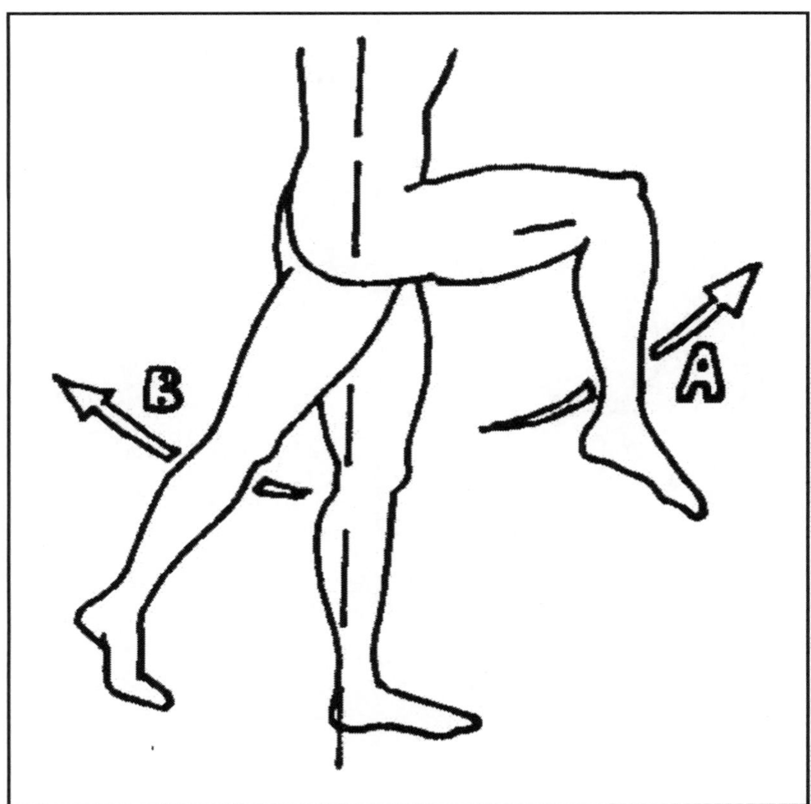

BONES
1. Femur
2. Pelvis

JOINT
1. Hip

ACTIONS
1. Hip Flexion
2. Hip Extension

HIP FLEXION

Iliopsoas
Pelvis to Femur

Rectus Femoris*
Pelvis to Femur

Tensor Fascia Latae
Pelvis to Femur

HIP EXTENSION

Gluteus Maximus
Sacrum; Pelvis to Femur

Hamstrings* (3)
Ischial Tuberosity to Tibia

1. Biceps Femoris
2. Semitendenosus
3. Semimembranosus

*2-Joint Muscle

MUSCLES/ACTIONS

(A) Hip Adduction and (B) Hip Abduction

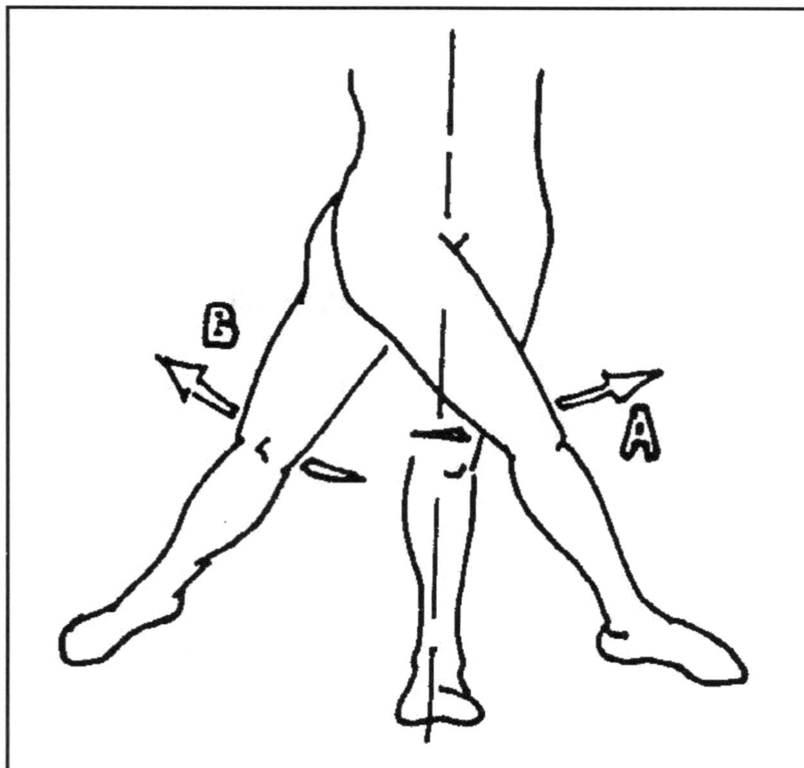

BONES
1. Femur
2. Pelvis

JOINT
1. Hip

ACTIONS
1. Hip Adduction
2. Hip Abduction

HIP ADDUCTION
Hip Adductors (4)
Ischial Tuberosity to Femur

1. Adductor Magnus
2. Adductor Longus
3. Adductor Brevis
4. Pectineus

HIP ABDUCTION
Gluteus Medius
Pelvis to Femur

MUSCLES/ACTIONS

(A) Knee Extension and (B) Knee Flexion

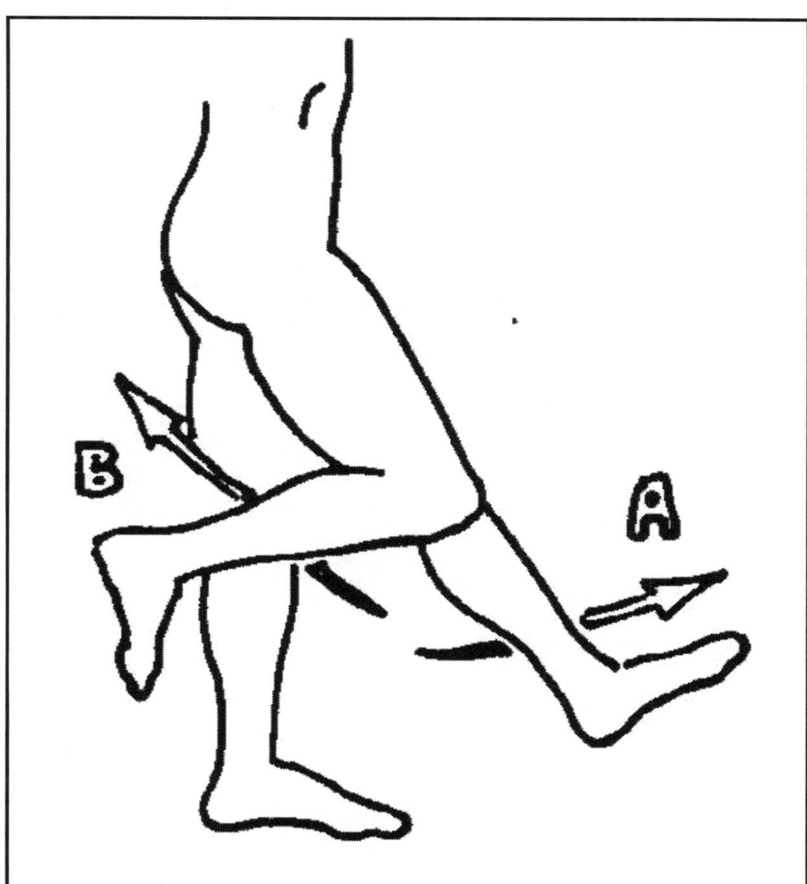

BONES
1. Femur
2. Tibia

JOINT
1. Knee

ACTIONS
1. Knee Flexion
2. Knee Extension

KNEE FLEXION
<u>Hamstrings* (3)</u>
Ischial Tuberosity to Tibia

1. Biceps Femoris
2. Semimembranosus
3. Semitendenosus

KNEE EXTENSION
<u>Quadriceps (4)</u>
Femur to Tibia

1. Vastus Lateralis
2. Vastus Intermedius
3. Vastus Medialis
4. Rectus Femoris*

*2-Joint Muscle

MUSCLES/ACTIONS

(A) Dorsi Flexion and (B) Plantar Flexion [Extension]

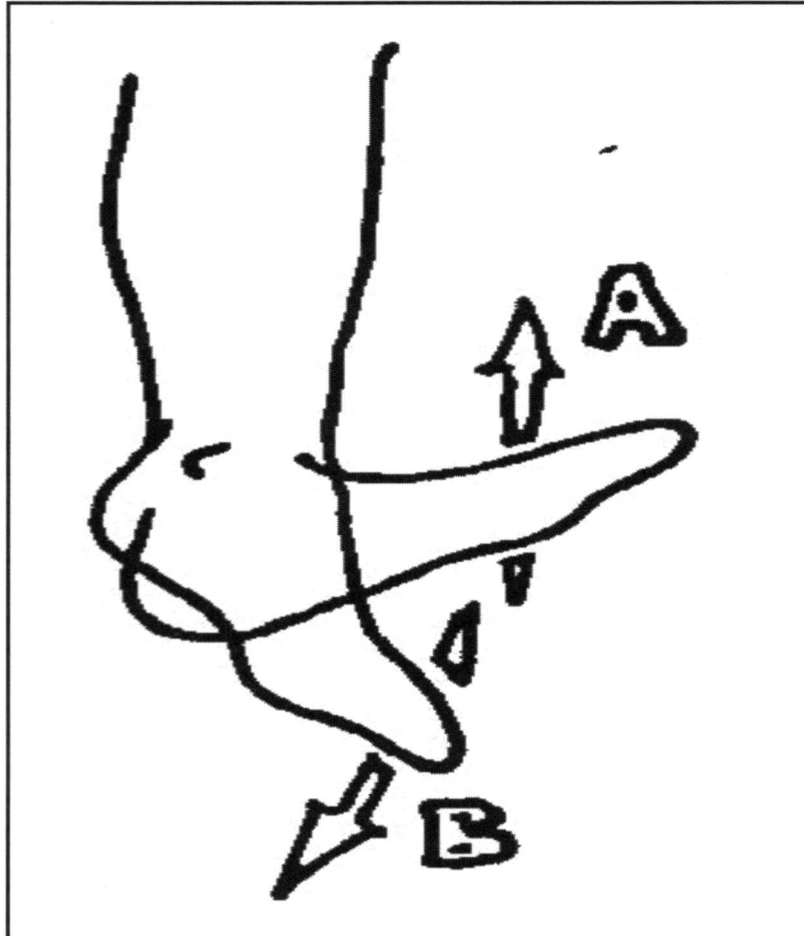

BONES
1. Tibia
2. Talus
3. Calcaneus

JOINT
1. Ankle

ACTIONS
1. Dorsi Flexion
2. Plantar Flexion

DORSI FLEXION
Anterior Tibialis
Tibia to Top of Foot

PLANTAR FLEXION
Gastrocnemius*
(Lower) Femur to Calcaneus

Soleus
Tibia to Calcaneus

*2-Joint Muscle

IV. IMPORTANT BONES/JOINTS/MUSCLES

- *Bones* – Calcaneus, Tibia, Fibula, Femur, Pelvis, Cervical Spine, Thoracic Spine, Lumbar Spine, Sacrum Spine, Coccyx Spine, Ribs, Clavicle, Scapula, Humerus, Ulna, Radius, Talus, Sternum, Ischial Tuberosity

- *Joints* – Ankle, Knee, Hip, Spine, Shoulder, Scapulo-thoracic, Elbow

- *Muscles* – Anterior Tibialis, Posterior Tibialis, Soleus, Gastrocnemius, Vastus Lateralis, Vastus Intermedius, Vastus Medialis, Rectus Femoris, Semimembranosus, Semitendinosus, Biceps Femoris, Tensor Fasciae Latae, Gluteus Maximus, Gluteus Medius, Gluteus Minimus, Erector Spinae, Rectus Abdominus, Obliques Externus, Obliques Internus, Transverse Abdominus, Latissimus Dorsi, Rhomboids, Trapezius, Deltoids, Pectoralis Major/Minor, Rotator Cuff, Biceps, Triceps, Sternocleidomastoid (SCM), Serratus Anterior, Pectineus, Iliopsoas

CHAPTER ONE

Definition of Personal Training

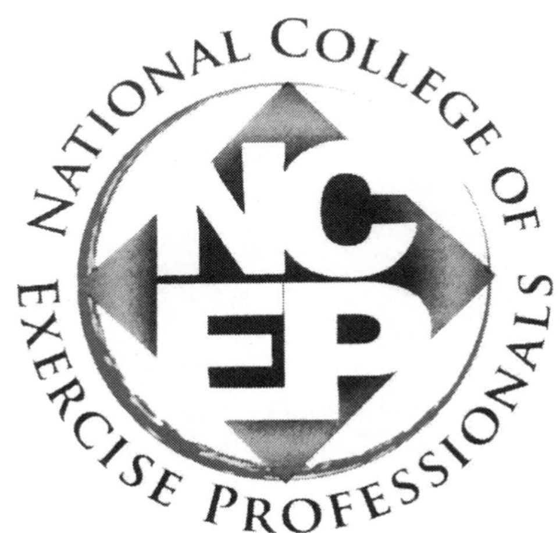

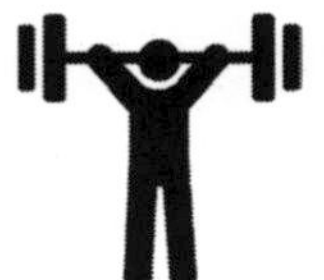 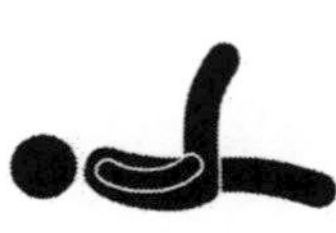 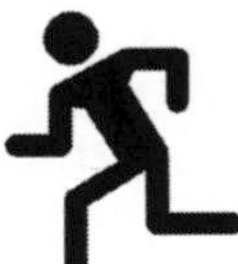  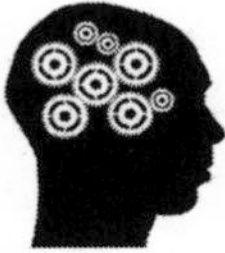

PERSONAL TRAINING

Before jumping into any discussion of personal training, it is first necessary to frame our understanding about health and wellness more generally. For decades now, medical errors in hospitals are the third leading cause of death in the United States, behind only heart disease (first) and cancer (second). While this statistic may be startling at first glance, in reality, it makes sense. In today's society, it is common—if not expected—to go to the doctor for the many minor health issues that occur that are often preventable. Instead of focusing on prevention, as a society, we only think about our health once we get sick. Thus, when individuals rely on doctors for every little symptom, the probability increases for things to go wrong—the more "issues" an individual has, the more medical visits he/she undergoes and the more medicine ingested. Although advances in Western medicine have been extraordinary and medical technology has improved exponentially, as a whole, Americans are less healthy overall. Our point is that a fundamental shift needs to happen when thinking about health: there must be a renewed focus on lifestyle, instead of relying on medicine, doctors, and procedures, in order to change the health conditions of millions on individuals. This is where you come in as a personal trainer, or what we like to call an "exercise professional." Although you may not be a doctor, you have the extraordinary opportunity to change peoples' health—and peoples' lives—in very significant in more ways than you could ever imagine.

The Personal Training Industry

Welcome to the wacky wonderful world of personal training. Unlike most professions, no one really knows what we do. In fact, many people who call themselves personal trainers have trouble describing to others what they do for a living. Currently, there are no national regulations that govern personal training, leaving this industry in a "free-for-all" state. Yet, despite these factors, the number of personal trainers (and the fitness industry in general) continues to grow dramatically. The fitness field is burgeoning and personal training has never been more popular. With no set industry standard of what a personal trainer does, and no set regulations of what a personal trainer must be, we hope to provide you our definition of personal coaching and help guide you on a path to success for you and your clients.

You may be asking yourself why you decided to take this course, or why you may have decided to be a personal trainer (or even to hire one). First, however, what we would like you to do is create a definition of what personal training is to you—it is most likely that you have chosen this journey to enter the field because of some prior experience with personal training and/or health and fitness. Before you create a definition of personal training, write down who you think the top five people in our profession are, and what characteristics they possess (see Part A and B on page 30). When you are through with the characteristics of trainers, then create your definition (see Part C). We hope you take this definition to heart, and post that definition on your refrigerator or locker or anywhere you will view it often. Read it every day before you go to work and before every client you see. And, please do use a favor: when you no longer live up to what you wrote on the paper today, please re-evaluate your definition of training and decide if you are still helping people make better choices for their lives. Since everyone defines personal training differently, peoples' only thought of personal training is their perception of you. When an individual decides to become a personal trainer, that person has entered something bigger than his/herself. For our industry to grow both in numbers and in respect, we need to hold ourselves to the highest standards possible—personal training today will be the definition of personal training tomorrow.

So, What Makes a "Good" Personal Trainer?

A surprise to most, one of the most successful personal trainers over the last couple of decades is Richard Simmons. Before saying anything, write down your honest thoughts of Richard. What you have just written down is many peoples' *perceptions* of him, without thinking about what he represents. There are some very endearing qualities of Richard Simmons that have made him so successful. Can you think of some of these characteristics? If you have more negative thoughts of Richard Simmons than positive, you may want to reconsider if personal training is right for you.

Richard Simmons is certainly not a trainer in the stereotypical mold, but his unique qualities and motivational style are why we think he is a great role model for those entering the profession. Richard Simmons has made out a career out of helping people feel good about themselves, and helping them get active in ways that are life-altering. Can you think of anyone who cares more about other people's well-being than Richard? Shifting someone's mindset from having given up on a more satisfying life because of obesity, depression or self-esteem issues to instead, helping that person feel hopeful about his/her life again is truly priceless! Richard Simmons, among others, have been able to motivate people to live healthier lives. If your view of personal training is about helping your clients get "big" or to look like the models, please reconsider your stance. Unfortunately, this ideology has remained a black cloud over the profession, and has prevented personal trainers from gaining legitimacy in the eyes of health care professionals.

Reiterating the Scope and Objectives of the NCEP Manual

The purpose of this manual is to introduce you to the wonderfully enriching profession of personal training, and to attempt to educate you on both the art and the science behind the most extraordinary creation: the human being. This manual is meant to help you to learn as much as you can about the way the human body works, within the context of personal training. We hope it provides cutting-edge exercise science, but in an easily digestible manner that you could explain to anyone regardless of educational background. We seek to take complicated material and frame it in a way that is both useful and practical in your career as a trainer and in your everyday life.

Everything in this book is based on both empirical evidence and practical application. If a concept makes sense to you, it is probably true. Believe in your common sense when it comes to the human body, and avoid believing a concept just because someone told you so. Unless someone can thoroughly explain the *why*, then he/she probably should not be sharing knowledge. We were given instincts and survival skills for a reason, and it is obvious when someone has a true grasp of a concept when he/she can "break it down" to a level that anyone can understand. Concepts should also be able to be applied immediately; if you cannot do what you have just read, it should not be in the book. We say what we mean, and we have done what we say. And, we want you to be able to do it, too. Once again, on behalf of the National College of Exercise, we would like to say thank you for making the choice to want to help others, and/or yourself, adopt a healthy lifestyle.

What is Personal Training?

A. *List 5 characteristics of a good personal trainer.*

1.______________________________

2.______________________________

3.______________________________

4.______________________________

5.______________________________

B. *Name the three most successful/recognized personal trainers.*

1.________________________

2.________________________

3.________________________

C. *Define what personal training is to you.*

____

____

____

____

____

Refer back to "your" definition of personal training to ensure you are meeting your standards.

BENEFITS OF EXERCISE AND PROPER NUTRITION

Often clients are unaware of all the benefits of exercise and proper nutrition. To know your product—health and fitness—you should be able to rattle off dozens of benefits of exercise and proper nutrition. Here are just a few of the many, many benefits:

Better Appearance

- Improves skin tone
- Improves posture, coordination and grace
- Improves muscular tone and definition
- May decelerate aging
- Look healthy, vital and alive
- Reduction of body fat

Improved Health

- Improved cardiovascular and respiratory efficiency
- Reduces risk of cardiovascular disease
- Improved circulation
- Reduces risk of high blood pressure (hypertension)
- Improves daily function
- Reduces stress and tension, both muscular and emotional
- Improves strength
- Improves/maintain range of motion
- Improves coordination, balance and reflexes
- Improves body awareness
- Improves sleeping and eating habits
- Improves respiration
- Improves function of internal organs
- Retards atrophy
- Strengthens the abdominal muscles relieving many cases of lower back pain
- Increases energy level
- Decreases likelihood of illness or injury

Feeling and Performing Better

- Stimulates greater mental activity
- Increases work capacity, energy level and drive
- Improves confidence and well being
- Eliminates inhibitions
- Improves vitality of life
- Relieves stress and tension

CHAPTER TWO

Five Components of Fitness

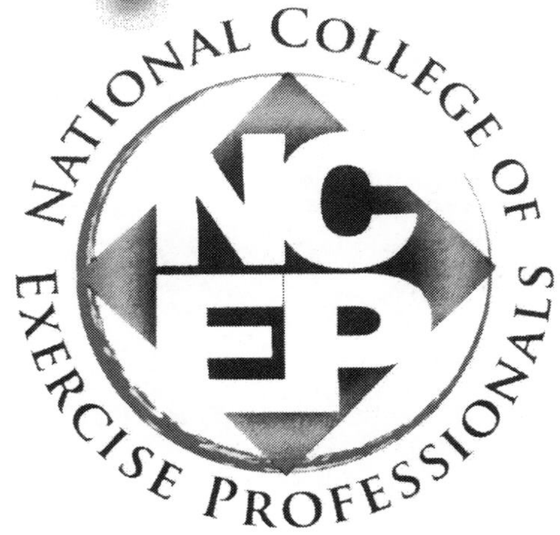

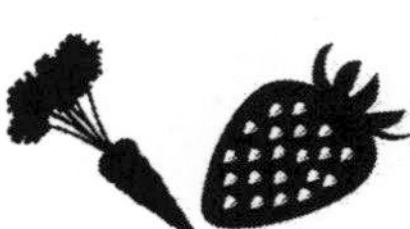

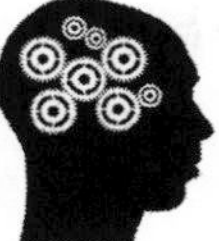

FIVE COMPONENTS OF FITNESS

1. **Nutritional Guidance** - *defined as a meal strategy that is both healthy and results oriented*

   A. **Calorie** - *unit of energy*

   B. **Gram** - *unit of weight used to measure nutrients*

2. **Flexibility Training/Range of Motion (ROM)** - *defined as creating optimal length/tension relationships*

   A. **Active** - *ability to move a bone around an axis using only internal force*

   B. **Passive** - *ability to move a bone around an axis with help from an external force*

   C. **Static** - *not continually moving*

   D. **Dynamic/Ballistic** - *in constant motion*

3. **Cardiovascular Training** - *defined as stress placed on the heart for it to become more efficient at pumping the blood through the veins*

   A. **Blood Pressure Definition** - *amount of pressure placed on the arterial walls during the pumping (systolic) and filling (diastolic) phases*

   B. **Normal** - *120/80 mmHg*

   C. **High** - *140/90 mmHg*

   D. **Resting Heart Rate** - *number of times the heart beats in one minute at rest*

   E. **Training Heart Rate** - *(220 - age) X % of max heart rate*

4. **Resistance Training** - *defined as stress placed on the muscular system for it to become more efficient at handling load*

   A. **Endurance** - *sub-maximal force repeated over time*

   B. **Power** - *work/time*

C. **Strength** - *maximal force produced in a specific environment*

1. **<u>max strength</u>** - *maximum amount of force you can produce in any environment (stable)*
2. **<u>relative strength</u>** - *maximum amount of force you can produce in situations relative to bodyweight (unstable)*
3. **<u>reactive strength</u>** - *maximum amount force that can be exerted after a force has been exerted on it*
4. **<u>stabilization strength</u>** - *maximum amount of force you can produce to keep a joint from moving in any direction*

***Core Stabilization Strength** - *defined as the ability to stabilize your spine and transfer load efficiently throughout the body*

5. **Attitude Training** - *defined as the ability to always have the mental fortitude to motivate yourself and others during exercise*

CHAPTER THREE

Health History

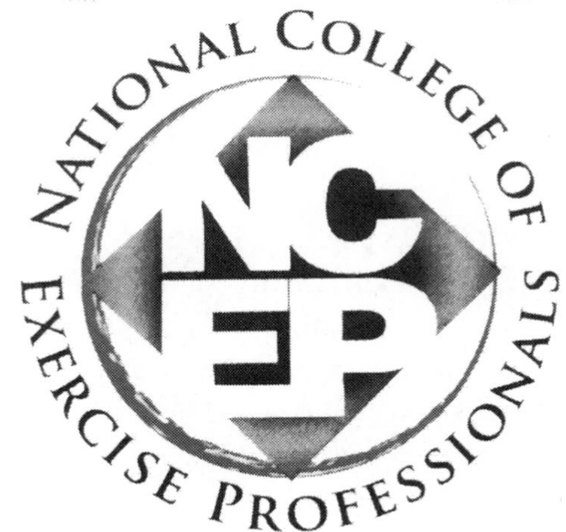

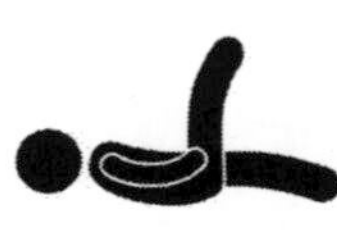
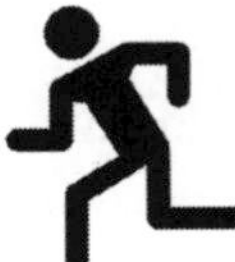
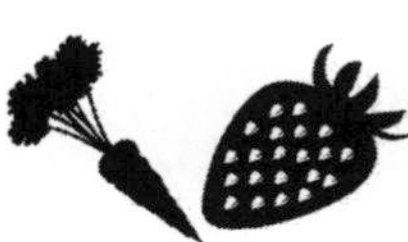
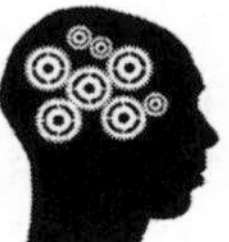

HEALTH HISTORY

Learning a Client's Basic Health History

Although learning about a client's health history may not seem important (or exciting), we believe, as an exercise professional, it is an essential first step to any client-trainer relationship. Every trainer should create a file for each client to follow his/her program and reach his/her desired goals, starting with detailed information on his/her health history. It is important that all of the client's information is thoroughly documented in this file. At minimum, every client should at least fill out what we call a "PAR-Q" before any physical activity to identify those individuals that may need a physician's clearance. A PAR-Q is a series of seven questions that qualify clients who may be at high risk of cardiovascular disease. These clients must receive a doctor's clearance before they start an exercise program. Although we prefer that trainers get even more in-depth with their new clients' health background than just those seven questions, it is a sufficient baseline.

Asking about a client's health history can be tough, and there is a level of sensitivity involved in doing so. Furthermore, based on the information gathered from the health history screening, you might determine that a physician's clearance is necessary at this time. You should have the doctor's clearance before you create the exercise program. In addition to the ACSM guidelines (discussed later in the chapter), any condition or assessment value that causes you to be concerned for the client's health or safety is reason alone to ask for a medical clearance. As alluded to, it is important for you to think about what the client may be feeling when you ask for a clearance. Most of the time, the client is anxious to get started with the program, and anything to prevent that can be disheartening. Thus, he/she may become upset when asked to wait for a clearance if you deem him/her unfit to start an exercise program without doctor's permission. However, a good presentation can minimize a negative reaction, and you must be direct in conveying your concern about his/her health. Instead of ending the session entirely, think of what you can do so the client will not lose enthusiasm. For example, you will still be able to perform all of the assessments, talk about goals and adherence factors, and design an eating strategy. To expedite the process, try to fax the clearance form to his/her physician or provide a copy to give to his/her physician. Schedule another appointment the minute you receive the clearance form. We believe understanding that, for some people, exercise involves some risk, shows your professionalism as a trainer.

Bottom Line: More Information Leads to Better Program Design

However, for most individuals, exercise is a safe endeavor. Accordingly, all clients should undergo a medical history screening if you design a workout program. When asking questions during this screening, if the answer is "Yes," always follow-up with more specific questions. Note that follow-up questions are the key to learning important information about your client. Example follow-up questions would be: when?, what?, how?, where?, why? Also, ask the client if he/she has seen a doctor for this "Yes" condition that he/she is describing, and if there are any known or understood limitations. The more information you know about a client's health history and ailments, the better you will be at being able to design a program that improves his/her quality of life.

MAJOR CORONARY RISK FACTORS

1. *Have you ever been diagnosed with hypertension or systolic blood pressure > 140 or diastolic blood pressure > 90 mmHg on at least 2 separate occasions, or on anti-hypertensive medication?*

   Yes No Initials__________ Date____________

2. *Do you have high cholesterol > 200?*

   Yes No

3. *Are you a cigarette smoker?*

   Yes No

4. *Do you have Diabetes mellitus?*

   Yes No

   If "Yes" - IDDM or NIDDM (please circle)

5. *Do you have a family history of coronary or other artherosclerotic disease in parents or siblings prior to age 55?*

   Yes No

If you answered "Yes" to any of the above questions, then please answer the following:

6. *Have you recently consulted your physician about increasing your physical activity and/or participating in a fitness evaluation?*

   Yes No Initials__________ Date____________

7. *If you answered "NO" to question number 6, will you agree to consult your physician prior to increasing your physical activity and/or participating in a fitness evaluation?*

   Yes No Initials__________ Date____________

MEDICAL INFORMATION

We strongly suggest that all people should consult a physician before starting any exercise program

1a. *When was the last time you saw your doctor?*

____

____

1b. *Why did you seek your doctor's advice?*

____

____

2. *Are you currently taking any medication?*

Yes No

Explain: ______________________________________

____

____

____

3. *Do you have any medical condition, such as diabetes?*

Yes No

If so, what? ___________________________________

____

____

4. *Have you had surgery in the past 6 months?*

Yes No

If so, what? ___________________________________

____

____

5. *Do you often experience fatigue and/or drowsiness?*

   Yes No

6. *Do you often experience headaches?*

   Yes No

7. *Do you have trouble sleeping?*

   Yes No

8. *Do you drink several cups of coffee to keep you going during the day?*

   Yes No

9. *Do you often experience digestive difficulties?*

   If yes, please explain: ____
   ____

10. *Do you eat foods high in fiber, such as whole grain bread, cereal, or fresh fruit or vegetables each day?*

    Yes No

11. *Do you eat foods high in fat and cholesterol, such as fatty meat, cheese, fried foods or eggs each day?*

    Yes No

12. *How many meals do you eat each day?* ________________

13. *Do you eat breakfast regularly?*

    Yes No

14. *What is your daily caloric intake? (estimate)*

____

____

15. *Do you often crave sugar?*

Yes No

16. *Are you currently taking nutritional supplements?*

Yes No

17. *Is there any reason why you can't exercise?*

Yes No

18. *In an average week, how often do you exercise?*

# of days______________ minutes/hours:_______________

19. *How long have you been exercising?*

Weeks/months/years__________________

20. *What kind of exercise do you do?*

____

____

____

21. *Have you ever participated in a diet and/or nutrition program before?*

Yes No

Explain:_______________________________________

____

____

22a. *Did you achieve your goals?*

Yes No

22b. *Was it permanent?*

Yes No

23. *Are you happy with your health and the way you look?*

Yes No

24. *What are your desired goals?*

____
____
____

25. *On a scale of 1 to 10, how serious are you about achieving your goals?*

Least 1 2 3 4 5 6 7 8 9 10 Most
(please circle)

26. *Have you experienced, or are you experiencing, any injuries or physical problems with your:*

- Neck?

____
____

- Upper Back?

____
____

- Lower Back?

____
____

- Shoulders?

____
____

- Elbows?

- Wrists?

- Hands?

- Hips?

- Knees?

- Ankles?

- Feet?

-Any other issues that were not addressed?

POSITIVE RISK FACTORS OF CORONARY HEART DISEASE

Based on the ACSM "Guidelines for Exercise Testing and Prescription" (1995), sets of questions were created to determine the client's risk of developing cardiovascular disease. If a client answers "Yes" to any of the following conditions, footnote the details accordingly.

- **Age** – *Record client's age. Age is a major coronary risk factor for men over age 45 and women over age 55.*
- **Family History** - *"Does anyone in your immediate family (mother, father, sibling) have any heart problems prior to age 55?" If so, this is considered a major coronary risk factor.*
- **High Blood Pressure** – *"Has a physician diagnosed you with high blood pressure?" Hypertension diagnosed by a physician greater than or equal to 140/90 is a major coronary risk factor. (RD/Nutritionist Referral).*
- **Diabetes** - *"Has your doctor diagnosed you with diabetes?" If yes, ask: "How do you control it?" Note that diabetes is considered to be a risk factor for CHD. Diabetes is a metabolic disease in which the body's ability to produce and use insulin for sugar metabolism is impaired; the individual is unable to utilize sugar properly to sustain muscular functioning. As having a metabolic disease the individual would be classified as "known disease" for risk stratification. Therefore, the member needs a medical clearance prior to beginning an exercise program. Document all information in detail including the medication they are taking. This is a major coronary risk factor. (RD/Nutritionist Referral).*
- **Cholesterol Level** - *"Have you ever had your cholesterol measured?" If yes, ask: "Do you remember what level it is?" A cholesterol reading of 200 or greater is a major coronary risk factor.*
- **Heart Disease** - *"Do you have any heart conditions?" Any problem with the heart including mitral valve prolapse, myocardial infarction, angina, dysrhythmia, or arteriosclerosis of the coronary artery" is a major coronary risk factor. (RD/Nutritionist Referral)*
- **Smoking** - *"Do you smoke?" If yes, ask: "How many per day? For how long?" Smoking is considered a major coronary risk factor.*
- **Sedentary Lifestyle** - *"Is sitting a large part of your day? Would you consider yourself sedentary with no regular exercise or active recreational activities?" Sedentary lifestyle is a major coronary risk factor.*
- **Obesity** - *If he/she has a Body Mass Index (BMI) of 30% or higher, this individual is considered obese. In 2013, the American Medical Association (AMA) classified obesity as a disease, and can be counted as a "known disease." Obesity is considered a major coronary risk factor.*

MAJOR SIGNS AND SYMPTOMS OF CARDIOPULMONARY DISEASE

There are many symptoms, most very serious, that suggest an individual may have heart and/or lung problems. As a personal trainer, we never diagnose diseases. However, below are a few more common symptoms that can discovered through questioning a client's health history:

- **Chest Pain** - *"Have you ever experienced chest pain?"*
- **Dizziness** - *"Have you ever experienced abnormal or unexplained dizziness?"*
- **Heart Murmur** - *"Have you been diagnosed with a heart murmur?"*
- **Shortness of Breath** - *"Have you ever experienced unaccustomed shortness of breath with mild exertion?"*
- **Irregular or Accelerated Heart Rate** - *"Have you ever been told that you have an accelerated heart rate?" (Either palpitations or resting heart rate of 100 beats per minute or more.)*
- **Medications** - *"Are you presently taking any medications? If so, are you aware of any of the side effects from the medication?" (The trainer should always refer to a Physician's Desk Reference book to become aware of possible physical reactions from the medication.)*

RISK STRATIFICATION

The information collected from the previous pages on

- **Positive Risk Factors of Coronary Heart Disease**
- **Major Signs and Symptoms of Cardiopulmonary Disease**

determines the client's risk stratification for metabolic and coronary heart disease. It is your job as a trainer to identify the appropriate risk stratification and determine whether you should ask him/her to get a physician's clearance before starting an exercise program. (ACSM Guidelines)

Apparently Healthy (AH) - *Individuals who are asymptomatic and apparently healthy with no more than one major coronary risk factor*

Increased Risk (IR) - *Individuals who have signs or symptoms suggestive of possible cardiopulmonary or metabolic disease and/or two or more major coronary risk factors*

Known Disease (KD) - *Individuals with known cardiac, pulmonary, or metabolic disease.*

NOTE: Any condition or assessment value that causes concern for the client's health or safety is the basis for a medical clearance.

All IR and KD individuals must get a medical clearance form signed by a physician before starting an exercise program.

REAL-LIFE EXAMPLES

Apparently Healthy (AH)

Man, age 43, **high blood pressure (140/90),** exercises frequently and plays basketball often

» *Only one major coronary risk factor (high blood pressure)*

Women, age 49, **smoker**, exercises on occasion, active mom, and enjoys spinning classes

» *Only one major coronary risk factor (smoker)*

Increased Risk (IR)

Man, **age 53**, **high blood pressure (140/90)**, exercises frequently and plays basketball often

» *Now, has two major coronary risk factors (high blood pressure and age)*

Women, age 49, **smoker, has office job and rarely exercsises**

» *Now, has two major coronary risk factors (smoker and sedentary lifestyle)*

Known Disease (KD)

Man, age 37, **diabetes**, retired semi-pro tennis player

» Diabetes is a "known disease" and this person's fitness level does not matter

PHYSICIAN'S CLEARANCE FORM

Physician's Name:____________________________

Address:____

Phone #:_________________Fax #:____________

Patient's Name:______________________________

Dear Dr. _______________________:

My trainer had a question regarding _____________________________________ on a Par-Q or fitness assessment. I am planning to begin an exercise program, which involves:

☐ Cardiovascular Training ☐ Strength Training ☐ Flexibility Training Other__________

Please help by providing the information below. I hereby give you my permission to release my medical information pertaining to my exercise program to the Club. Thank you.

______________________ ________________________

Patient Release Signature Date

Does your patient have any limitation to participation in an exercise program? □ Yes □ No. If yes, please explain.

____

Is your patient on any medications which might affect his/her heart rate or blood pressure response to exercise?

Medication ____

Type of Effect ____

Please indicate any restrictions to exercise participation

☐ None

☐ Limit activities to ____

☐ Exercise program is not medically advisable._

______________________ ________________________

Physician Signature Date

Please fax to:________________________________

CHAPTER FOUR

Assessments

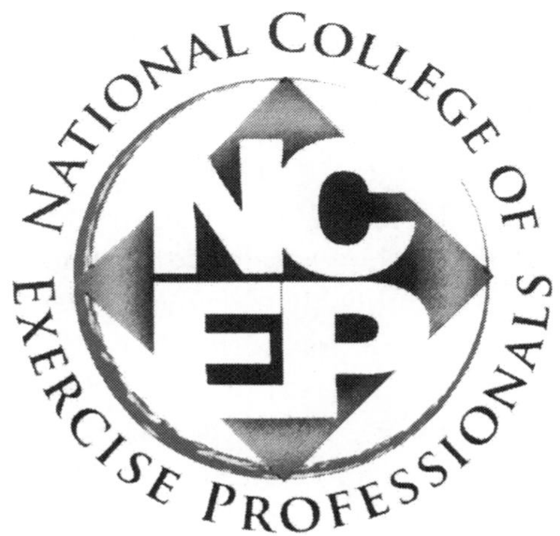

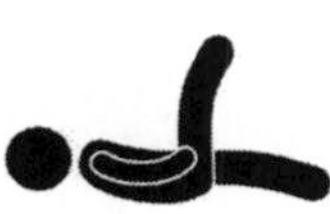
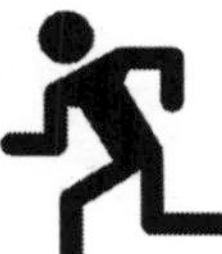
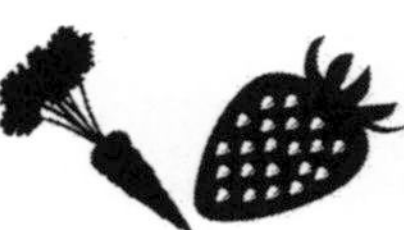
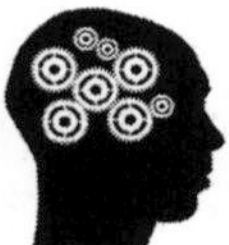

CLIENT ASSESSMENT

Understanding the Importance of Assessments

After acquiring a client's health history, assessing his/her movements and posture, among other things, is the next important step. To start this assessment process, we suggest you introduce your client to exercise by having him/her peform some dynamic movements. Dynamic just means that a person is moving (see Chapter Six). Far too often we sit and ask the client so many questions, and talk for so long, that the hour appointment goes by without the client leaving his/her chair. Provided your client is considered "Apparently Healthy," we want to counteract the effects of being sedentary by having the member perform some movements using only his/her own bodyweight. This will give the trainer a clear picture of how well the client can control his/her body and how well the neural system is working.

Thus, the first step of any program should be to gain neural control. Without neurological efficiency, the muscle cannot work well or, in turn, grow effectively. This is an important step that tends to be left out in many traditional exercise programs. We do not want to fall into the trap that intends to ignore this critical component of body functionality. While the client is answering the health history questions, keep in mind the characteristics of common postural distortions and the implications that are involved with them. When you have become very familiar with the three patterns outlined in Chapter 11, you can predict or even ask the member if he/she is feeling anything in areas before he/she tells you! This will add to your credibility as an exercise professional—it will separate you from other trainers—and eventually add to the sale of your services.

The next step is to perform a quick postural assessment, which can happen immediately as the client is walking toward you. In that brief instant certain blaring characteristics may (and usually do) jump out at you. This could set the stage of how this member may answer his/her health history and lifestyle questions. After extrapolating the health history, orthopedic, and lifestyle questions, it is time to have your client undergo dynamic assessments that go beyond just posture.

Dynamic Assessments and Progression

This chapter outlines numerous dynamic (i.e., moving) assessments, organized by movement. Generally, it is useful to perform a few core assessments before progressing to the seven primary movement pattern assessments described in the following pages. Having your client undergo these assessments will be invaluable in helping you identify strengths and weaknesses with your client. Note, however, that we ***do not diagnose*** or even tell the client there is anything wrong with him/her. Instead, communicate to the client that all we want to do is assess his/her body movement, determine what muscles may be tight or loose, and give an appropriate program for that member. Although there are hundreds of assessments that can be used, the first assessment of any program, as alluded to, is for posture, generally followed by the overhead squat. By understanding posture, you can then use the overhead squat—often considered the cornerstone of any body analysis—to assess almost every joint in the kinetic chain, along with the other assessments.

STANDARD BODY ASSESSMENT CHECKLIST

There are many very specific assessments that you, as an exercise professional, can use to examine your clients' weaknesses/strengths and muscular deficiencies. However, there are seven main body parts of the body to pay the most attention to, as your clients will often have many of these very common issues below. A quick look at your clients' movement will illustrate many of these deficiencies:

1) Head and neck

Neutral position: *Neck not tilted, rotated, forward or back*

2) Shoulders

Level: *Not elevated, depressed rolled forward or back*

Scapulae

Neutral position, medial borders essentially parallel; about 3 to 4 inches apart

3) Thoracic and Lumbar Spines

Straight, without scoliosis

4) Pelvis

Level: *No anterior or posterior tilt*

5) Hip Joints

Neutral position: *Not adducted or abducted*

6) Knees

Straight

7) Feet and ankles

Parallel or toeing out ever so slightly

CORE ASSESSMENTS

TVA Breathing Tests:

Position 1 - **Standing**

1. Have your client stand in good posture
2. Place two fingers over umbilicus and other fingers in the small of their back
3. Note the distance between your two fingers during inhalation and exhalation
4. The distance between the umbilicus and their spine should increase during inhalation and decrease during exhalation

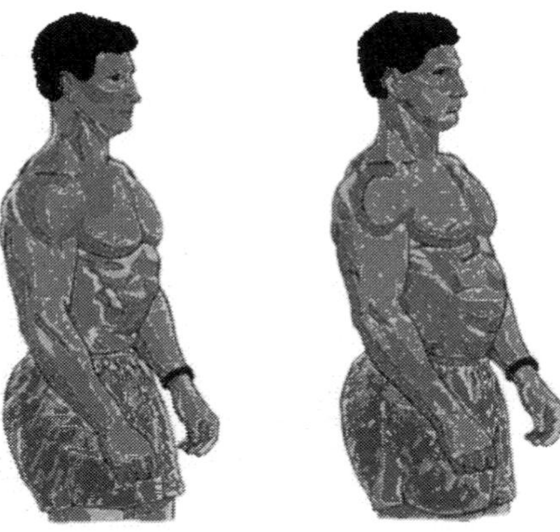

Position 2 - **Four Point Kneeling**

1. Have your client on their hands and knees maintaining a good posture
2. Repeat steps 2-4 of Position 1

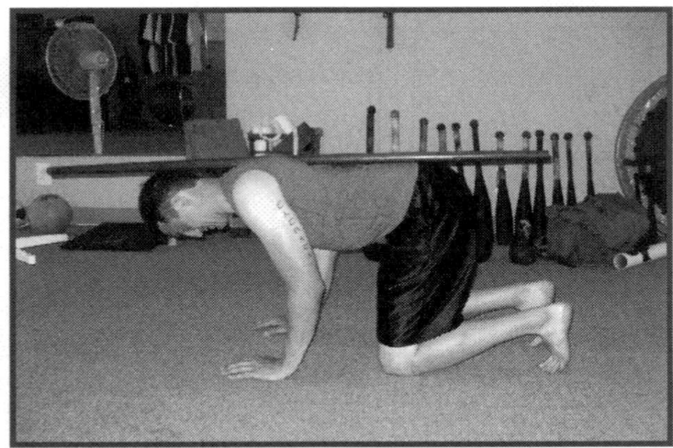

Position 3 - **Supine**

1. Have your client lie on their back
2. Place your fingers under their back where your fingers will be on their spine
3. Have the client place pressure on your hand as if to flatten their back
4. Ask client to hold that pressure on your hand, continuing to breath from diaphragm

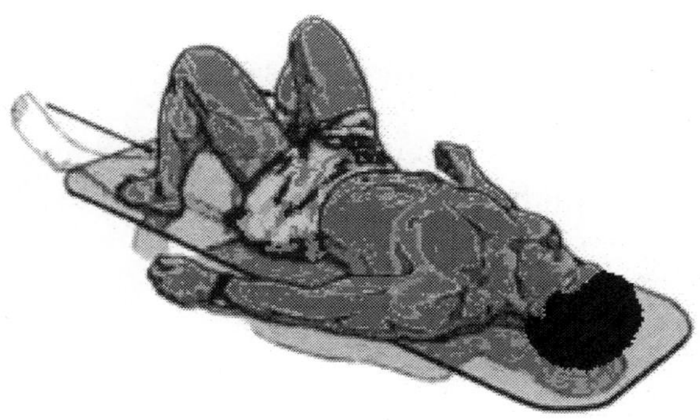

Leg Lowering Test:

How to perform: Have client lie supine holding their hips and knees at 90 degrees. Have them contract their TVA with your hand or blood pressure cuff underneath. Ask them to lower each leg without releasing pressure from your hand/the cuff.

What to look for: The belly will start to protrude which in turn lets you know they have re leased tension in the TVA and transferred it to the rectus abdominus. A normal reading is down to 15 degrees or so. Don't be alarmed if your client cannot drop their legs at all without releasing tension. Have them practice position 3 from the previous section.

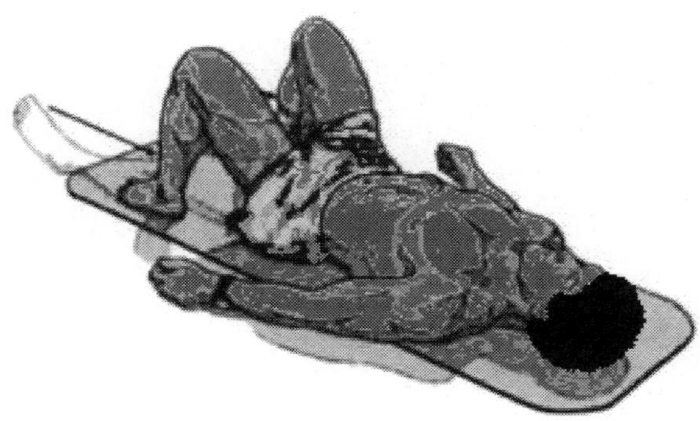

NOTE: Have client flex hips to 90 degrees and flex knees to 90 degrees

GAIT ASSESSMENT (BALANCE)

Balance in Gait (walk)

NOTE: *All one-legged exercises should be performed on both legs to determine if a client has a dominant side. It is common for this to be the case and any difference should be noted.*

How to perform the Gait test (for all positions):

1. Analyze client's posture and balance
2. Note any swaying or compensations
3. Especially note client's foot and ankle

Position 1

1. Ask client to take one normal step forward
2. Have client hold that staggered stance
3. Ask client to look left/right
4. Note time client is able to hold cbalance

Position 2

1. Ask client to lift one leg (i.e., stand on one foot)
2. Ask client to look left/ right
3. Note time client is able to hold balance

Position 3

1. Ask client to lift one leg
2. Have clienttry to 'walk in place' using the raised leg
3. Note time client is able to hold balance

SQUAT (FLEXIBILITY)

Overhead Squat

NOTE: The overhead squat is one of the most powerful assessments, primarily because it works almost the entire kinetic chain. By examining a client's overhead squat, you will be able to determine multiple weaknesses and areas of muscle tightness that can help you, as an exercise professional, design an appropriate exercise program. If there is only one assessment that can performed, we recommended the overhead squat because it can tell you a lot about what a client needs to work on to be stronger and feel better. As you become more experienced, you will notice some of the same patterns (i.e., deficiencies) among your clients that are common to the general population.

How to perform: Flex your shoulders up to your ears. Instruct your client to squat down as far as they can while keeping their shoulders flexed maximally.

What to look for:
Feet - if the feet rotate externally or the heels pop up, there is an inherent tightness in the calves (gastrocnemius and soleus muscles)
Knees - if knees fall inward, check tight IT band and weakness in the glutes
Low Back - if the lower back region hyper-extends it is a good indication of tight hip flexors
- if lumbar region flexes, then overactive external obliques and weak inner unit
Arms - if arms cannot stay flexed, then tight lats and anterior shoulder girdle and weak posterior shoulder girdle and external rotators
Head - if head juts forward, then it usually means the deep neck stabilizers are weak

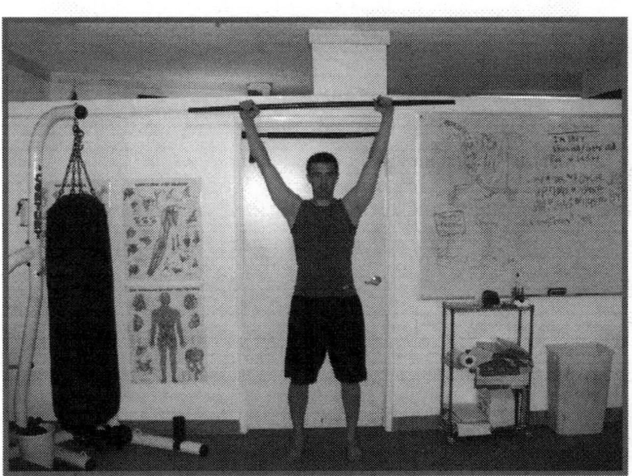

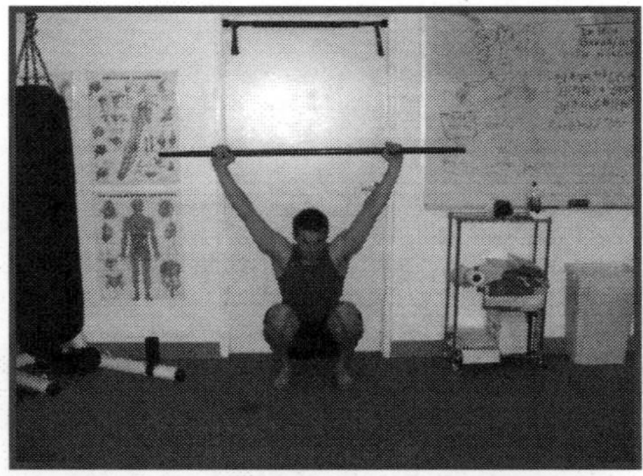

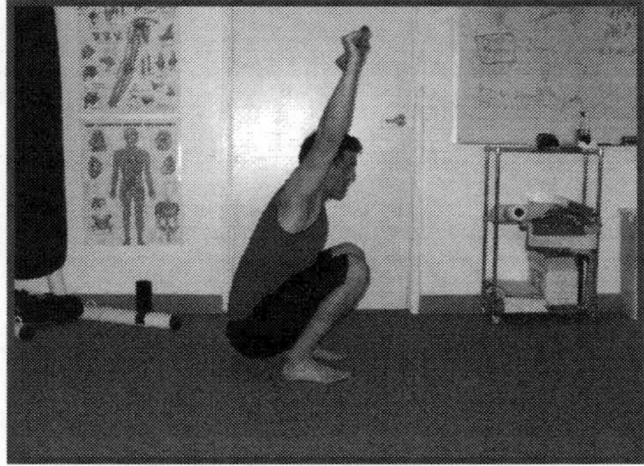

PUSH (STRENGTH)

Push-up Hold

How to perform: Have client assume push-up position and hold. Place dowel vertically on back.

What to look for:
Entire Body - should stay in alignment for the duration of the assessment
Head - if cervical region hyper-extends, then the sternocleidomastoid is dominant
Scapulae - if they stay abducted and winged it indicates a weak serratus anterior and possibly inhibited rhomboids
Low Back - if lumbar region hyper-extends, then the inner unit is suspect (i.e., weak)
- if low back flexes, look for overactive external obliques and weak inner unit

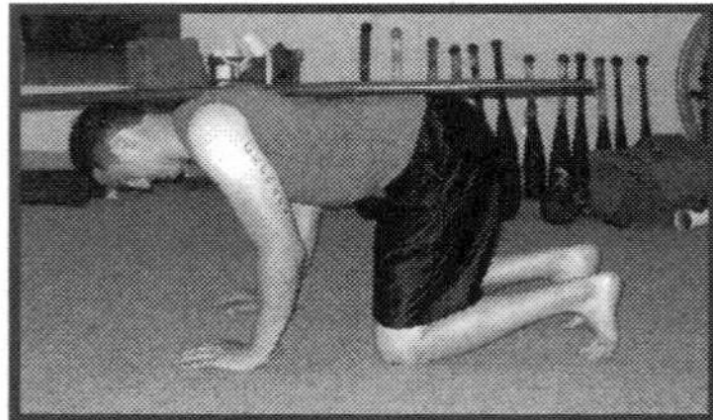
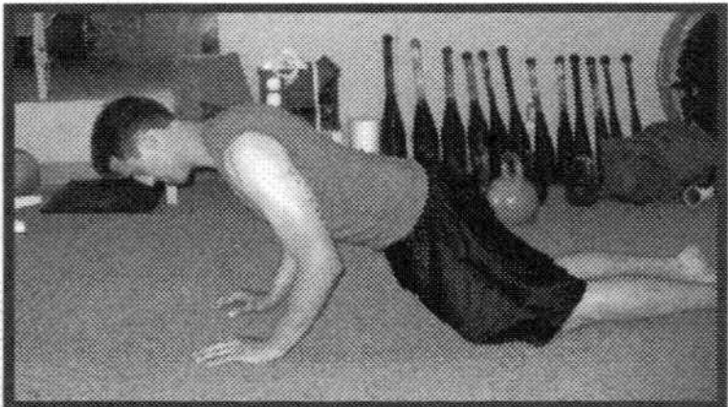
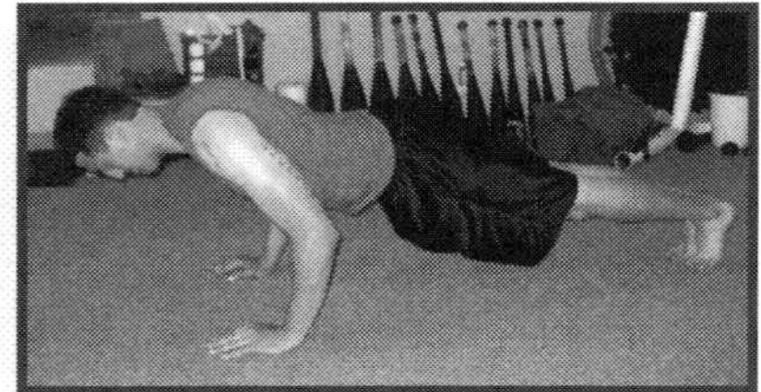

PULL (STRENGTH/POSTURE)

Cobra

How to perform: Have client stand with good posture. Then, have client slowly externally rotate his/her arms while simultaneously adduct the scapulae.

What to look for:
Entire Body - should stay in alignment for the duration of the assessment
Head - if cervical region hyper-extends, then the sternocleidomastoid is dominant
Scapulae - inability to stay adducted indicates weak rhomboids and possibly tight pectoralis
Low Back - if lumbar region hyper- extends the inner unit is suspect.

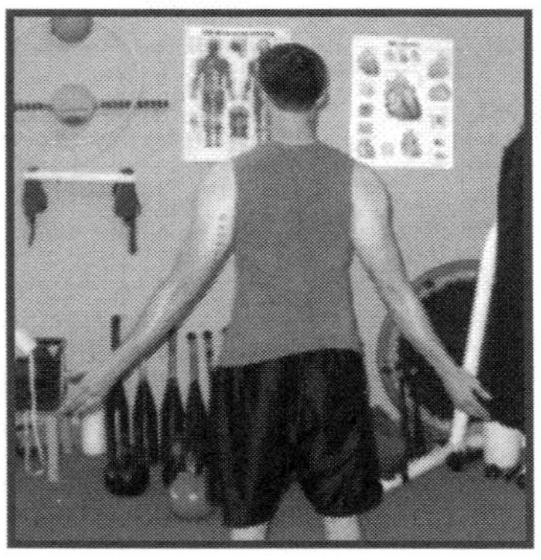
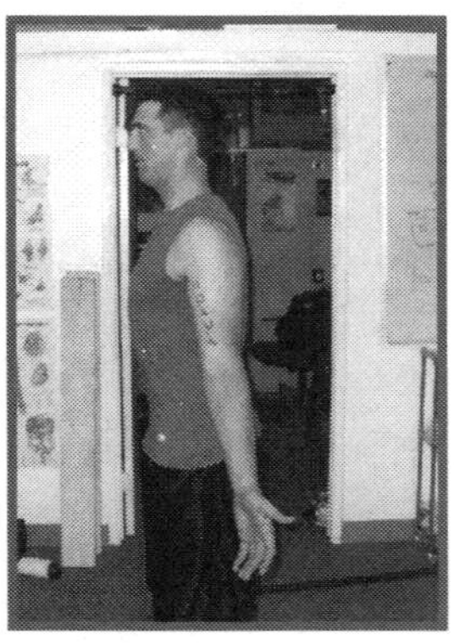

BEND (FLEXIBILITY)

Toe Touches (Spinal Flexion)

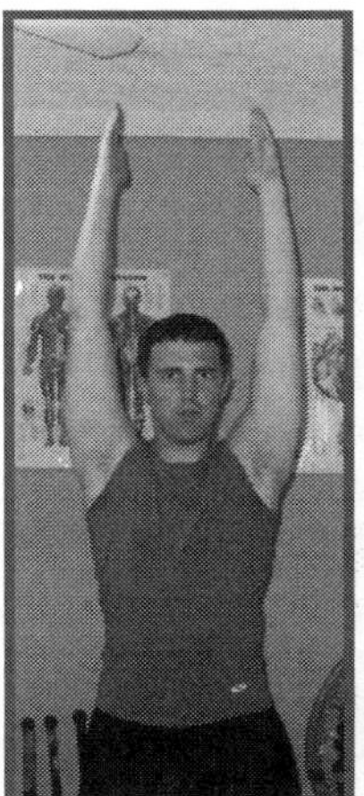

How to perform: Have client stand with good posture. Then, have client slowly bend down and touch his/her toes, or as far as he/she can.

What to look for:
Entire Body - should stay in alignment for the duration of the assessment
Head- if cervical region hyper-extends, then the sternocleidomastoid is dominant
Scapulae - they should abduct and elevate while bent over
Low Back - lumbar region should flex uniformly throughout the assessment
Feet - should stay pointing forward; feet that rotate our indicate tight external rotators at the hip, most likely periformis

---

Side Bends (Lateral Flexion)

How to perform: Have client stand with good posture. Then, have client slowly bend to each side as far as he/she can without hurting his/her muscles.

What to look for:
Entire Body - should stay in alignment for the duration of the assessment; if body tends to fall forward, client is flexor dominant; if client tend to fall backward, he/she is extensor dominant
Head - make sure it stays in alignment with shoulders
Shoulders - client should stay neutral and not rotate either way while bending to the side
Low Back - Lumbar region should laterally flex uniformly throughout
Feet - should stay pointing forward; if they rotate out, it indicates tight external rotators at the hip, most likely periformis.

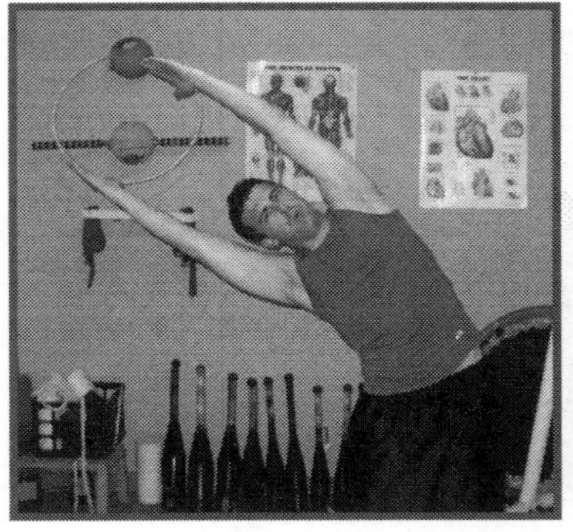

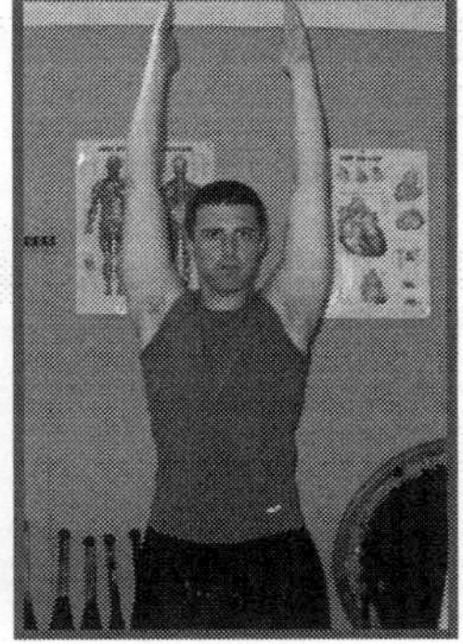

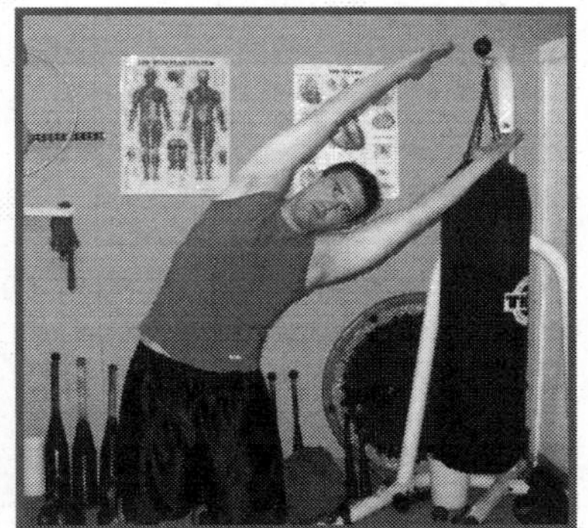

Back Bends (Spinal Extension)

How to perform: Have client stand with good posture with their arms crossed over their chest. Then, have them slowly bend back as far as they can without hurting themselves. Keep chin tucked throughout!

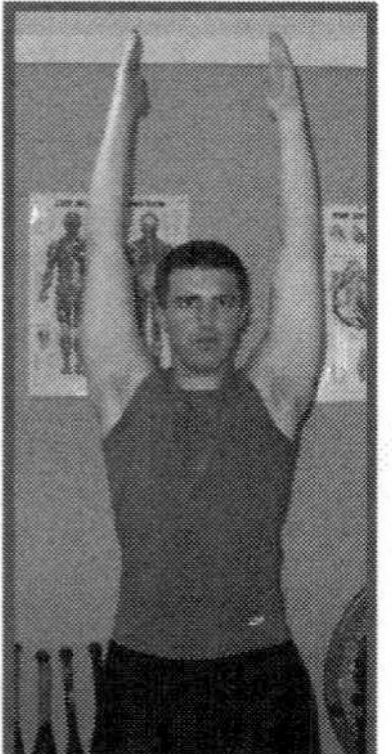

WARNING: *Closely monitor TVA! If it does not stay contracted, STOP assessment.*

What to look for:

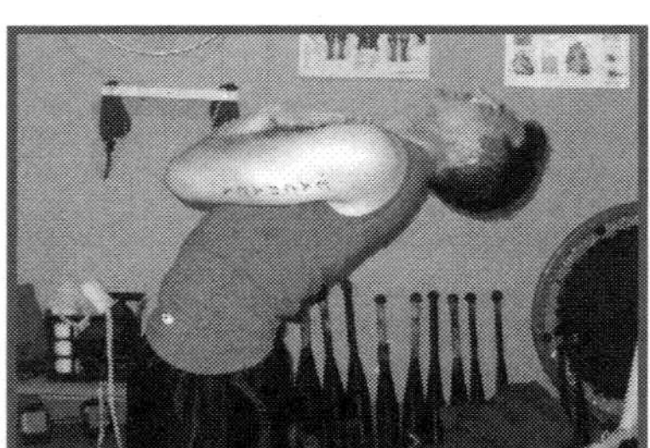

Entire Body - should stay in alignment for the duration of the assessment
Head - if cervical region hyper-extends, then the sternocleidomastoid is dominant and they have weak hyoid muscles
Upper and Lower Back - should extend uniformly throughout
Feet - should stay pointing forward; if they rotate out, that indicates tight external rotators at the hip, most likely periformis

---

TWIST

Wood Chops and Reverse Wood Chops (Spinal Rotation)

How to perform: Have client stand with good posture. Then, have them reach toward the upper right side and then slowly bend and rotate down and towards the left side and vice-versa. (Reverse Chops just start at the bottom and rotate to the top.)

What to look for:
Entire Body - should stay in alignment for the duration of the assessment
Head - should be extended when in the "up" position and tucked at the bottom
Scapulae - they should abduct and elevate while bent over
Upper and Lower Back - should flex and extend uniformly throughout
Feet - should stay pointing forward throughout the movement; if they rotate out, that indicates tight external rotators at the hip, most likely periformis

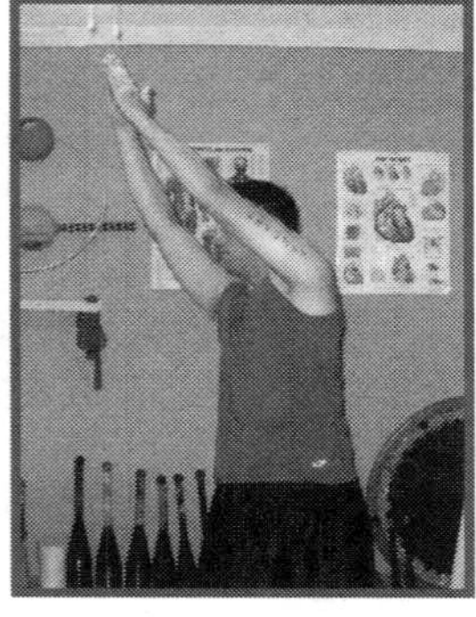

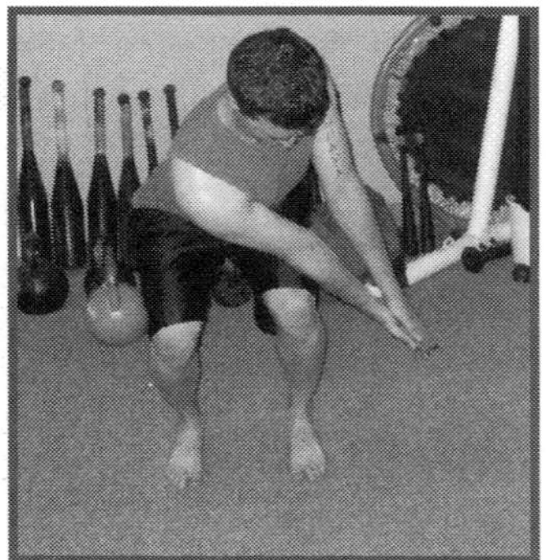

LUNGE

Front (Sagittal) Lunge

How to perform: Have client stand with their feet spread 2 feet apart and both pointing forward. Then, have them slowly bend their knees until just before the back leg knee touches the floor.

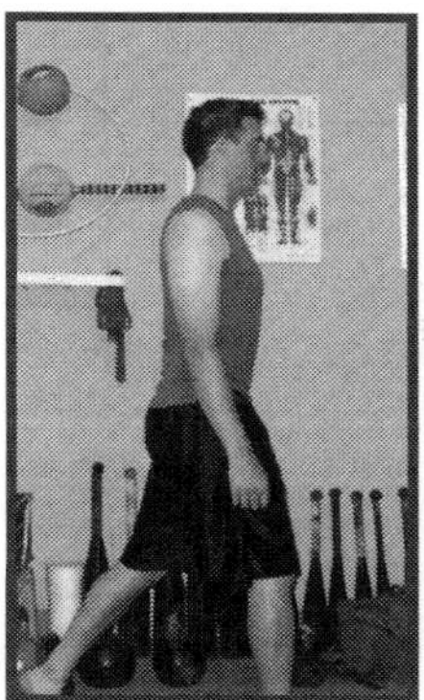

What to look for:
Entire Body - should stay in alignment for the duration of the assessment
Head - should stay in neutral position for the duration of the movement
Scapulae - should stay in neutral position for the duration of the movement
Low Back - lumbar region should stay in neutral position for the duration of the movement
hip, most likely piriformis
Feet - should stay pointing forward; of they rotate out, that indicates tight external rotators at the

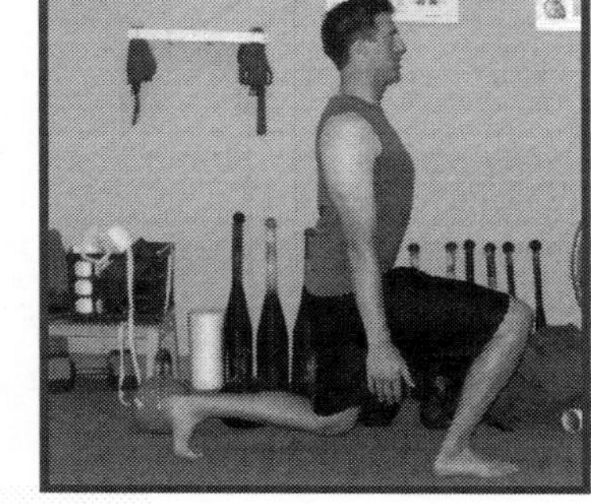

Multi-Planar Step/Hop/Lunge and Hold (Coordination)

How to perform: Have client take a normal step, hop or lunge in each plane (i.e., Sagittal, frontal, and transverse and have them stabilize that position.

What to look for: Pay attention to the client's ability to stabilize at the ankle and all other joints throughout the kinetic chain. There should be little or no instability after impact.

NOTE: *These pictures below only show the lunge in each direction. Remember to have your client transfer his/her weight to the lead foot, and stabilize on that foot.*

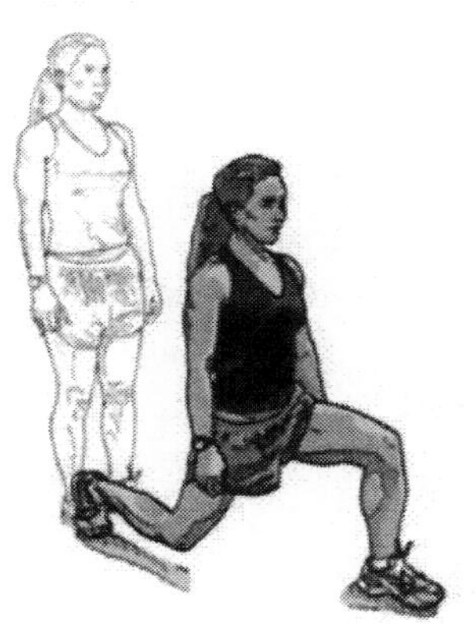

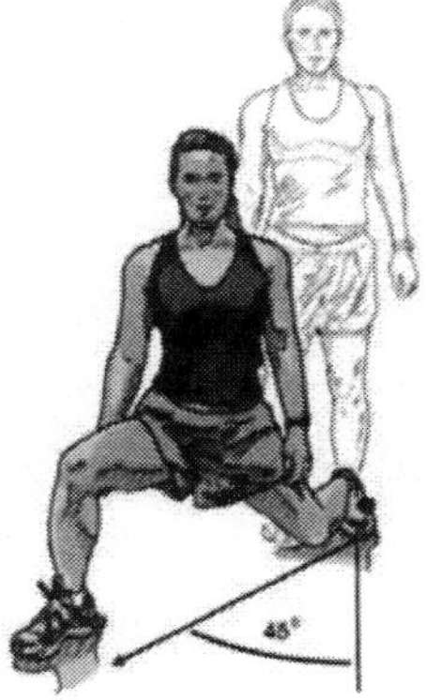

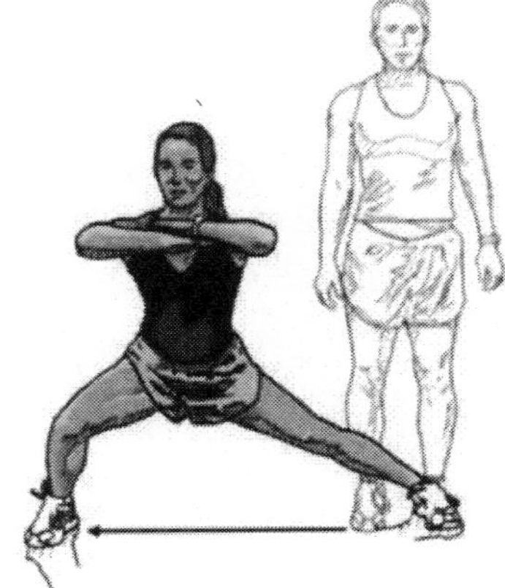

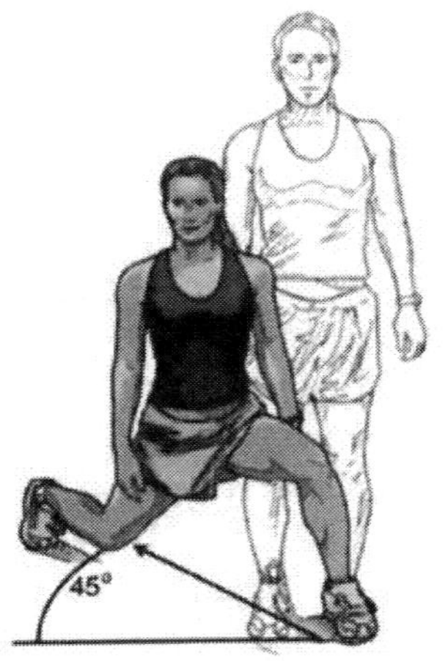

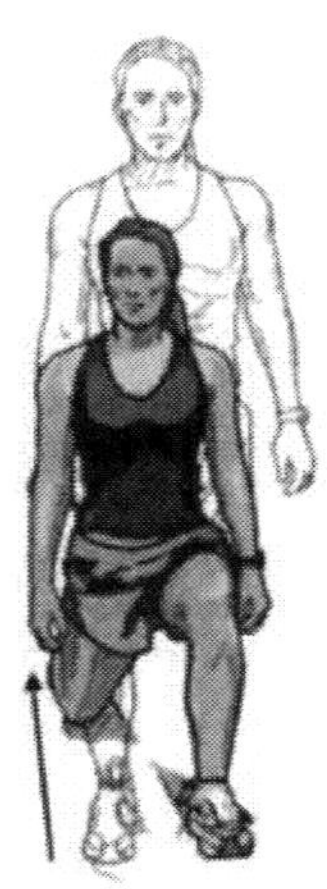

CONCLUSION

Assessments are an important aspect of any quality exercise program, and being able to adequately assess your clients' movement is essential to your success as a trainer. In order to design a program that will help your clients move (and feel) better, we must first understand *how* they move. This includes muscle weaknesses and areas of tightness, as well as imbalances that can hinder their daily activities and general quality of life.

Of course, do not be surprised if many of your clients are unable to perform these above assessments very effectively. Let the client know they are not meant to be discouraging. In fact, these movements were meant to be encouraging; your job as an exercise professional, after all, is to get him/her moving. No matter how the client does with each movement, you should tell him/her that he/she is doing well and to keep up the good work. The less you describe how the movement should be performed, the less the client will know if he/she performed it poorly. For example, if you instruct a client to raise his/her arms to the side of their heads and squat, provided he/she can go down at all, your client will feel as though he/she completed the movement well. Your skills as a trainer will allow you to recognize all the irregularities as your client performs the squat that will help guide you in designing an exercise program. This specially designed exericse program will in turn help your client improve his/her daily movement. For example, when a person's chin juts out and the cervical spine becomes hyper-extended, you know this individual has a rounded shoulder, forward head posture. Yet, just because you notice this does not mean you must share this information immediately with your client. Instead, please be tactful and socially aware with your responses.

CHAPTER FIVE

Nutrition

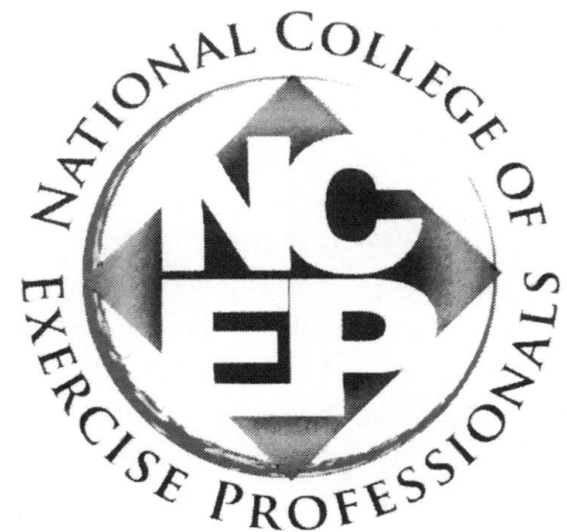

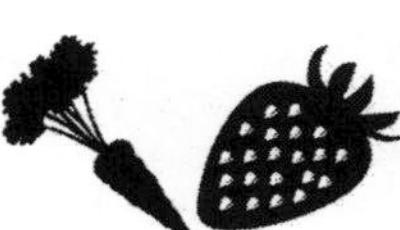

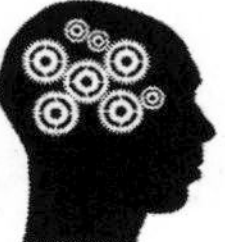

NUTRITION

Even the best designed exercise program will not get the results your client desires without proper nutrition. We believe that nutrition is not just a separate field of study in its own right, but an intricate a part of fitness—which is why we consider it one of the five main components *of* fitness. In fact, it is so important that every client should receive a personalized exercise program with at least some guidance on nutrition. However, nutrition has become a subject ripe with misinformation and confusion. Thus, this chapter provides our five basic guidelines for discussing nutrition with your client. We believe that, above all, your advice should easily fit into any client's lifestyle and that you should always keep the health of the client as the first priority when giving any nutritional advice. Before discussing our strategy for discussing nutrition with clients, it is important to first briefly outline general misconceptions, and the role that food plays in our society.

A Nation "Obsessed" With Eating

In modern society, we have been conditioned and socialized to do things that are unhealthy. Believe it or not, some of the eating behaviors we might think are healthy actually do us harm and cause us to store fat. For instance, how many of us willingly starve ourselves all afternoon so that we may earn the reward of a big dinner later that night? Certainly many of us are guilty of these social rules. Yet, this common behavior (both the starving part *and* the big dinner part) is often responsible for much of our total excess stored body fat. For example, you should be able to communicate to clients that an alternative—and pleasurable—way exists for him/her to still feel "satisfied" at dinner while cutting back on that "big" meal without any major sacrifice.

As a nation, we are obsessed with eating. Some people eat in response to stress, anger or frustration; others eat as a reward for being "good" about not eating at other times. But, with all the other things going on in our lives, eating does not have to be another "thing" that is stressful or complicating. In reality, eating is simply a means by which we obtain fuel. Our bodies can either burn this fuel immediately for energy, use it to build muscle, or store it as fat (to be theoretically used for energy later). Which of these routes our food takes is entirely up to us, because when and what we eat determines what happens to that fuel. With that in mind, many sports nutritionists and dieticians suggest to "eat now for what you plan to do later." Albeit simple, this is sound advice; in other words, refrain from eating as a reward for something you already did. Instead, eat for what you *will* be doing in the next few hours or tomorrow. For example, it is much better to eat before your workout, so you will be properly fueled, than to starve first and then eat a huge meal after your workout as a reward for all the calories you just burned. That is not how the body works, and as we will explain, these basic principles should be communicated to your clients.

Still, with all the diets that come out every year, it is no wonder most people are confused. From the high protein diets to the low carb diets, every diet leads you to believe it has the answers to all your problems. But, most of these overnight sensations are based on monetized media campaigns or pseudo-science that have no real scientific basis. In fact, statistics show that most people who begin some sort of diet will gain back their original weight (and often a few extra pounds) within a year. With statistics like that, what can a person do? What is the right amount of calories to eat in a day? Are carbohydrates the enemy or the answer? If fat is so bad, why are some people promoting high-fat diets? Do we really get enough protein? (How does a reasonable person sort this all out?) Even if you knew all the variables, how could you possibly stick to any one program long enough to create a lasting lifestyle?

While all the hoards of information thrown at us can seem overwhelming, good news exists: there are a few components that should cut across any diet or eating pattern, if followed correctly. Essentially, any eating pattern should divide calories among more frequent, smaller meals, cut back on sugar, try to eat good fats instead of trans fat, and include drinking plenty of water. Thus, without going into elaborate detail about whether the body is better suited to a high carbohydrate diet or a high protein type diet or the specific ways your body utilizes different sources of fuel, we can still offer guidelines that allow your client to have success on any plan. And, most importantly, that allows your client to meet his/her goals without worrying about specific foods—guidance that should probably come from a certified dietician instead.

As we will explain, ultimately, the single biggest common denominator throughout all truly successful eating programs is to eat small, well-balanced meals more often. This is true whether you are trying to lose fat or gain muscle, or both. You cannot just instruct your client to stop eating; such an approach is both unhealthy and antithetical to helping him/her adopt a healthy lifestyle (plus not effective in keeping weight off). We believe, as part of a total fitness program, you should help clients develop a healthy lifestyle by observing the following guidelines in this chapter.

The crux of proper nutrition and a healthy eating strategy is composed of 5 parts: (1) eating "balanced" meals and snacks every 2-3 hours; (2) eating "healthy" unprocessed food; (3) watch fat intake; (4) drink plenty of water; and (5) proper supplementation. We will explain what these mean in practical terms in ways that you can explain and discuss with your clients.

COMPONENT 1:
EAT AT LEAST 5-6 SMALL MEALS PER DAY
(AND AVOID CALORIE RESTRICTION)

The most important of the five components is eating every 2-3 hours. Every time you go on a diet, reduce the amount of food you eat, cut calories, skip meals, or do anything else that "threatens" your body's food supply, such actions actually stimulate your body to store more fat through the following channels: (a) loss of muscle mass; (b) slowing of your metabolism; and (c) biochemical changes that encourage your body to hang onto its fat stores *and* create new fat stores.

Understanding the Body's Metabolism

First, (a), understanding muscle mass: the simple formula to remember for diets (i.e., cutting calories, excessive cardio, etc.) is that much of the weight you will lose on a diet will be muscle. (This is because in a calorie deficit, your body will inevitably need to use, or "burn," some muscle as energy.) Understand that since muscle is your greatest source of metabolism, it requires more energy than any other macronutrient (i.e., more than fat). While the exact amount of calories burned per pound of muscle varies per person, losing muscle mass cuts down on the amount of calories your body needs at rest. Essentially, every person has a set number of calories he/she burns at rest. While this is determined by a lot of factors, such as genetics, it also it based on body composition. Thus, people who lose large amounts of weight on a diet are also losing muscle mass; not only is this unhealthy and makes individuals weaker, but when a person resumes his/her "normal" eating habits, he/she has less calories to consume before gaining weight. Most studies show that people who lose weight on a diet gain that weight back *plus* extra weight, too.

In connection, (b), losing massive amounts of muscle mass is one of the ways in which eating *infrequently* will slow your metabolism, such as through two or three big meals a day. When you reduce your caloric input, within about three hours or so, your body thinks it is starving. Thus, the body will quickly attempt to perform its basic life support functions—keep your body temperature about 98.6° F, pump blood to the heart, attack germs and viruses, etc.—with as little energy as possible (i.e., using fewer calories). Thus, if muscle requires more energy (calories) than fat, it makes the most sense for your body to get rid of, or "burn," muscle first! As your body begins to slow down performing all of its functions when you go on a diet, it enters a quasi-survival mode, or sometimes referred to as "starvation mode." Basically, your body enters a state of sympathetic nervous system—stress or "fight or flight"—dominance. In lay terms, what this means is that your body believes that it is in a crisis, since it does not have enough energy (i.e., not enough food) to perform the body's necessities, and thus, prioritizes its activities. For example, your core body temperature decreases (especially in your extremities), your digestion slows down, cellular repair slows, etc., meaning that your body cannot fully recover from activity. Basically, your body has to perform other "budget cut backs" to survive on fewer calories—and remember, one of those cutbacks is to use (i.e., "burn") muscle for energy (inefficiently). Both avoiding calorie restriction, but more importantly, eating small meals constantly throughout the day will help prevent the "starvation mode" from switching into effect.

Finally, weight loss aside, (c), there are also biochemical changes that occur in your body when you restrict calories. For example, there are changes in your thyroid's secretions (T3), which will mean lower body temperature, and changes in your adrenal gland's secretions, causing sympathetic nervous system dominance. One interesting biochemical change is that the surface structure of your fat cells actually changes. On the surface of your fat cells are receptors that, if stimulated will release fat, and receptors that will store fat. Normally, or in non-emergency times, your fat cells' surface has a relative balance of release and storage receptors. The problem when you go on a diet is the number of storage receptors, particularly in women, increase significantly, making it much easier, and much more efficient, for your body to store fat. This change is pretty slow to return to "normal" post-diet, which is one reason why it is difficult to lose as much weight as fast the second, third, fourth, etc., time that you go on a diet.

Solution: Frequent Eating Leads to Active Metabolism

Our solution? Make your body comfortable with its food supply by eating frequently enough to supply adequate nutrition (and stabilize your blood sugar levels, discussed next). Although it varies per person, most peoples' bodies go into starvation mode somewhere between three and five hours after the most recent ingestion of food. Therefore, eating a meal or snack every 2-3 hours keeps your metabolism active and ensures that you *can* actually access your stored body fat and retain a high metabolism.

When you are eating every 2-3 hours, strive to eat balanced meals and snacks that are full of nutrients. Nutrients are the life sustaining compounds that we get from food, and they can be divided into two basic groups: *micro*nutrients and *macro*nutrients. *Micro* equals the nutrients that we need in very small amounts that are measured in milligrams, and even micrograms (one millionth of a gram), and provide no calories. These are vitamins, minerals, and while official dietary minimums have not been established for enzymes, and phytonutrients, most cutting-edge nutritionists would agree that they are essential. *Macro*nutrients, on the other hand, are needed in much larger quantities and are usually measured in grams or ounces (see the end of this chapter). These include *protein, carbohydrates, fat,* and *water*. With the exception of water, these all provide calories or fuel for our body to perform its vital and non-vital functions.

A quick note about the macronutrients: again, with the exception of water, each of these macronutrients have, at one time or another, come under fire as being "evil" or the "enemy" in terms of weight loss or even general health. While discussing health trends by various popularized doctors is beyond the scope of this manual, we subscribe to what a majority of decades of research has shown: that a well-balanced diet is most effective for promoting general health. Furthermore, it is our belief that there are no "evil" macronutrients, just better or cleaner sources from which we must chose each of them. Decades of research has shown that each of the macronutrients are necessary for lasting health. Avoiding fat, protein, or carbohydrates all have the potential to cause very serious health problems, and the avoidance of any will cause a deprivation or deficiency in your body.

Overall, a balanced meal or snack means that it contains all three calorie containing macronutrients: fat, protein, and carbohydrates. Every individual will have a need for different ratios of one nutrient to the other throughout his/her life depending his/her activities (this is what we call substrate utilization, which is beyond the scope of this manual). If you are interested in learning more about nutrition, please inquire about our Holistic Nutrition course.

COMPONENT 2:
DO NOT EAT REFINED FOODS, ESPECIALLY SUGAR

The second component of a healthy eating strategy is, quite simply, to eat "healthy" food, or what we consider to be minimally processed whole foods that are close to their natural state. It may surprise you to find out how processed some foods really are, as a thorough understanding is critical when undergoing conversations with your clients.

Processed Foods Versus Whole Foods

"Minimally processed whole foods" are the foods that you will find on the perimeter of the grocery store: fresh meats, dairy products, fresh fruits and vegetables, and some whole grains. Processed foods are often the foods that you will find on the interior of the grocery store: Pop Tarts, boxed cereal, flours, minute rice, cookies, preserves, and just about everything else that comes in a jar, can, box, or plastic wrapper.

One of the greatest examples of the tremendous difference between a whole food and a processed food is what happens to wheat flour. When kept at room temperature for long periods of time, whole wheat flour will begin to be occupied by a host of mealy bugs. Yet, if (refined) white flour is similarly left out, no bugs will ever appear; essentially, white flour has been so thoroughly processed that it *has very little nutritional value.* The mealy bugs have no interest in this white flour! If bugs do not want this flour, imagine what this "food" will do to a human being who eats 200 pounds of this stuff per year.

White flour is describned on ingredient lists as "wheat flour," "enriched wheat flour," "unbleached wheat four," or "unbleached enriched wheat flour." Unless it explicitly says, "whole wheat flour," you are eating a processed version of white flour. All that is left by the time the wheat grain is processed into white flour are purely refined carbohydrates that are absorbed as fast as white table sugar into your blood stream. Refined and concentrated carbohydrates, such as sugar and white flour are probably the number one threat to your health (and your waist-line). Recent studies have shown that sugar—and not fat—is the biggest cause of growing obesity in this country. Thus, to understand the refined carbohydrate-body fat connection, you have to first understand the insulin-blood sugar relationship.

Understanding the Body's Response to Glucose

Whenever you eat a food that contains carbohydrates—grains, fruits, vegetables, baked goods, sugar, and even most dairy products—they are converted during the process of digestion into what is known as glucose, or what is referred to as blood sugar. Blood sugar is one of your body's primary sources of fuel. Your brain can only function using glucose, while the rest of your body can use a mixture of fuels (and if you do this right that mixture will be largely made up of stored body fat). The post-lunch "sleepies" are what happen to your when your blood sugar dips low.

How blood sugar is used and absorbed depends on the food itself. For example, some carbohydrate foods such as sugar, flour products, candy, etc., are absorbed extremely quickly into the blood stream. Minutes after your consume one of these high "glycemic index" foods, your blood sugar levels increase to very, very high levels. The Glycemic Index (GI) is just a scale that measures how fast a food affects, or raises, your blood sugar. Foods like meat essentially have no affect whatsoever on your blood sugar and are considered low GI foods because they do not contain any carbohydrates. Also considered low GI foods are most "whole" foods—remember foods that are not in a refined state—such as grains, yams, all berries, and almost all vegetables. This term just means that they have a very slow, long lasting effect on your blood sugar levels. On the other hand, foods such as flour and sugar skyrocket your blood sugar levels almost immediately.

Insulin is the primary hormone, or chemical messenger, responsible for the regulation of your blood sugar levels. High levels of blood sugar stimulate high levels of insulin (what you often hear in regards to Diabetes) in the blood, which is a storage hormone. This just means that insulin first stores your blood sugar (or blood glucose) as glycogen—which your body then stores in your muscles and liver. This glucose, which is converted to glycogen, is stored in each muscle in your body for future activity. However, since your capacity to store glycogen is rather small, instead of converting (and then storing it as muscle glycogen), your body very quickly begins to store the glucose in your fat cells (and increasing your fat). And, why does this matter? Well, too much blood sugar, with no where to "go," converts into fat—a process which is slowed down by whole foods, because they take longer to digest and enter your bloodstream in the first place. Here's this process in diagram form:

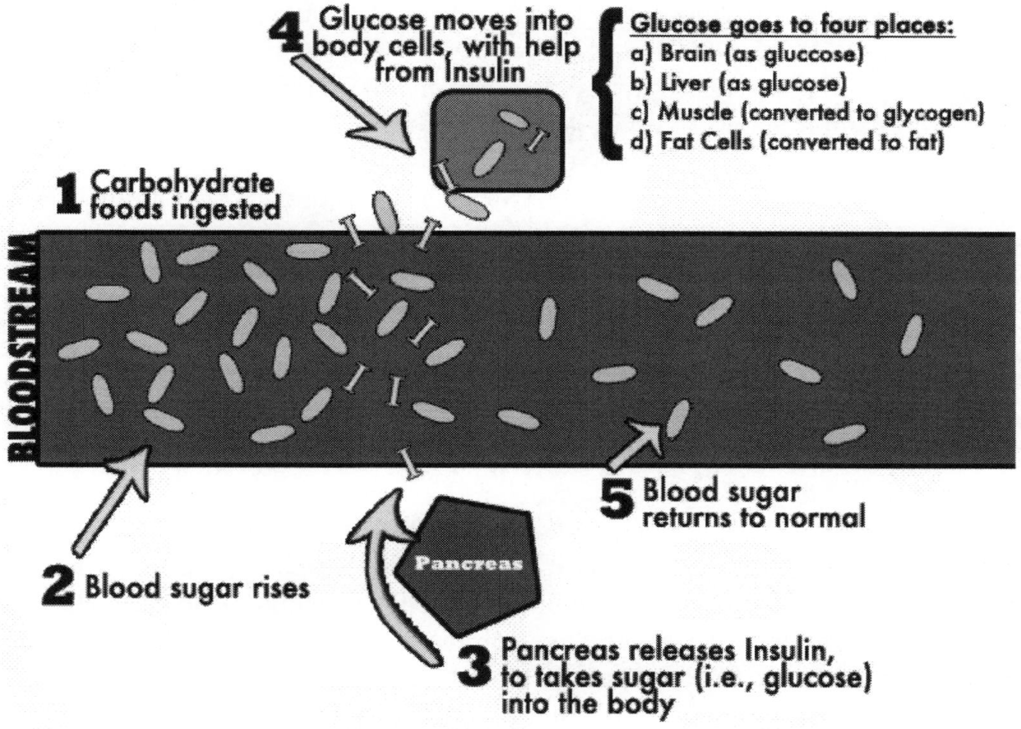

Insulin's opposite hormone is called glucagon. Glucagon is a release hormone, as in it "releases" fat. When insulin levels are high, glucagon levels drop automatically. So, whenever you consume a high GI food, you rapidly raise your blood sugar levels. This triggers your body to store fat, and physically shuts off your body's ability to even access your stored fat. Therefore, the more stable you keep your blood sugar—by eating food low on the GI scale and eating every 2-3 hours—the more you keep your storage hormone, insulin, in check. This, in turn, keeps your glucagon, or fat-releasing hormones high, allowing you to burn fat for fuel constantly throughout the day. Furthermore, high insulin levels caused by high GI foods actually inhibit muscle growth by suppressing the production of human growth hormone (HGh), which is integral in helping your muscles grow. High insulin levels thereby limit the capacity and efficiency of your fat burning furnace: muscle tissue. To recap, high GI foods actually encourage fat storage in three ways: high insulin levels, low glucagon levels, and low HGh levels. Eating whole, natural foods that keep your blood sugar levels stable is both healthy—remember whole, natural foods have the most beneficial nutrients, vitamins, and minerals—and conducive to maintaining a healthy weight for your clients.

Basically, if you stick to the foods available at a farmer's market, or on the perimeter of a natural grocery store such as organic meats, dairy, some whole grains, fresh fruits and vegetables, you are consuming the right types of foods. Although you should not be suggesting certain meals for clients, giving them general shopping tips about picking out, and eating, natural foods as written here, is highly encouraged and appropriate.

The Importance of "Natural" Animal Products

One final note about eating natural foods: the importance of eating organic animal products. Ideally, it is critical for you to eat animal products that are raised in an environment where they are given free space to move, exposed to sunlight, fed something that closely resembles their natural diet, and given a minimum of drugs—only what is necessary for truly medicinal purposes. Sadly, the majority of animal products, which we characterize as dairy, eggs, poultry, meat, etc., come from facilities where animals are raised in caged, extremely toxic environments. Essentially, instead of living outdoors in freedom, animals—primarily chicken and cattle which are both most commonly consumed—live cradle to the grave inside of a what looks a lot like a factory, hence the term "factory farm." Inside of these factories, chickens, for example, live crammed 10, 20 or 30,000 chickens deep in a space that does not allow them to do much of anything; these animals cannot move, and are raised, and thus covered during their life spans, in their own feces. Thus, to combat these conditions and the wrath of diseases that fester inside these farms and within these animals themselves, they are commonly injected with high doses of antibiotics to keep them alive. As you can imagine, these animals—diseased, raised in unnatural settings, and unhealthy—are full of toxins that they develop over their putrid life-span.

As you may have seen at a health food store, we believe it is very important to eat animal products that are free of antibiotics and injected hormones, and thus, that are cage-free and/or "free-range" raised and most importantly, grass-fed. The best characteristic, which covers these components and other more stringent criteria such as non-GMO animal feed, would be to eat certified organic meat. Basically, the food industry has created two completely different types of the same food. This difference comes from how the food is both grown and processed. On the one hand, we have what we will refer to as "conventional" food, and on the other hand there is certified organic, grass-fed food. While it is beyond the scope of this course to discuss the vast amount of literature written on the dangers of eating "conventionally raised" animal products, we believe that the latter—eating organic animal products—is an important part of developing a holistic eating pattern.

COMPONENT 3: WATCH YOUR FAT INTAKE

The third component of a healthy eating strategy is to watch your fat intake. Specifically, you should help your clients watch both the amount of fat they get in their diet *and*—but maybe most importantly—the type of fat they are ingesting. All fat is not created equal, which is discussed in this section. Broadly, there are three types of fat: *saturated*, *unsaturated*, and the worst of all, *trans*. One of the biggest problems with understanding fat intake (including high-fat diets) revolves around the misunderstanding that all fats are (incorrectly) created equal. Simply put, there are many different kinds of fat, and both the quality of the food (i.e., free-range chicken vs. conventially-raised chicken) and the way it has been processed and cooked, can affect the fat content of food (and its cholesterol levels).

The "Good" Fat: Omega-3 Fatty-Acids

Understand, first, that the term "fatty-acid" is only a fancy word for "type of fat." To explain this phrase, we can look at the Inuit Eskimos. This population group consumes a diet composed almost entirely of fat, oil and protein with tons of cholesterol, and tons of animal fat, yet they still have remarkably low levels of heart disease. Their lifestyle is possible because they consume animal products that are natural (i.e., closer to organic meats) and mostly, have high levels of Omega-3 (from fish, discussed below).

It is important to know that Omega-3's are considered the "good" fats—the type of fats that raise your HDL (the "healthy" cholesterol) and decrease your LDL (the "lousy" cholesterol) in your body. These particular fatty-acids protect the heart nicely; high levels of Omega-3's have also been shown to help in the prevention of inflammation, improve skin, and possibly even help chronic illnesses such as allergies and diabetes. Most Omega-3 fats are considered *unsaturated fats.* What you need to know for this course, and for your general knowledge to share with clients, is that our ancestors (like the Inuit Eskimos) ate a diet with a ratio of 1:1 or 2:1 Omega-6 to Omega-3. Today, however, we in Western cultures consume a diet of 20:1 or 25:1, which is really, really bad for our bodies on many levels—heart disease, high cholesterol, etc., not to mention unhealthy weight gain. Most animal foods produced via conventional methods that involve feeding animals very unnatural and unhealthy diets, such as grain, drastically alter the fatty-acid ratios in their meat, milk and eggs. (Conversely, and not coincidentally, eggs from free-range chickens can have a fatty-acid ratio close to 1:1.) In reality, while the chemical structure of fats is quite complex and beyond the scope of this manual, understanding that the ideal ratio of Omega-6 to Omega-3 is 1:1 and that all fats are not equal, is seminal knowledge. Quality sources for Omega-3 include fatty cold water fish (i.e. salmon, mackerel, herring, etc), flax seed oil, and most nuts (like walnuts).

Reviewing the Types of Fats

Consuming foods with high levels of Omega-3's, which are *unsaturated fats*, promotes good health while consuming animal products that are high in *saturated fats* are unhealthy, and a major issue among many Americans. Unlike unsaturated fats (many of which are Omega-3's) that lower your cholesterol, saturated fats do not. Further, trans fats are even more dangerous; trans fats are essentially man-made, in that they are not found in foods alone. Instead, processing certain types of foods, such as baked sweet goods, snack chips, and in some margarines, create this type of fat. Unfortunately, most food nutrition labels inaccurately state a (junk) food's trans fat content; labels can be calculated prior to cooking, and if a food develops trans fat during the cooking process, this may not be reflected. Essentially, if you stay away from what is considered "junk" foods and, as referenced in the prior pages, refined foods, you can avoid foods that have trans fat. Overall, educating your clients about the differences among fats—and that they should limit their intake of the "bad" saturated and especially trans fats—is a straight-forward, yet important piece of advice.

COMPONENT 4: DRINK PLENTY OF WATER

"[Water] is nature's miracle medicine: simple, safe, free… and effective!"
- Dr. F. Batmanghelidj

Water is considered an essential nutrient for a reason. Yet, we often do not consume enough of it. Among many potential issues, a lack of water may promote kidney and liver disease, high blood pressure, cataracts, ugly skin, inability to effectively lose fat, to look fatter than you are (the water held under your skin when you are chronically dehydrated looks and feels like fat), muscle cramps, respiratory illness, low energy, etc. Conversely, water helps you lose fat, have beautiful hydrated skin, may lower your risk for diseases, have more energy, and even have an enhanced ability to concentrate and focus. Simply put, every organ, every cell, every single life supporting the biochemical reactions that occur inside of your body requires water; you are approximately 60% water (men slightly more) and your brain is approximately 85% water. You will die in just two to three days without water intake!

Every day your body runs a six to ten glass water deficit through breathing, perspiration, normal metabolism and elimination—and that does not take into account any additional activities or exercise. Many people chronically do not drink enough water, and studies show that even having a 2% water deficit in your body (note that the scientific definition of "dehydration" is a loss of body water greater than 2%) can affect athletic performance. It is also noteworthy to mention that cups of coffee, tea or soda generally *costs* your body water, and may not help hydrate you.

The Important Role of Water for Body Functionality

There are many ways that water is essential for your body to function. First, among many reasons, water is vital in helping your body eliminate waste and other toxins so that you do not die of autointoxication, or self-poisoning. Fat cells are one of the primary places your body stores toxins and extra waste because remember, the body always prioritizes its resources. For example, if you have the flu your body puts immune function at the top of the list for energy usage; it spends all of its energy fighting off the illness and eliminating waste through mucous, diarrhea, etc. When your body is using all of its energy to fight disease, it does not have much left over to do anything else—a reason why you feel so tired when you are sick! In connection, loosing body fat, from a hunter-gatherer survival stand point, is just about as unimportant to your body as anything could possibly be. From this survival perspective, your body wants to hang on to as much fat as it can for as long as it can, as losing body fat requires that you release the toxins stored in your fat. Here's our point: if you do not have sufficient water supplies to eliminate this extra waste, then your body is not going to let you lose that fat, or at least not as much of it. Drinking enough water is both important for general health and for general fat loss.

Furthermore, when you run a water deficit, your body comes up with creative ways to keep the vital life-sustaining biochemical functions occurring in your body. Essentially, your body needs "free-water," or water that is not doing anything else such as being in the liquid of your blood, the liquid in your brain cells, or the fluid that lubricates your joints (which if they hurt could definitely be helped through adequate hydration). During chronic dehydration, your body hoards "free water" under the surface of your skin. The fluid under your skin is soft, squishy and can affect the appearance of muscular definition—dehydration can actually make your body look like it has more fat from an aesthetic perspective.

Tips for Drinking Water for Life and Exercise

To recap above, adequate hydration can decrease bloat, and thinking about your clients, it is quite common for individuals to begin an exercise program (and start to drink more water), and subsequently drop 5-10 pounds in the first week or so by shedding the "free water" under the skin. While this weight was not fat, again, it still often appears as if it is. More specifically to exercise, drinking water also has many, many benefits while causing issues for those people who are dehydrated. For example, staying hydrated has been shown to positively affect athletic performance, particularly aerobic activities—remember, most of your muscles are made up of water—while conversely, dehydration reduces your work capacity and increases your perceived rate of exertion (i.e., an activity may seem harder if you are dehydrated).

As an exercise professional, we suggest that you encourage your clients to drink more water, which can be easier said than done. Encourage them to drink a bit more each day (i.e., modest goals), such as by bringing a water bottle with them to work each day, and asking them to "sip" throughout the day. The act of "sipping" water slowing is like putting your body through a filter—imagine drip irrigation occurring as your body flushes out the toxins. This is preferable over bulk drinking. We like to suggest to clients that just as they take showers when they are physically dirty, it is useful to flush out the toxins and take a "shower on the inside." And, of course, for physical exertion, water is essential for all extra activity—for you and your clients!

How Much Water Should I Drink?

To support fat loss:

- half your body weight in ounces/day (200lbs = 100oz), or
- 3-6 Liters/day
- keep a bottle with you all day, and sip often

Where Should I Get My Water?

Water equivalents:

- herbal tea (without sugar)
- sparkling water
- water with lemon
- regular water (variety is limited)

Avoid/Enjoy in Moderation:

- coffee
- black tea
- sodas
- juice

Notes About Other Beverages

We also should comment about other popular beverages, most notably coffee and juice/sodas. Although coffee as a "pick-me-up" has become a staple of peoples' busy lives, we believe that staying hydrated, combined with an active lifestyle and healthy food (not to mention the emotional "buzz" of living life on your own terms) will give you more energy than ever before. Remember, caffeine, and thus coffee, is considered what is known as a "diuretic," which is substance that can exacerbate dehydration. In regards to juice and soda, believe it or not, it is quite common for juices to have *more* sugar than does soda (although the latter is certainly full of sugar, too). As discussed as part of Component 2, consuming sugar and refined carbohydrates as a regular part of your diet is one of major factors for weight gain among Americans. Thus, consuming juice (or soda) is not a fill-in for drinking water.

One final note about water quality: we believe that you should avoid tap water as much as possible. Of course, this can be very difficult to do, but depending on the regulations of each state (they vary), tap water generally contains significant amounts of chlorine. Municipalities add chlorine to our water to kill microbes, and it works very, very well. However, chlorine can cause imbalances in your gut, and subsequently can disrupt your many digestive processes. Most of all, natural spring water and other water sources usually taste better than tap water—and the better your water tastes, the more eager you will be to drink it!

COMPONENT 5: PROPER SUPPLEMENTATION

We will be honest: adding this fifth, and final, component can be seen as controversial. There are a wide range of existing opinions across the health industry both in terms of the necessity of supplementation itself and the types of supplementation. We acknowledge this and want to make sure you understand that as you approach your client about nutritional guidance, you recognize the varying opinions. However, we are not alone in understanding supplementation's potentially important role in health: in 2002, the Journal of the American Medical Association (JAMA) officially reversed its long standing position against vitamin supplementation. In this significant shift, they concluded that: "we recommend that all adults take one multivitamin daily."^ Of course, in a perfect world, you would not need supplementation at all—in theory, you would be able to satisfy all your vitamin and mineral requirements through food. Yet, for most people, this generally does not happen, and thus, we agree that a multivitamin may help.

A Deeper Look at Vitamins and Minerals

We believe that not all vitamins and minerals are created equally. Although careful research is still needed in the field of supplementation and debates remain, we have come up with a few guidelines based on our own experiences and review of the available research:

1. *All vitamins and minerals should come from whole foods with at least 100% of the Recommended Daily Allowances, and never synthetic replications*

^Fletcher, R. H., & Fairfield, K. M. (2002). Vitamins for chronic disease prevention in adults: clinical applications. *JAMA*, 287(23), 3127–3129.

2. *All vitamins and minerals should come from organic sources that have been cold pressed, and never heated*
3. *Be sure you consume adequate vitamins, minerals, and phytonutrients (nutrients from green plants)*
4. *Consider taking an Omega-3 supplement (sometimes referred to as fish oils), particularly if vegan*

With these guidelines in mind, we believe that one of the main reasons why many people are not getting the needed amount of vitamins and minerals is because our food is less nutritious than it used to be. Conventional food in the grocery store often has less vitamins and minerals, as well as higher concentrations of metals and certain chemicals. While research between organic and conventional produce is still ongoing, below is a table from one such study showing the difference in nutrients between organically grown and conventionally grown produce. (Remember, even if the percent difference varies, it can only be a benefit to eat organic!)

Average Nutrient Differences Between Organic and Conventional Produce

Nutrient	% Difference Organic vs. Conventional Produce
Vitamin C	27% more
Boron	37% more
Calcium	31% more
Chromium	86% more
Copper	11% more
Iodine	49.8% more
Iron	22% more
Magnesium	28% more
Manganese	15.2% more
Molybdenum	17% more
Phosphorus	15% more
Potassium	12% more
Selenium	37.2% more
Sodium	19% more
Vanadium	9% more
Zinc	8% more
Nitrates (poison)	**15% LESS**

Source: Worthington, V. (2001). "Nutritional Quality of Organic Versus Conventional Fruits, Vegetables, and Grains." *The Journal of Alternative and Complimentary Medicine, 7* (2), 2001, 161-173; See also, Smith, B.L. (1993). "Organic Food vs. Supermarket Foods: Element Levels," *Journal of Applied Nutrition, 45*, 35-39); See originally, Schuphan, W. (1974). "Nutritional value of crops as influenced by organic and inorganic fertilizer treatments, *Qualitas Plantarum – Plant Foods for Human Nutrition, 23*: 333-358.

Although these deficiencies may not seem like a lot, over time, they add up. For example, what if you suddenly lost 27% of your income? Or, if you had 27% fewer hours in the day (about 18 hours instead of 24 hours)? For individuals who already eat few fruits and vegetables, combined with the fact that the food they eat may be less nutritious, can lead to vitamin and mineral deficits that need to be addressed.

Recommendations and Suggestions

With all this being said, the world of supplementation is quite overwhelming. Although beyond the scope of this manual, one of these reasons is that the supplement industry has expanded in recent decades, exponentially increasing the amount of products. Specifically, the *Dietary Supplement Health and Education Act of 1994* contributed to this boom; essentially, because of this law, companies were no longer (and still are not) required to prove any health claims of their product prior to selling it as long as they issue a disclaimer. You have probably read this disclaimer many times before, which declares that: *"This statement has not been evaluated by the Food and Drug Administration. This product is not intended to diagnose, treat, cure, or prevent any disease."* Taking this factor into account combined with the growing popularity of health and fitness in general, there is no shortage of supplements to choose from.

Again, with so many products available, NCEP has painstakingly come up with certain companies and certain supplements to support. One particular company that we believe produces quality supplements is Nutrilite. Founded by Carl Rhenborg in 1934, this company was one of the first companies to invent a multi-vitamin/mult-mineral and has been producing multi-vitamin/multi-mineral supplements derived from living plant sources since its founding. Both their multi-vitamin/multi-mineral as well as their fish oil supplements (refer back to Component 4 about the need for a proper fatty-acid ratio) are good choices. Of course, we do not feel that Nutrilite is the only good vitamin company on the market, as there are certainly many others. We only chose to support them because they invented the concept of a multi-vitamin/multi-mineral, have been doing it the longest, and are the number one selling vitamin in the world today. As an exercise professional, we believe you should have the knowledge and wherewithal—using our tips and your common sense—to recognize other quality, all-natural supplements.

We also think it is very valuable to brainstorm less "traditional" notions of supplementations, such as the H.O.P.E. Formula, put forth by an individual named Brenda Watson. Supplementation does not always have to be pills alone; instead, think about supplementing your diet with certain foods, too, to reach a specific goal. No matter how good a supplement may be, nothing can imitate the nutrients (and their absorption by the body) of whole food. For example, in this program, H.O.P.E. merely stands for **H**igh fiber, **O**mega-3, **P**robiotics, and **E**nzymes (primarily for digestion). Eating foods that help your body supplement these things is also useful, and this is merely one example of this strategy.

Overall, explaining supplementation to your client can be a challenge, particularly because it may antithetical to our holistic lifestyle philosophy. Ultimately, we can sum up our stance (and what you can explain to clients) via three points:

1. *In theory, you do not need supplements because you are eating adequate whole foods*
2. *But, food is less nutritious and diets are less diverse, so people are not getting full nutrition*
3. *So, while controversial, research shows that a quality supplement can be helpful*

SIX ESSENTIAL NUTRIENTS

1. **Proteins** - *4 calories per gram*; used mostly in your body for tissue and organ repair (i.e., muscle synthesis; 12-25% of total calories/day

2. **Carbohydrates** - *4 calories per gram*; used mostly by your body for energy (i.e., main source of fuel); 50-60% of total calories/day

3. **Fats** - *9 calories per gram*; used to protect organs, for energy, and to aid in the absorption of vitamins; 10-30% of total calories per day

4. **Vitamins** - *0 calories*; necessary for proper growth and maintenance and health

5. **Minerals** - *0 calories*; vital for physical and mental well being

6. **Water** - *0 calories*; water consumption is vital for the conversion of fat into energy; helps clean the body of toxins; should drink about 96 ounces of water/day

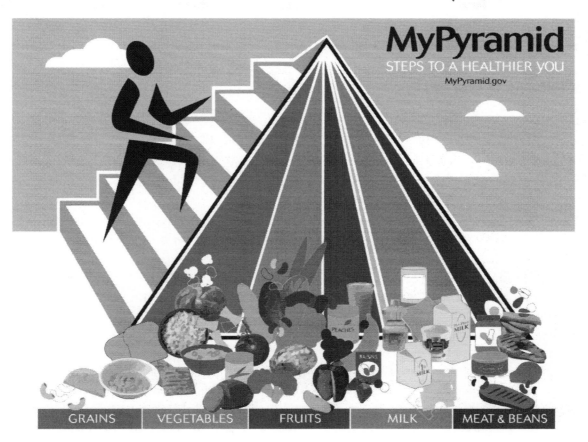

The UDSA's updated food pyramid from 2005, entitled "MyPyramid" (United States Department of Agriculture)

BODY COMPOSITION

A. % fat vs. % lean body mass (LBM)

B. What is Muscle?

- Active fat burning tissue
- Five pounds of muscle burns an extra 6 pounds of fat per year at rest
- Pound for pound, half the volume of fat

C. What is Fat?

- Non-active tissue, burns zero calories
- Pound for pound, twice as big as muscle
- Hides muscles with an unattractive and dimply covering

D. Methods of Body Fat Measurements

- Skin Calipers
- Electro-Impedance
- Hydro-static weighing
- Bod Pod

E. Why Do We Measure a Client's Body Fat?

- To get a starting point of reference
- Often times a good determiner of overall conditioning
- It is expected that trainers will do it (i.e., some other train did it)

F. Understanding Body Fat Accuracy

Even though we believe an initial assessment of a client's body fat percent exemplifies professionalism and serves an important purpose, also understand that these measurements are highly inaccurate, no matter the method. Most measurements have a SEE (Standard Error of the Estimate) at +/- 2.7%, meaning that a person's measurement can vary as much as 2.7% higher or lower. For example, if your client has a 13% body fat measurement, he/she could actually have 10.3% body fat or 15.7% body fat. We have no way of knowing where, within that range, that person's body fat actually falls. Furthermore, 1/3 of all measurements are even more inaccurate above or below the +/- 2.7% SEE. (Using our example, there is even a chance that a person's body fat is actually above 15.7% or below 10.3%!) Thus, use this knowledge at your discretion. For example, if a client reacts very poorly to a measurement, you can explain to him/her that these measurements are not always accurate. Conversely, for others, the number is useful and no further explanation is needed.

CHAPTER SIX

Program Design

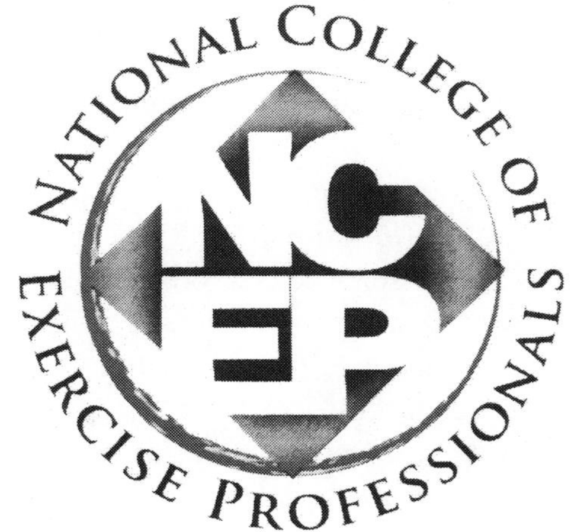

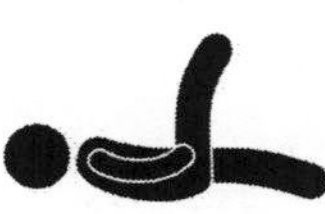

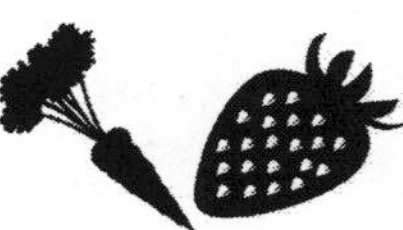

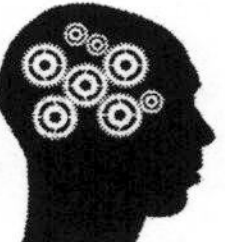

PROGRAM DESIGN

Introduction: Understanding the "Art" and the "Science" of Program Design

The goal of every trainer should be to help each client develop a balanced exercise program that will help create a lasting lifestyle change. Each program should consist of all five of the components of fitness. Since we addressed the nutritional component in the previous chapter, we now need to address the other components: cardiovascular training, resistance training and flexibility (also called ROM or range of motion programming). Each program should take into account the client's specific needs, goals, lifestyle, and limitations—thus, we believe that there is both an *art* and a *science* to creating the best possible program for your client.

The first key to your success as a trainer is to have the ability to apply the science of a particular program, considering all aspects of fitness such as nutrition, physiology, anatomy, health history background, human motivation, and many other variables. We also cannot forget that an important part of personal training is the word personal. Personal means that you work with a variety of clients, each with different goals, needs, likes, dislikes, lifestyles and limitations. Yet, this is where the "art" portion comes in; if you create the best program for a client's needs based on the science you have learned, but the client never carries out the prescribed program because he/she does not like it, then the program is not useful after all. Understanding the science of programming will lead you to choose the best exercises for an individual's physical needs while the art of programming will help you choose the best exercises in accordance with what the client wants to do and will adhere to. *It is your job as a trainer to blend these together to create the best possible program.*

The NCEP Programming System

We have designed a unique system to meet the needs of any client that a fitness professional will encounter. *Our programming system allows for the trainer to add or cut whatever he/she feels is in the best interest of the client while also providing the trainer structure and guidance in implementing a quality, individualized exercise program.* This chapter details our programming system across the three main training aspects: resistance training, cardiovascular training, and flexibility (or range of motion) training. Each component will have a defined "level" system that breaks down proper progression for the client, and that is unique to our fitness philosophy.

A Quick Primer: Understanding the "Modern" Client

Before delving into the specific programs, we need to first look at the client of today to understand why our programs make the most sense. One thing that can be said for sure is that Americans are gaining more weight. It is widely known across multiple health organizations that over one-third of America can be considered obese. One of the reasons for this, among many, is due to the lack of movement in society more broadly. Most Americans work in a job where they sit down for a great part of the day, as the Center for Disease Control (CDC) and the United States Surgeon General estimate that more than 60 percent of American adults are not regularly active. Unfortunately, since sitting for long periods of time each day has become so common, key postural muscles become less active which causes a decrease in the body's ability to stabilize during any type of activity. Thus, when thinking about designing a fitness program, the *last* thing we want to do to an individual who sits for a large part of the day is to have them sit and do exercises.

Designing a Program to Help Improve a Client's Quality of Life

As a result of prolonged sitting, certain muscles tend to become shorter and others tend to lengthen. These shorter muscles tend to affect the rest of the kinetic chain when introduced to an unstable environment such as walking, running, lifting free weights, etc. These imbalances create predictable patterns of dysfunction throughout the kinetic chain called **Serial Distortion Patterns**. Three of the most common patterns of dysfunction are ***Rounded Shoulder Pattern, Pelvic Tilt Pattern*** and ***Pronation Distortion Pattern***. (These are explained in much greater detail in Chapter Twelve on Postural Dysfunctions.)

As an exercise professional, we want you to rely on your questioning and listening skills to find out all you can about each client—particularly identifying these common patterns of dysfunction. Only after you know as much information about a client's life and movement patterns will you be able to use your technical knowledge and experience to develop a safe, effective and enjoyable program for that person. Of course, after completing this first class, or just reading this book, you are not expected to be able to assess all the intricacies of each postural deviation. You are, however, expected to see gross irregularities in the way your client performs certain movements and be able to put them into one or more of the three categories outlined. For each category there are certain corrective stretches and corrective exercises that should be done. With proper exercise programming, you can maximize the client's benefits and minimize the risk of injury. Keep in mind that sometimes there is conflict between what the client wants and what the client needs—or, as we like to say, where the "art" and the "science" intersect. In these situations try to educate your clients and help them understand the importance of accepting alternate exercise selections, if only for a little while. By adding the appropriate exercises to the program you will decrease the chance of overuse injuries and keep the client healthy enough to continue working out (both of which you should communicate often to your client). Your goal should not be shortsighted, merely placating the member with short-term solutions. Rather, you should aim to help each member make a lifetime commitment to proper exercise. In fact, this broader perspective should always guide you in developing programs for your clients.

The guidelines for exercise design are based on a solid foundation of scientific information. Remember, however, the program design guidelines outlined in this manual are principles, not laws; these guidelines presented should be utilized with flexibility and with special emphasis placed on the goals and needs of each (unique) client. The secret is to give the client what he/she needs wrapped in the package of what he/she wants—*the "science" and the "art."* For example, if your client has a rounded shoulder pattern, heavy bench presses are probably not the best thing for him/her to do. If you discuss with your client that he/she cannot perform bench presses, that person may not want to train with you. The trick is to give them a pressing exercise on an unstable surface. This way the client gets to press, but the load is so low that it will not worsen his/her condition.

Assessing the Client for Program Design

Before you can suggest what exercises might be best for your client, you should first put the member through a series of assessments to determine how his/her kinetic chain is functioning and where the weak links are located. For beginning trainers, you may feel that this activity is too complicated for someone new to training. Remember, however, that it is a process, and you will get better over time. Thus, we have created a system for Program Design that will work for any client you may encounter. After working with many clients and with more education you will be able to conduct more assessments—and be proficient in identifying individuals' dysfunctional patterns—while your program designs will improve exponentially. Doing these assessments will separate you from the rest of the industry; most trainers do not even think about each client as an individual and rarely consider what exercises may be best suited for each client's needs.

The process starts with studying the kinetic chain through a series of static and dynamic assessments. A static assessment is performed when the client is not moving. Conversely, a dynamic assessment is performed when the client is involved in some activity such as walking or performing an exercise. Dynamic assessments are sometimes referred to as *Bio-motor Ability Assessments*. Therefore, the next step is to determine what muscles might not be working efficiently in these assessments. What we mean by not working efficiently is that the muscle is either weak, or tight, or does not have enough endurance, or is even too strong. After you have found what is not "working" efficiently, you can then design a program to isolate that part to make it stronger, more flexible or whatever you found to be the issue. After you isolate the muscle and get it to perform better in isolation, you then design a program to integrate that part back into the kinetic chain for it to become a functionally efficient part of the whole body.

As always, we need to always keep in mind that the physiological and perceptual responses to exercise vary considerably from person to person. People adapt to training at varying rates and levels. What works for one person may not work for another! The most appropriate exercise program for a particular client is one that is most helpful to change his/her lifestyle, improve his/her health, and help reach his/her goals. This chapter, and our course, will teach you how to create a great program using our system of programming. The key to a balanced program design is to address all of the bio-motor abilities given to all human beings and then focus on the ones that the individual client wants or needs more of. If every trainer were currently adhering to this practice, the training world would be a much better place for clients and trainers alike.

In summary, the best program designs will take into account all the components of fitness, based on a client's muscular needs and personal goals. *It only makes sense that before we can truly make the best program for any client we must first 'test' or assess him/her in each category.* We will attempt to show many different assessments for each component, and illustrate some reasonable choices based on the outcomes of these assessments. (Refer back to Chapter Four for many of the assessments that you would perform as a trainer.)

STANDARD POSTURE (ANTERIOR VIEW)

The first assessment you should do is to examine overall posture. You should start by having your client stand and face you. Start at the head and assess each check point. You should note any gross irregularities that may jump out at you. There are notes to the right of each joint to help illustrate with what a standard posture would look like.

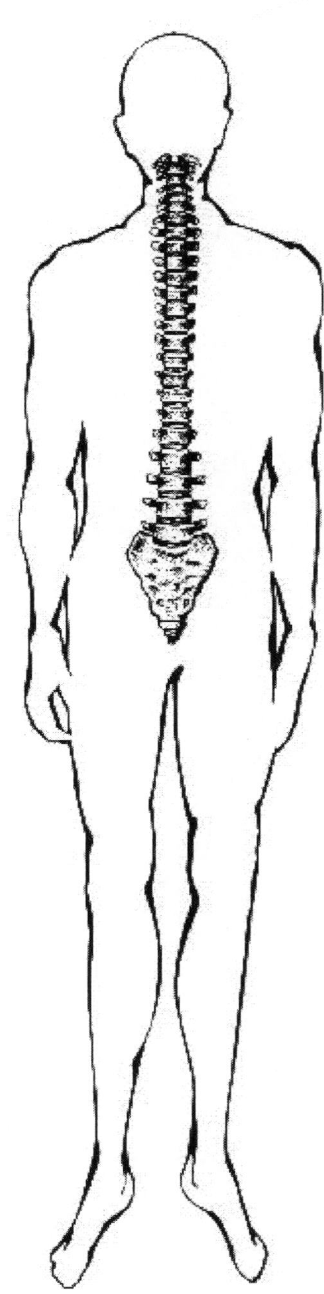

CHECK-POINTS

Head: Neutral position, neither tilted nor rotated

Cervical Spine: Straight

Shoulders: Level, not elevated or depressed

Scapulae: Neutral position, medial borders essentially parallel and about 3 to 4 inches apart

Thoracic and Lumbar Spines: Straight, without scoliosis

Pelvis: Level, both posterior superior iliac spines in same transverse plane

Hip Joints: Neutral position, neither adducted nor abducted

Lower Extremities: Straight

Feet: Parallel or toeing out slightly

STANDARD POSTURE (LATERAL VIEW)

When you have completed the anterior assessment, have your client turn to the side (so you can assess them from the lateral position. Once again, we have noted the check-points that you should look for when examining this person's standard posture.

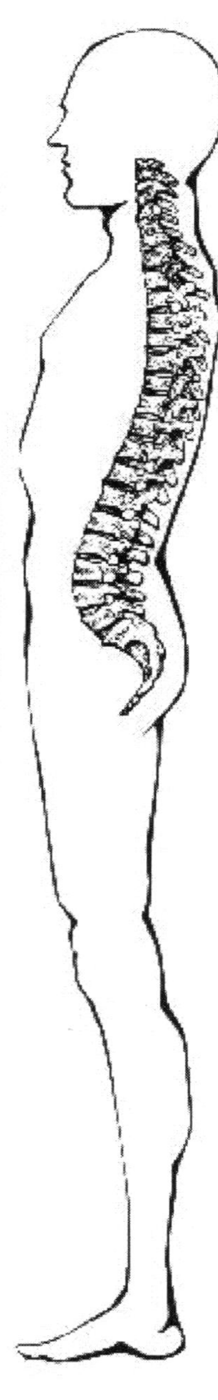

CHECK-POINTS

Head: Neutral position, not tilted forward or back

Cervical Spine: Normal Curve, slightly convex anteriorly

Scapulae: Flat against upper back

Thoracic Spine: Normal curve, slightly convex posteriorly

Lumbar Spine: Normal curve, slightly convex anteriorly

Pelvis: Neutral position, anterior superior spines in same vertical plane as symphasis pubis

Hip Joints: Neutral position, neither flexed nor extended

Knee Joints: Neutral position, neither flexed nor hyper-extended

Ankle Joints: Neutral position, leg vertical and at right angle to sole of foot

What Do We Mean by 'Posture'?

Posture, by definition, means the way you normally hold yourself. Posture affects every aspect of our being and our life writ large. As an exercise professional, having the ability to identify faulty posture can have an immediate and long-term lasting affect on your client. In fact, it may be the single most important assessment you make for your client because when the skeletal system becomes misaligned it cannot adequately support our bodies. This, in turn, will require the muscular system to help, which then causes predictable patterns of dysfunction throughout the entire kinetic chain. Here's an example to internalize the effects of bad posture: stand up, roll your shoulders forward, jut your chin out and slouch slightly. You will feel tension develop at the base of the skull because of the forward head. This will limit blood flow to the brain and decrease its functional capabilities. The forward head will also cause the mandible (the jaw) to retract, placing a stress on the tempo-mandibular joint which can lead to dysfunction. The forward slouch will cause restricted breath and limited oxygen flow. Less oxygen in leads to a lower ability to clean the blood and remove the waste products that build. The lessened ability to clean the waste leads to increasing toxicity of our cells and a more toxic body. These negative effects continue all throughout the entire kinetic chain. Thus, we believe that it is important to focus on the skeletal system and muscular system. We want to create an optimal length tension relationship between the muscles surrounding a joint. Muscles work most efficiently when they are certain lengths, and these optimum lengths will be created by having good posture.

The law of reciprocal inhibition states that when the agonist contracts, the antagonist must relax to some degree to allow motion at the joint to occur. When an agonist becomes continually shortened, the antagonist becomes continually lengthened rendering it much less functional. This predisposes an individual to certain orthopedic conditions that can be exacerbated through improper program design. It is important to be able to correctly assess posture and design the best possible program for your client. While some exercises should be given to certain members, other exercises would not be in the member's best interest to perform. We believe strongly, as you can see, that posture assessments can be a powerful tool in determining what exercises would be most beneficial for your client. Yet, assessments can usually be performed most efficiently when the client is *not* concentrating on his/her posture. For example, we know that when people are being watched—even if they just have this perception—they tend to hold themselves differently. Remember that the key to an effective program design is giving your clients the proper exercises; we cannot do this unless we know the way in which individuals hold themselves normally (after all, that is the definition of posture). Thus, make sure to assess their "normal" posture *before* asking them to try to get into "good" posture. Even as you do this, you should try to cue them as little as possible and let them find it (whatever "it" may be) on their own. Remember, you should always start with posture because it directly aligns with Level 1 of the NCEP resistance program design system, discussed next.

Stabilization Strength: The Key to Posture and the Six Primary Positions

Once you are satisfied that your client has put himself/herself in "good" posture, try to have this individual hold it. This is the first test to measure his/her STABILIZATION STRENGTH and depending on your client, it may be quite a challenge for him/her to hold that new posture. Of course, there are postures in regards to every position you can think of, which is why we have broken up these postures into six primary positions. The 6 primary positions are: *lying, sitting, kneeling, standing, squatting, and lunging*. All exercises in the gym are basically performed while being in one of these primary positions. We use the same checkpoints for each position as we did for the standing posture. Then, we should monitor these checkpoints during every exercise—in essence, turning every exercise into an assessment. Since there are both static and dynamic assessments, there are both static and dynamic exercises as well. Yet, before we can truly get a good picture of the clients' movement capabilities, we should first get a picture of the client's stabilization abilities. You will never go wrong in your practice if you always remember this saying: *stability must precede mobility.*

Seven Primary Movement Patterns

Along with the six primary positions there are seven primary movement patterns. These patterns are: *pushing, pulling, bending, twisting, squatting, lunging, and gait (i.e., walk).* (Note that some of these movements, like squatting and lunging, can be done both as a movement or a static position.) These movement patterns are combined with the primary positions to make exercise. Instead of calling an exercise a lying push, someone made up the term bench press. The problem with exercise names is that they are not descriptive enough and it is just another thing that can confuse your client.

Still, as we discussed earlier in Chapter Four, our first dynamic assessment is always the squat. With virtually every joint in the kinetic chain being used in the squat, it is often regarded as the cornerstone dynamic assessment. We use this movement to assess the overall flexibility of our client. After we learn more about the anatomy and functions of muscles we can see how each muscle in the kinetic chain is affected and then determine which muscles are not working as they should. (We will continue to discuss this even further in the later chapters.)

- 7 PRIMARY MOVEMENTS -
PUSH
PULL
BEND
TWIST
SQUAT
LUNGE
GAIT

Every physical movement deals with at least one of these primary movements, and the best trainers are able to design a program that has the client perform as many as possible in ways that are most conducive to his/her lifestyle and activities.

RESISTANCE PROGRAM DESIGN PRINCIPLES

There are **five possible applications of force** that can be applied to each of the *seven movement patterns*, which we can assess from any of the six positions. The goal is to try and choose the position most appropriate for the individual, based on need and abilities. **NCEP** only focuses on three of the five possible applications of force because we feel they are the 3 most needed for general health and conditioning. These applications are noted as **Level 1, Level 2 and Level 5 in our "Resistance Training Chart"** (on page 88). *Level 1* type application is an isometric hold, or, more simply, when an individual is in 'good' posture via what we call Core Stabilization Training. We start by putting the client in good posture in various movements and have them hold it. For example, we have them do a squat and try to hold it for 30 seconds or more. In ***Level 2*** training, we have them do the movement very slowly, concentrating on the eccentric contraction, going down very slowly and controlled (discussed in the Physiology chapter). Lastly, in ***Level 5***, we have them do the movement, but their base of support must lose contact, and then must *react* to a new base of support. In using the squat pattern, that would be a squat jump for Level 5 training. After we have coordinated the movement, we try to add in **speed and movement in all planes of motion**.

We have created a resistance training chart that notates each of the 5 levels of resistance training. **Levels 3 and 4,** not discussed above, are very specific and intended only for a small group of people after they have become efficient in Levels 1, 2 and 5. This is because we at the National College of Exercise Professionals believe in training the total person through a holistic lens. As such, we take the approach that as a personal trainer, we are not just training muscles—we are conditioning the nervous system that activates the muscles and develops pathways, discussed below.

Neuromuscular Facilitation or Developing "Neuro Pathways"

A key component of the NCEP system revolves around the concept of neuro pathways. To understand neuro pathways, we will use deer trails in the countryside as an analogy. As the deer walks through the forest, it develops a pathway where the brush, bushes and grass gets worn down and opened up. For the deer to go down this trail, it takes very little effort or energy. Conversely, when the deer goes through another area of the forest where the brush, bushes and grass are fully grown, it takes great effort to push its way through—the deer cannot rely only on memory. When the deer gets spooked, it will immediately run down the worn-down trail as it takes less energy and is easier and faster for the deer. However, if the deer continues to go through the deep brush, it will eventually build a new trail. In turn, if the deer does not go down the old trail, eventually the brush, bushes and grass will grow back. The old trail will then become difficult to go down, and the new path will become the preferred way for the deer to go when it gets spooked.

The nervous system works this way, too. For example, when a person first learns a new dance, it feels awkward and is difficult to perform. However, after practicing the dance, it becomes smoother and easier to perform. The science behind this is simple: as this person develops a neuro pathway for this movement, the movement becomes both efficient and more recognizable by the body. Going further, if a person is walking down the sidewalk and has to jump out of the way from a biker, this person's movement pattern will happen instinctually. Like the deer, he/she will perform the movement pattern that he/she is used to performing, and not necessarily the most efficient movement to avoid the biker. In fact, when people have poor movement patterns, it can lead to injury and they can get seriously hurt. To change movement patterns, individuals must regularly move with new (i.e., better) neuro pathways while having restraint to avoid the old inefficient movement patterns. Eventually, these new pathways will be established and the old patterns will be less efficient, instinctually making the body be less likely to utilize it.

Inside the gym, this process is commonly called **"Muscle Memory"** while the scientific term for this process is **neuromuscular facilitation**. Once you understand this process, you will be able to assist your clients tremendously because you will no longer be just training muscles—you will be training the nervous system and thus, the total body in a more holistic (and functional) way.

As you carefully choose exercises, you will want to match the exercise movements with the movements of your clients' chosen sport(s) and for their daily life activities, because life itself is a sport. The ancient activities of Tai Chi and Yoga are perfect examples of neuro pathway development training. The movements are slow (30 seconds to 3 minutes) and/or held in a specific position. One of the world's greatest martial arts experts Leo Fong created the terminology of the 4 Stages of Development:

- **Develop the tools.**
- **Polish the tools.**
- **Dissolve the tools.**
- **Express the tools.**

First a person must learn the movement (develop the tools), then he/she must perfect the movement pattern (polish the tools), eventually through regular training he/she can learn to stop thinking about the correct movement (dissolving the tools), and finally, he/she will automatically perform the ideal movement pattern (express the tools). Like the deer, this person will go down the new pathway without thinking because it is more efficient, and, in some sense, more instinctual.

Introducing Athletic Performance Enhancement

Now that you understand the principles of neuro pathways, you will understand that, as an exercise professional, you are not just training muscles, but training the nervous system and training movement patterns. We keep reiterating this important principle because it is what is unique about our NCEP philosophy. We also want to (re)acknowledge that most people in modern society sit at their job, they sit at home while relaxing, and even often sit going between their work and home in the car. As a reminder, we do *not* want to have them sit during their training, and the reasons for this are also connected to postural issues created from excessive sitting discussed in previous chapters. Furthermore, the lack of regular and functional movement patterns results in poor nuero pathways. While choosing exercises, we like to incorporate complex and integrated movements, not segmented and segregated movements. One way to do is through athletic training, or what we call "Athletic Performance Enhancement." Athletic performance is directly related to complete movement, agility, balance, explosiveness, and reaction speed. We train these abilities in an integrated fashion, while also identifying specific needs for the client's development. Some of the tools for Athletic Performance Enhancement training include the agility ladder, agility rings, balls, cones, and many, many others.

With the agility ladder, for example, the client can work on simple steps that develop excellent movement patterns. We can also work on lateral and transverse movement and go beyond moving only in the frontal plane. Once the person can move effectively, this person can then train with speed and explosiveness. Next, we can add tossing a ball as he/she moves, challenging this person's proprioception—or more simply, the ability to identify an object moving in space and adjust to it. For example, as an individual moves through the agility ladder, we can toss him/her a ball to catch and throw back. You can also use a deck of playing cards to force your client to move in unexpected directions. Remember the science *and* the art? These exercises serve both many functional purposes (increase heart rate by keeping clients moving, develop coordination through new neuro pathways, mimic common movements, etc.) while generally being very fun and stimulating for the client to engage in.

Another term often thrown around in fitness settings is "plyometrics." Simply put, plyometrics refer to when a person leaves contact and then makes contact again. Any type of jump is an example of this. The ability to make contact with proper body positioning and balance comes from the neuro pathways; controlling, and redirecting, and then changing force is the essence of explosiveness. In scientific terminology (and dicussed later), the muscles must *eccentrically* control the force and then *concentrically* produce force in the opposite direction or a new direction. The shorter the time between the controlling and redirecting the force, the more "explosive" the action. As a trainer, we want to make sure that the client has proper movement patterns to absorb the force and then train him/her to produce force with a shorter amount of time between the two. For this reason, the key is training the force reduction and then the quick force production in a variety of directions. A common application are box jumps. In this exercise, the use of box jumping will be enhanced by jumping down from a short box and then quickly exploding in a new direction—back to the top of the box—as fast as possible.

Putting It All Together

In conclusion, we want to identify the movements of our clients' chosen sport(s) and then *match* their movements in the Athletic Performance Enhancement training exercises. Ideally, the resistance training exercises mimic the appropriate sport movements and in particular, work on force controlling (or eccentric phase). If the client does not play a specific sport, that is no problem—a great exercise professional can match the basic movements of an individual's functional life activities to movements on the gym training floor. We wholeheartedly believe that life itself is a sport and therefore, that we are all athletes. (The next page details, specifically, our resistance system training chart for all clients, following the principles dsicussed above.)

NCEP RESISTANCE TRAINING SYSTEM

Intensity Progression Chart

Level	Goal	% of 1 RM	Rep Range	# of Sets	Rest
Level 1	Develop Neural Pathways	BW-light	30 sec to 3 min	Not to exceed 2	Time required to set-up next exercise
Level 2	Endurance	50-70	12-20	1-3	20-30 sec
Level 3	*Hypertrophy*	*70-80*	*6-12*	*2-6*	*30-90 sec*
Level 4	*Strength*	*80-100*	*1-5*	*3-5*	*2-5 min*
Level 5	Power	BW-40	1-5	3-5	2-5 min

*BW = body weight

Resistance Training Requirements:

*Level 1 is CORE STABILIZATION TRAINING. It should be a part of every resistance training program.

*Levels 1, 2 and 5 are **mandatory and must be completed in sequential order.**

**Levels 3* and *4* are entirely goal specific and should be performed after Levels 1, 2 and 5 if you decide to use them.

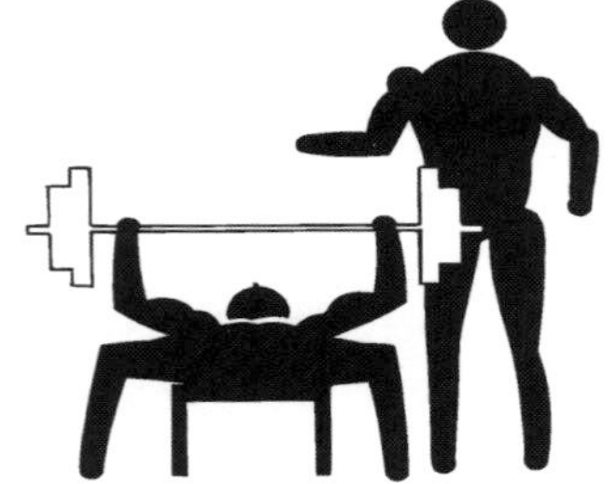

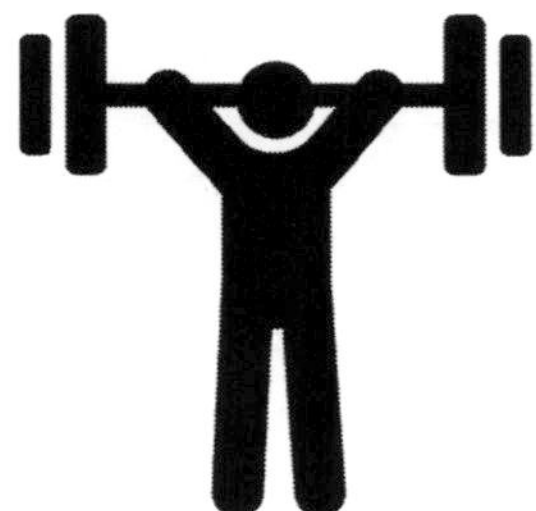

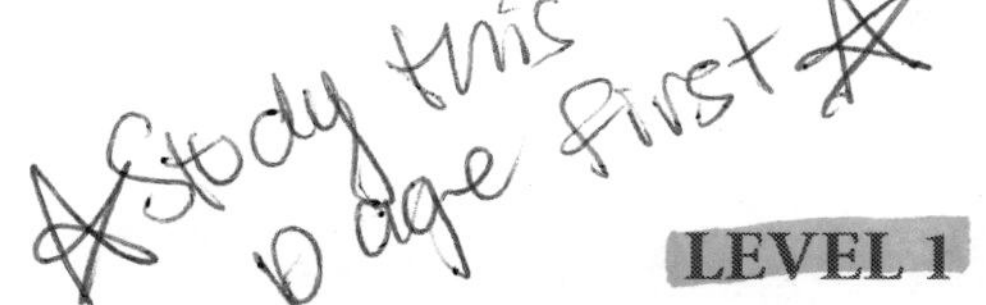

LEVEL 1

Goal: *Develop Neural Pathways (Start a Training Program)*

In **Level 1,** the training goal is to awaken the nervous system by developing neural pathways and turning on the intrinsic stabilizer muscles that protect the spine. This level focuses on increasing **stabilization strength** by using ***static exercises*** focusing on **BALANCE and CORE STABILITY**.

LEVEL 2

Goal: *Obtain Muscular Endurance*

In **Level 2,** the training goal is to create **muscular endurance strength** by using ***dynamic exercises*** with special focus on ECCENTRIC STRENGTH.

LEVEL 3

Goal: *Obtain Muscular Hypertrophy*

In **Level 3,** the training goal is to create the most amount of cellular adaptation to make size increases in the muscular system by using ***stable exercises*** focusing on using the appropriate load to exhaust the muscle within 6 to 12 reps.

LEVEL 4

Goal: *Obtain Muscular Strength*

In **Level 4,** the training goal is to create **max strength** adaptation in the muscular system. Use ***stable exercises*** much like those in Level 3, except using appropriate loads that would exhaust the muscle within 1 to 5 reps.

LEVEL 5

Goal: *Increase Coordination, Speed and Power*

In **Level 5,** the training goal is to increase **reactive strength** through better coordination. An increase in reactive strength and coordination will increase an individual's ability to use more speed and to generate greater power. Do plyometric-type exercises slowly until coordination is developed, and then progress to doing them as fast as possible, with quality control, always having ***safety*** as a concern.

CARDIOVASCULAR PROGRAM DESIGN PRINCIPLES

Cardiovascular training is training that increases the functional capacity of the heart, lungs, and blood vessels that transport oxygenated blood to the working muscles. Maintenance of even average levels of cardiovascular fitness can reduce one's risk for coronary heart disease. Other benefits of cardiovascular exercise include weight control, hypertension control, better lipid control, and possibly, assistance in controlling the stresses of life. The NCEP follows the basic guidelines of the American College of Sports Medicine (ACSM) when designing the aerobic component of the exercise program. *In order for an activity to qualify as aerobic exercise, it must involve a continuous, rhythmical, and sustained movement using large muscle groups.* Such activities include walking, swimming, running, cycling, aerobic dance, roller-blading, ice skating, rowing, cross country skiing, rope skipping, stair climbing, and various recreational and even weight training if you use light weights and is performed in a continuous manner with few or no rest periods.

When creating the cardiovascular portion of program design it is important to match the client's aerobic activities to his/her fitness level, exercise goals, orthopedic history, and personal preference. For example, the beginning or overweight client may find walking, swimming, or circuit weight training more comfortable than impact options such as jogging or rope jumping. Clients who are interested in improving their aerobic fitness will find any of these exercises suitable. The client may want to try cross-training or alternating between two or more aerobic activities as a way to add variety and fun, and reduce the risk of injuries from over training. If a client is training for a specific sport, such as a marathon, you should focus most of his/her training in that sport (this is an example of the law of specificity). In other words, the runner should run, the cyclist should cycle, and the swimmer should swim. Although any aerobic exercise will enhance cardiovascular fitness, muscles tend to adapt specifically to the type of exercise performed.

Before designing a program you should always test the client's ability to perform aerobic exercise. We have designed three tests to conduct before creating a program: *talk test, leveling test,* and *recovery heart rate test* (see page 92). After clients pass each test, they are ready for you to design a program. First, however, you should teach the client how to monitor the intensity of the exercise. It is often difficult for the beginning client to gauge exercise intensity correctly. Use of individualized exercise target heart rate zones, subjective ratings of perceived exertion, and the talk test will assist the client in achieving his/her goals in the safest and most efficient manner possible.

Understanding the Importance and Meaning of Cardiovascular Health

It is important to communicate to your clients that they should get some physical activity every day—even low intensity activities provide health benefits. A bevy of recent research has demonstrated that even walking at a moderate pace increases cardiovascular fitness and reduces the risk of heart disease by increasing the "good," HDL-cholesterol and strengthening the heart. In fact, walking and running have similar positive effects on HDL-cholesterol and for decreasing the risk of heart disease. Thus, your clients do not have to do vigorous activity to receive health benefits. Also note that individuals do not have to do all their activity in one session. Studies show that you can get almost the same benefit from three 10-minute exercise bouts as one 30-minute bout of equal intensity. We believe that most people can find time to take a brisk walk for two, five, or ten minutes several times during the day.

Just about everyone could benefit from being more active. It should be your goal to create a program that will help your client make the choice to adopt a healthy lifestyle full of exercise. Yet, don't confuse the term cardiovascular training with weight loss. Nowhere in the definition of cardiovascular training does it say weight loss. This is a common misconception in the fitness community. Keep cardiovascular training for getting the heart in better shape and let the weight get controlled through nutrition and the adaptation to a healthy lifestyle.

NCEP CARDIOVASCULAR TRAINING SYSTEM

F.I.T.T.R. Cardiovascular Components

	Level 1 Testing	Level 2 Improvement	Level 3 Maintenance
Frequency	3 days per week	3-7 days per week	3-5 days per week
Intensity	40-60% of predicted max HR	50-85% of predicted max HR	70-85% of predicted max HR
Time	Up to 15 minutes	20 min per session	20-30 min per session
Type	Sustained large muscle group rhythmic activity	Sustained large muscle group rhythmic activity or interval	Sustained large muscle group activity or interval
Rate of Progression	10% every other week or as client is able	10% every other week or as client is able	10% every other week or as client is able

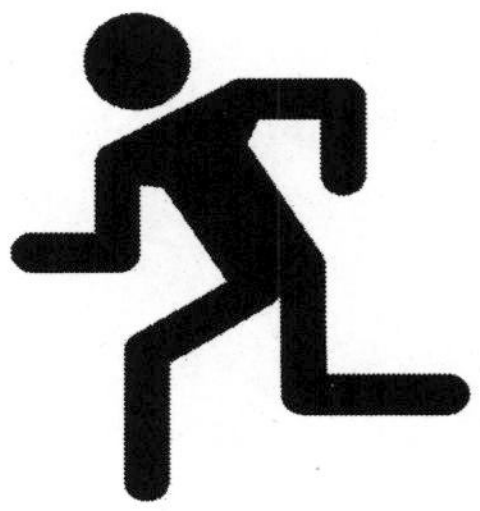

TESTING PHASE

All clients must test out of Level 1 on the F.I.T.T.R. chart by successfully fulfilling the requirements of these tests below. Even if an individual says that he/she is in great shape, it is your responsibility as an exercise professional to administer these tests to prove that he/she is indeed in satisfactory cardiovascular health before advancing a client to Level 2.

- ✓ ***Talk Test*** - Have your client perform a cardiovascular enriched exercise and have him/her carry on a conversation with you. We do not expect him/her to be able to quote Shakespeare, but we do need him/her to be able to at least answer your questions without being out of breath.

- ✓ ***Leveling Test*** - Your client's heart rate must level off somewhere within his/her heart rate range or the exercise is deemed too intense for that individual. If you are having your client exercise at very low rate and his/her heart rate will not level in the target range, we suggest you have this person see his/her doctor to get the heartbeat examined.

- ✓ ***Recovery Test*** - Your client should be within 10 beats a minute of his/her normal resting heart rate within 1-3 minutes after stopping the exercise. If this person's heart rate does not drop within the stated range, we recommend that him/her do not proceed to Level 2.

NOTE: *The Talk Test and the Leveling Test should be performed about midway through a cardiovascular activity, such as during a walk/jog on a treadmill.*

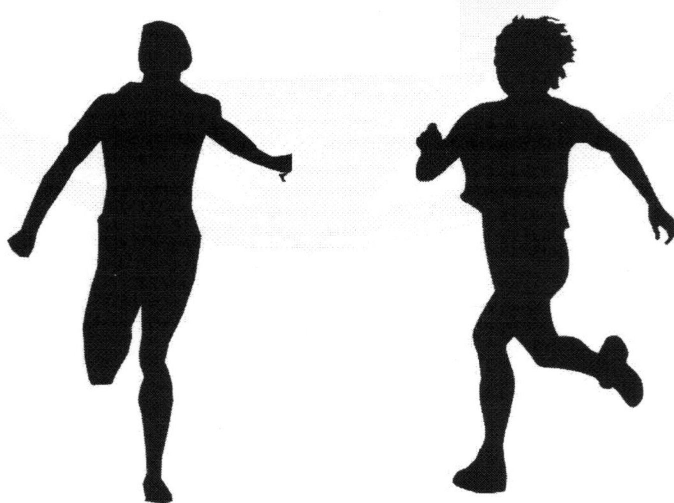

FLEXIBILITY PROGRAM DESIGN PRINCIPLES

Flexibility may be the single most important component of any program design. Yet, while flexibility is considered one of the five components of fitness, it often remains one of the least understood. An individual who is not flexible will often have problems completing any exercise routine, as a lack of flexibility in any muscle will cause muscle imbalances throughout the entire body. These muscle imbalances will affect normal length-tension relationships around the affected joint, which, in turn, will eventually lead to altered movement patterns and over time to joint injuries. Often times a joint injury occurs because there are muscles around that joint that are tight and other muscles that are loose. These imbalances ultimately lead to dysfunctional movement patterns, which then cause altered movement patterns, which *then* create altered wear patterns and unnatural stresses placed on the joint. Each of these issues combined make the joint wear down and can eventually cause a serious injury. As you can see, flexibility is extremely important!

When people refer to flexibility, in reality, what they mean is the range of motion (ROM) at a certain joint and the musculature surrounding that joint. Lack of flexibility is often attributed to the muscles, although, there are other factors that contribute to a joint's flexibility that are overlooked. Believe it or not, muscles account for **only 40 percent** of joint flexibility! Therefore, ROM is also affected by bones, ligaments and tendons—all of which are not inherently flexible and do not possess characteristics that allow them to become more flexible. This is why muscles are the main component of flexibility (even if they are not the only factors in an individual's range of motion).

Breaking Down Range of Motion

Although the muscles surrounding a client's joint may have a "normal" range of motion, these muscles can be improperly stretched, under the trainer's direction, because the trainer did not do a thorough postural assessment and dynamic movement assessment before designing the flexibility program design. The following basic information should be considered when incorporating flexibility into the client's exercise program:

1. Always do a postural assessment and a dynamic movement assessment before creating a flexibility program. In this case, the dynamic movement assessment is the overhead squat.

2. Remember that passive-assisted stretching where the trainer is forcing the client to increase the stretch is something that should only be done by a *trained specialist*.

3. Remind the client that there are three things they can do each day to maintain and improve flexibility:
   *Drink plenty of water: keeping the body hydrated can make a big difference
   *Proper nutrition: this has a daily and cumulative effect
   *Stretch every day if possible: using your ROM will maintain it

4. Muscles and tendons stretch better when warmed up. Have the client stretch after 5-10 minutes of light aerobic warm-up and/or cool down at the end of the training session.
   *One form of warm up and cool down would be self-myofascial release. This is

done by 'rolling' on a foam roller. Until the adhesion in the muscle is 'broken up', the knot in the muscle will remain.

5. When static stretching and active stretching, the client should stretch to the point of feeling tension in the muscle but not pain.

6. Whenever possible, try to perform active stretches and ballistic stretches before the workout and save the static stretching for the end of the workout.

Introducing Dynamic Flexibility

The foundational ideas of this principle are as old as the study of human physiology. As a result, Dynamic Flexibility is not a new fitness fad or a repackaged version of some other movement system. Instead, it is a complex, holistic, and scientific approach to the rehabilitation of injury and the development of movement excellence. Many of the movements that we are teaching come from ancient warrior training from the Slavic and Russian military. We would be remiss not to mention that the two pioneers that have helped us form our unique NCEP system that we have adapted are Scott Sonnon and Dr. Eric Cobb.

Mobility Warm Up

This sequence is designed to set up your body for movement. To start, you will need a comfortable surface since some of the movements require you to place most of your weight on sensitive areas of the foot. A yoga mat for this job does very well. To further enhance the effects of the warm up, use a foam roller on your tension areas before you start the drills. All of the motions are done in a rep range of 3-5. As you become more comfortable with these motions and the sequence, you and your clients will easily be able to do this "Mobility Warm Up" in 10 minutes.

This sequence is set up from the ground up (i.e., bottom to top), to mimic the body's natural support structure. Yet, this sequence can be reversed and done head to toe, though the training result is much different. Play with it and find what works best to wake your client's body up.

START

Medial/Lateral Foot Tilt
Toe Pull Middle
Toe Pull Out
Ankle Circles
Hip Circles (4 Direction)
Hour Glass Hips
Thoracic A/P Glide
Thoracic Frontal Glide
Side Shoulder Circles
Back Shoulder Circles
Wrist Circles
Hand Circles
Big Wave Finger Ext/Flex

Neck Tilt
Neck Twist
Neck A/P Glide
Egyptian
Jaw A/P Glide
Jaw Frontal Glide
END

This may seem like a lot of movements, but this list is actually a very fast and abbreviated sequence when you consider the total amount of body movements available. Take your time at first, and make the movements slow and deliberate. This will enhance your mobility and will allow you to push through larger ranges of motion with little to no pain. (If you would like to learn more about our system of Dynamic Flexibility, please inquire about one of our advanced courses, the Exercise Therapy Program, which has a Flexibility Specialist certification.)

NCEP FLEXIBILITY TRAINING SYSTEM

Frequency	3-7 days per week	Only done by a trained professional	3-7 days per week	3-5 days per week
Intensity	1-2 sets X 10 reps	Determined by professional	1 set X 3 reps	1-2 sets X 10 reps
Time	Hold each rep 2-10 seconds	Determined by professional	Hold each rep 30 seconds	No hold at all, controlled motion
Type	**ACTIVE STRETCH**	**PASSIVE STRETCH**	**STATIC STRETCH**	**BALLISTIC STRETCH**
Rate of Progression	Hold at tension, no pain	Determined by professional	Hold at tension, no pain	As client is able

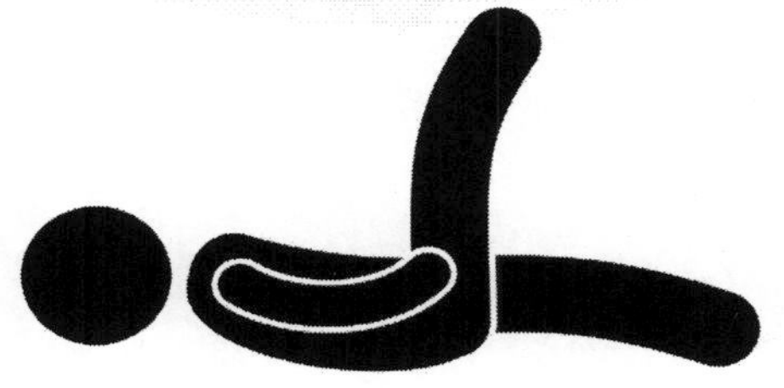

NCEP PROGRAM DESIGN

To recap, creating a successful program for your clients is what will separate you from other trainers in the field. Your goal is to become a true "exercise professional" that, coming full circle, captures both the science and the art of program design. A program must be fun and engaging for clients, but also be very individualized in a way that specifically improves your clients' movements and daily life activities based on their postural deficiencies and/or muscle weaknesses, for example. While you will become more experienced as you design more programs, below is our general suggestions for an hour-long session with any client—with the resistance section being the most adaptable to each client.

*__Pre-session:__ Self Myo-Facial Release (SMFR)/foam rolling, light core exercises, warm-up

1. **Attitude Training** - Meditation, Affirmations, Visualization, Power word & action for anchoring; work out attitude theme of the day (example: Wooden Pyramid of Success and Rainbow Warrior Principles)

2. **Movement Prep** - Stretching/ROM Training: Active & Dynamic Stretching; match the movements of the client's sports, activities and life

3. **Resistance Training**
   a. Level 1: *Nuero Pathway Development*
   b. Level 2: *Endurance*
   c. Level 5: *Power*
   d. Levels 3 (Hypertrophy) and Level 4 (Strength) are goal specific and should be performed only after levels 1,2, and 5 are completed
   e. 7 Primary Movements: *pull, push (ratio of 3:1 or 3:2), bend, twist, squat, lunge, gait*
   f. May want to start with squat, then upper body, and finish with lunge and gait
   g. Integrate Coronal Plane (lateral movement), and Transverse Plane (twisting movement); do not just perform Sagittal Plane (Frontal Plane) exercises
   h. Focus on multi-joint/compound movements.
   i. Name Exercises by movements, not muscles (i.e., standing row)
   j. Train the neuro pathway: *match the movements to the client's sports, activities, and life. Remember you're training movements not just muscles*
   k. Challenge the stability and balance of client not just the resistance level and speed of the movement; also, remember to adjust the resistance and speed when changing the difficulty of the stability level
   l. Ideally, train the clients standing up, not sitting down
   m. Ideally, choose exercises involving body weight and not machines

4. **Athletic Performance Enhancement Training**
   a. Match the movements of the client's sports, activities, and life
   b. Include agility training, hand-eye coordination, and spacial awareness
   c. Tools include: *agility ladder, agility rings, plyometric boxes, rebounder/mini tramp, medicine balls, reaction balls, cones, etc.*

5. **Core Training**
    a. Stability, balance, and core
    b. TVA, Rectus Abdominus, Obliques, Erector Spinae, etc.
    c. Bridging, twisting, mat work, stability balls, balance boards, etc.

6. **Cardiovascular Training***
    a. Level 1: *Testing Phase (Perform Talk Test, Leveling Test, Recovery Test)*
    b. Level 2: *Improvement Phase*
    c. Level 3: *Maintenance Phase*

7. **Post Work Out**
    a. Post-stretching: Static Stretching, Passive Stretching (matched with active stretching to reduce the naïve range of motion)
    b. Cool down
    c. Attitude training recap

**Generally, you will not have time to do cardiovascular training with clients within an hour-long session, as often cardiovascular programs are assigned for clients to perform on the days they do not meet with you.*

CHAPTER SEVEN

Enhancing Mobility (via Stick Mobility™)

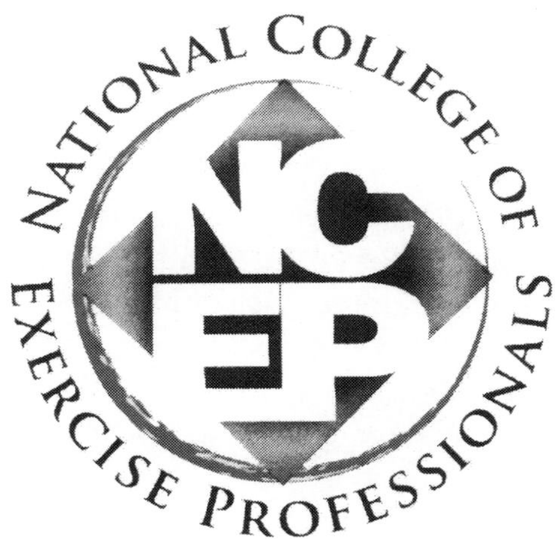

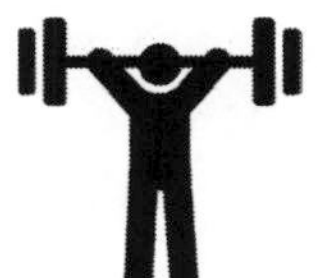
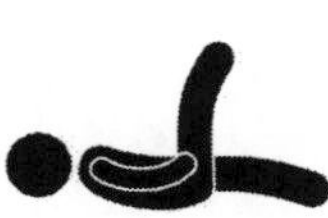
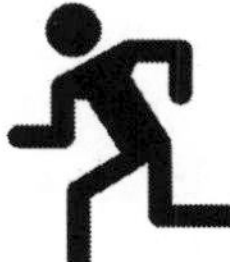

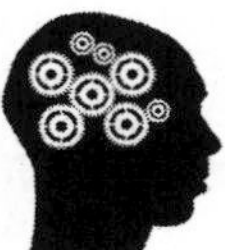

Enhancing Mobility (via Stick Mobility™ System)

Introducing Stick Mobility™ and Our Flexibility Philosophy

NCEP is proud to partner with the fitness enthusiasts at Stick Mobility™, who have developed an innovative, yet refreshingly simple, mobility system using a stick object (such as a dowel) to increase clients' mobility and overall Range of Motion (ROM). Stick Mobility™ connects seamlessly with our philosophy on how we conceptualize flexibility—again, increasing a person's Range of Motion, or ROM—via personalized movements based on his/her assessments. As you know by now, we at the NCEP believe strongly in the importance of movement and Stick Mobility™ provides a system that can help you, as a trainer, help your clients move better.

This chapter provides a sampling of important principles for creating and enhancing mobility, written in partnership with our friends from Stick Mobility™. The goal of this type of training is to achieve and control optimum range of movement on every segment of the kinetic chain. However, as we have alluded to throughout this manual, "optimum" is different for every client. Mobility training must be specifically designed for people depending on their history, activity levels, or sport. We will use the information that we gathered during our postural and movement assessments to identify our client's ability to produce and control optimum range of movement.

Reiterating Why Clients Need to Move More

Mobility, as most commonly defined, is the ability to move freely and easily. For most people, as we discussed, that is not always the norm. For example, we wake up in the morning, from sleeping, and then proceed to sit in our cars, trains, or planes on the way to work. Once there, we commence to sitting in our cubicles hovering over our keyboards. Only every once in a while do we get the privilege of moving in order to go sit once again in a meeting, or sit for lunch. When work ends, we sit once more via our commute home. Some of us go to the gym where we have been socialized to use machines to sit or lay down on (although, we all know now at this point in the manual that there are better ways to exercise). Finally, once we have arrive at home we kick our feet up and enjoy dinner while we watch TV—this pattern is quite common, right? According to a Nielson Family Study, the average American watches 5 hours of TV per day, which certainly aids to the problem as to why the average person is incapable of harnessing their ability to be physically mobile.^ This would also lend credence as to why so many people are injured in daily life when they exceed the limits of their body's regular movement parameters. The overall lack of the whole body's physical activity prevents us from moving quickly and easily.

The fitness industry has given the trainer a vast array of tools to help with the battle against immobility. We have foam rollers, balls, straps, tape, massage therapists, stretching, corrective exercises, and many more. The role of the trainer is to figure out which method works for that

^Nielsen Company, *The Total Audience Report,* 2015, http://www.nielsen.com/content/dam/corporate/us/en/reports-downloads/2015-reports/total-audience-report-q1-2015.pdf

particular client—and selecting the right tool or method is key. Yet, to know what method to use you have to understand the principles of creating true mobility, even beyond what we discussed in our previous section on flexibility training. Unfortunately, many trainers do not possess this knowledge, as these trainers may hurt their clients more than they can help.

The Basic Concepts of Mobility

Here are a review of important terms and principles that we have discussed in the manual that are essential to know in order to understand mobility training:

- **Mobility** is not just flexibility; it is the ability to move and a combination of flexibility, strength, and motor control.
- **Flexibility** is the ability to passively achieve range of motion and the ability to bend without breaking.
- **Strength** is the ability to withstand or exert great force (in a specific environment).
- **Motor Control** is the process by which humans use their brain to activate and coordinate the muscles and limbs involved in the performance of any movement.
- **Active Flexibility** is the ability to move a bone around an axis using only internal force. (i.e., reaching your arms overhead as far as you can control).
- **Passive Flexibility** is the ability to move a bone around an axis with help from an external force (i.e., having a partner pull your arms overhead as far they can).
- **Static Stretching** means the body is not continually moving.
- **Dynamic Stretching** means the body is in constant motion.
- **Proprioceptive Neuromuscular Facilitation (PNF)** is "a manual resistance technique that works by simulating fundamental patterns of movement, such as swimming, throwing, running, or climbing. Methods used in PNF oppose motion in multiple planes concurrently."^[1] (This is similar to our explanation of "Neuro Pathways" in Chapter Six.)

In addition, we must grasp other important principles and concepts in order to expand on our knowledge of creating better mobility for our clients. In 1993, Yuri Verkhoshansky and Mel Siff authored the book *Supertraining*.^[2] At the time, this book was filled with cutting edge knowledge that, unfortunately, still is not widely instituted in training programs over 20 years later.

The first idea we will look at is joint Range of Movement/Motion (ROM), first discussed in the previous chapter. To review, human bodies were designed with joints that can flex, extend, rotate, and glide. Having control of these motions at each particular joint is the key to mobility. There are certain cases where structural limitations will prevent a joint's ability to move through its full range. Greater neuromuscular control of your joints through a larger range of movement strongly coincides with improved resistance to injury. That said, we know that our passive flexibility is the key component to protecting a joint if it is stressed past its normal limits, but having controlled mobility is the key to better movement and performance. Traditional static and passive stretching exercise develop mainly passive flexibility, whereas combined strength and stretching exercises are considerably more effective in developing controlled mobility.

^[1]Chaitow, L. (2013). *Muscle Energy Techniques & Website*. Elsevier Health Sciences: 13.

^[2] Verkhoshansky, Y. V., & Siff, M. C. (2009). Supertraining, 6th Edition. (M. Yessis, Trans.). Rome, Italy; Michigan: Verkhoshansky.com.

The next thing we want to address is the aspect of transverse and frontal movement, or the lack of, in personal training. (Although we previously discussed how it is important to make sure clients move in all three planes of motion, this idea is expanded upon here via Stick Mobility's specific system.) We live in a world of rotation, yet we refuse to include that ingredient in our training protocols. Take a minute and think of all the movements that you and your clients perform, on a daily basis, that require rotation. Getting out of bed, showering, entering/exiting a car, walking, running, and playing sports all require rotation. Thus, we *cannot* forget to include this into our client's programming. Using Proprioceptive Neuromuscular Facilitation (PNF) techniques in spiral and rotational movement will enhance your client's multidimensional functional ROM.

Neuromuscular activation is essential for obtaining peak mobility performance. Your body needs to be strong in the beginning, middle, and end ROMs. Always note, however, that a client's pain threshold can be a limiting factor when attempting to increase these end ranges. Your joint health is dependent on your active flexibility. Passive flexibility is merely a joint's protective reserve. Can you produce internal force throughout the whole movement that you are attempting to accomplish? The ability to have neuromuscular control, along with joint stability, will aid with how much strength you can obtain over a joint's ROM. Including an isometric aspect will also aid in greater flexibility. Over time, slowly resisting against a fixed point, in different ROMs, will supplement your mobility.

Breaking Down the Stick Mobility™ System

Our NCEP philosophy, as discussed, uses primarily body weight as a training mechanism, but also incorporates many Stick Mobility techniques. We use these systems because they are the most accessible and practical for you and your clients. *So, what is Stick Mobility and why does it work so well?*

On its most basic level, Stick Mobility is a system developed using a stick to help us increase our functional ROM. It is very practical, efficient, effective, and safe. The stick provides us with a tool to help access greater ranges of movement. Using a stick maximizes mobility training, turning two-dimensional stretches into a four-dimensional training system that promotes full body enrichment. You are able to combine passive stretching, active stretching, PNF stretching, positional isometrics, and strength training all at the same time.

Using a stick as a tool also makes mobility training more accessible for all body types, especially for those that are not naturally flexible. For starters, it will provide your clients leverage to access ranges of motion they normally cannot reach and will enable them to easily apply tension to strengthen those ranges. Best of all, it can be done anywhere without an expensive training apparatus. The movements that can be performed mobilize multiple joints at the same time, maximizing mobility work and saving time; the techniques used with the stick incorporate positional isometrics and applying force into the ground will allow your clients to maintain stability and tension while taking the joints and body through rotation. This allows them to control all aspects of multi-planar movements.

The Stick Mobility™ system incorporates 4 stances: **full kneeling, half kneeling, horse stance,** and **staggered stance.**

- **Full kneeling:** both knees on the floor with full hip extension to start
- **Half kneeling:** lunge position with back knee on the floor
- **Horse stance:** standing wide base (hip width or wider) with pelvis tucked under so that head, shoulders, and hips are stacked on top of each other; drop hips down approximately 3-4 inches to activate the hip muscles
- **Staggered stance:** stand with shoulder width apart and step one foot straight back; distance of stride can vary depending on the exercise and heel may or may not be elevated depending on the exercise.

The rest of the chapter will illustrate bodyweight and Stick Mobility™ techniques to help fix postural and movement dysfunctions. These two modalities are the most accessible and practical forms of mobility training. Here is a simple formula to remember:

Joint Range of Motion + Joint Stability + Neuromuscular Control = Mobility

The formula to create mobility can be described, more specifically, as:

1. *Soft tissue work to excite the nervous system for the short term to help access more range of motion (ROM)*
2. *Passive stretching to access deeper ranges of motion (2 minute holds +)*
3. *Applying Isometrics in these ranges to lock down the range (10 second holds 3-6 reps)*
4. *Putting it all into motion, strengthening the movement pattern you're trying to fix*

This formula can be combined with the following stretches and activations to access and unlock your client's lost mobility. Your clients will be able to access better, controlled ranges of motion which will allow for safer and more efficient movement(s). Use the method and progression that is applicable to your client based on your findings from their movement and postural assessment.

Note: The following two pages illustrate an example of how using the Stick Mobility principles and tools can be used for a dynamic warm-up. For many more additional stretches and postural fixes, please contact us and we would be happy to provide you with pictures and instructions for additional stretches that may be useful for your client(s).

SAMPLE DYNAMIC WARM UP

Before we begin any mobility work or strength training you have to get the body warmed up and ready to go. The warm up below will prep your body from head to toe. You will need a short stick: 4ft for someone 5' 9" and below or 5ft for someone 5'10" and up. If you have really long arms and are under 5' 9" you may need a 5ft stick. The sequences listed below are listed in segments but are to be done in a flow sequence for 5 to 10 minutes.

Wrist/Elbow/Shoulder Warm Up

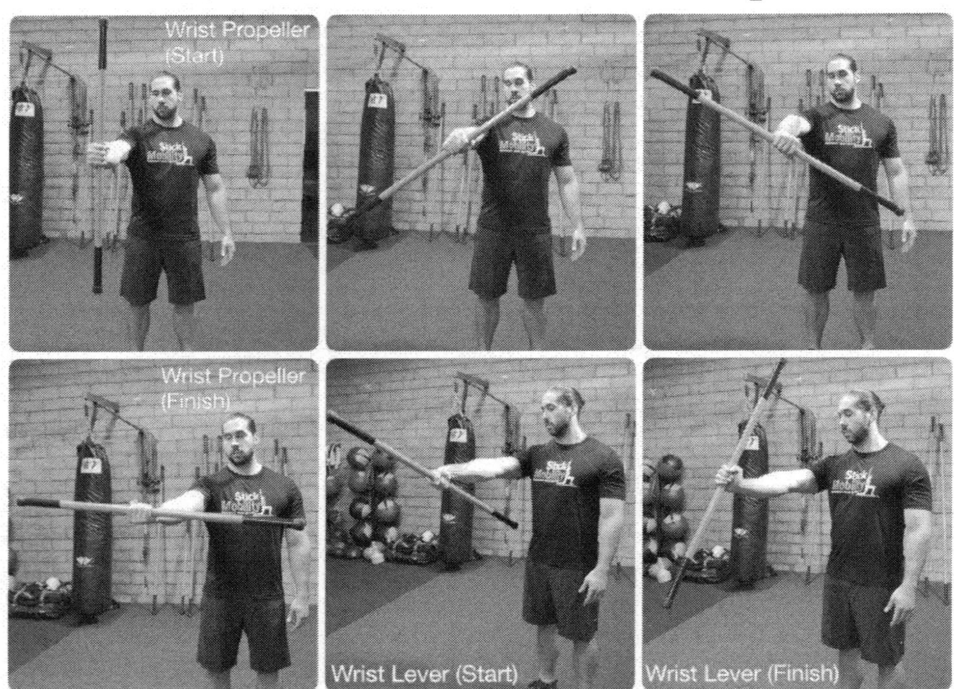

Instructions Wrist Propeller: For this you will need a 4 foot stick. Grab hold of the middle of the stick. Extend the arm out while keeping the elbow straight. Palm should be facing your midline with the thumb in top position. Begin turning the wrist in a clockwise rotation until end ROM is reached. Reverse direction and continue motion until end ROM is reached. Repeat for 20-30 seconds.

Instructions Wrist Lever: Begin with the same stick, and hand/arm position as the Propeller. Drive the thumb forward to lengthen the superior aspect of the wrist until end ROM is reached. Reverse the motion and pull the thumb back towards the elbow until end ROM is obtained. Repeat for 20-30 seconds.

Shoulder Complex/Thoracic Spine Warm Up

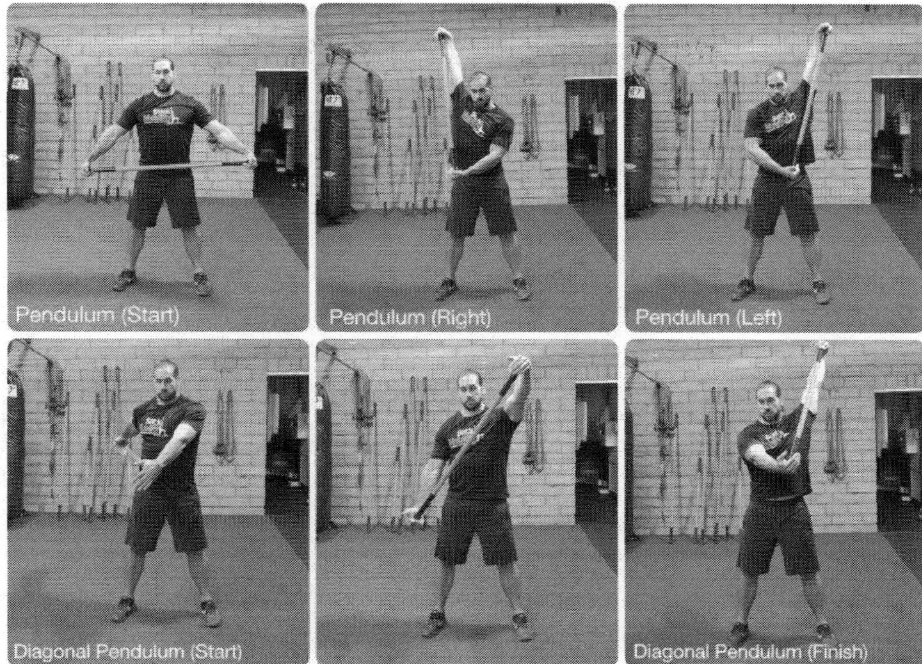
Pendulum (Start) · Pendulum (Right) · Pendulum (Left) · Diagonal Pendulum (Start) · Diagonal Pendulum (Finish)

Instructions: Grab either a 4ft or 5ft stick depending on height and arm length.

1) Pendulum: Start in horse stance, placing both palms against the ends of the stick. Apply light tension into the stick. Begin to push the stick side to side in front of body up overhead. Apply a bit more force with bottom hand to increase the stretch in the shoulder of top hand. Gradually find your end ROM. Perform repetitions for 20-30 seconds.

2) Diagonal Pendulum: In horse stance, apply light tension into both ends of the stick. Start with the stick in a horizontal position just outside your right hip. Begin to push the stick in a diagonal motion up over the left shoulder. Apply a bit more force with bottom hand to increase the stretch in the shoulder of top hand. Gradually find your end ROM. Perform repetitions for 20-30 seconds. Repeat on opposite side

Thoracic/Hip/Ankle/Foot Warm Up

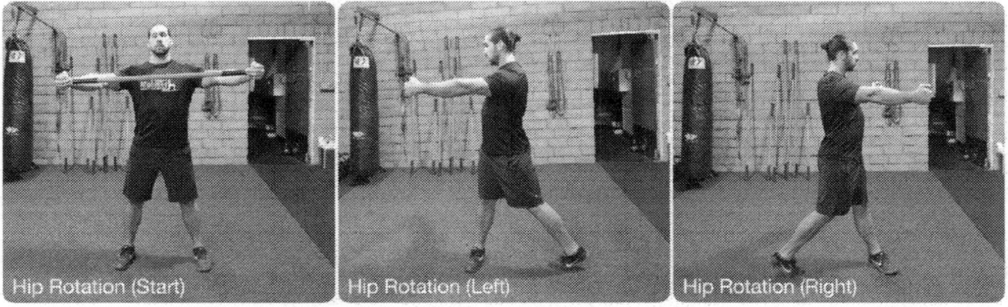
Hip Rotation (Start) · Hip Rotation (Left) · Hip Rotation (Right)

Instructions: Start in a stance just wider than hip width with a slight bend in the knees. Hold the stick with arms straight at chest height. Slowly rotate the hips either right or left making sure to pivot the back foot. You may push the arms across the body as far as they can go. Flow from side to side in a controlled manner and do this for about a 60-90 seconds.

Concluding Thoughts

We would like to leave you with this final message: the gift of mobility is the most powerful tool that you can give your clients. The amount of weight that your client can push, pull, lift, or throw is irrelevant if he/she does not have ability to move easily or freely. Your client's long term health and fitness is directly impacted by how well he/she can move. Limited mobility will lead to injuries, hindering your client's fitness goals. You, the trainer, have the ability and responsibility to help people achieve their optimal health and fitness levels. Yet, at the same time, you also have the ability to hinder their progress and cause great physical harm if you are irresponsible with your training techniques. Remeber, the client has put their faith and trust in you, as an exercise professional, to do what is best for them—and the Stick Mobility™ system is excellent way to help your clients look and feel better. As we have stressed throughout the manual and is central to our NCEP philosophy, allow this thought process to always be at the forefront of your training and you will change lives for the better.

To learn more about our friends at Stick Mobility, you can contact them on Instagram/Twitter (@StickMobility), YouTube (Stick Mobility TV), and Facebook (Stick Mobility), as well as via e-mail at Stickmobility@gmail.com for information about attending workshops or how to become a certified Stick Mobility™ practitioner. Furthermore, please contact us or our friends at Stick Mobility for additional stretches and postural fixes.

CHAPTER EIGHT

Attitude Training

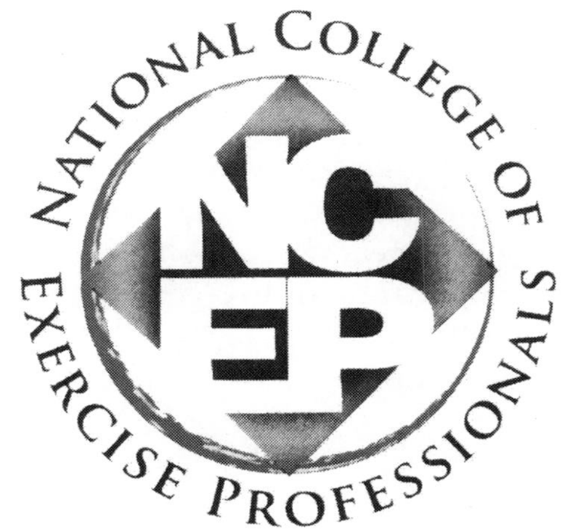

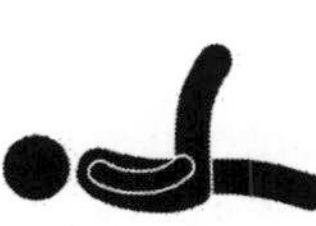
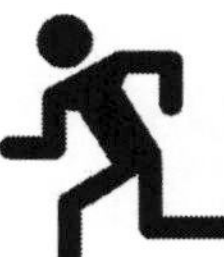
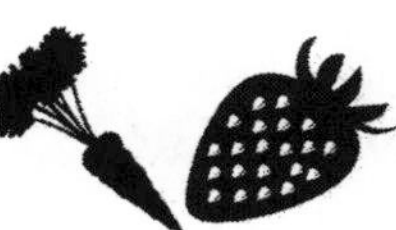
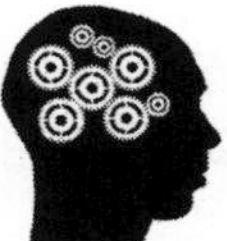

ATTITUDE TRAINING

One of the most important components—but universally the least discussed and explored—is *attitude training*. Rarely do trainers think about attitude training, or the mental state of their clients, when designing programs or during sessions. Conversely, we believe that incorporating attitude training and being innovative in the way you approach motivating your clients can be another way to separate yourself from other trainers. There are decades worth of social science research illustrating that people perform better when they are in a positive state, and finding strategies to keep clients motivated, happy, and engaged can be just as important to your success as the exercises they perform. Furthermore, as a trainer, you also want to help clients train not just their body, but their mind in ways that will contribute to their fitness and their life.

Keeping Clients Motivated and Basic Attitude Tips

When talking with other trainers in the industry, you will often year trainers say that their job is to motivate the client, but in reality, clients are *already* very motivated to come to a gym or health club in the first place. Instead, we must make sure to keep them from getting *de-motivated* as they progress in their exercise program (and hopefully, in their sessions with you). To do this, you need to identify what motivated a person in the first place and help the person stay connected to this reason. Remember that clients often live busy lives, and the last thing you want is for exercise to feel like work—it should be anything but!

Most people respond best to positive reinforcement and we believe strongly in training with this philosophy. One basic strategy we like to suggest is to use the so-called **"positive sandwich"** technique. As you coach clients, offer a positive comment, followed by a constructive criticism, and end with another positive comment or words of encouragement. Using positive words and imagery will help clients feel good about themselves and their training. However, this simple strategy helps avoid the "folly of praise." When you give excessive praise for efforts and performance that are not worthy of it, the client will naturally not give their full effort on the next attempt. Since every effort is "awesome," there will be no motivation for the client to give a greater effort and perform better. Using encouragement and positive reinforcement mixed in with honest and candid constructive feedback is a great recipe for success.

Another valuable technique in attitude training is to keep fitness fun and to "make it a game." When people are sluggish and having a hard time finding the mental energy to perform well, you can make training fun by incorporating games into the workout. This is particularly valuable when your clients participate in Athletic Performance Enhancement training; for example, playing catch, hopscotch, etc., will help a client connect to the childlike feelings of exercise being fun and not feeling like "work." It will also help them develop a competitive spirit, and a higher level of focus and concentration.

The M.A.V.A. Technique

While these tips are valuable, we also want to offer a few "tools" that you can use with your clients to both keep them from getting de-motivated and most importantly, help them improve their mind and general focus abilities. One such tool is the **M.A.V.A.** technique:

Meditation (or **M**indfulness)
Affirmations
Visualizations
Anchoring

Remember, the mind is like a computer—what comes out depends on the programming put in. To reprogram a computer, you delete the old programs and install new software. Therefore, with M.A.V.A., start by explaining to your clients that you will incorporate basic elements of Sports Psychology and if they are receptive, these elements will improve their focus and concentration (which, in turn, will positively affect their training results).

The first step is *meditation, or mindfulness.* Although this component is often viewed as a complex process, it is actually quite simple. Meditation is the process of clearing the mind and it is very beneficial for preparing mentally for a task at hand. One effective technique to induce a client in meditation is to have him/her focus on breathing and to tell the person to "relax his/her mind" while performing deep TVA breathing. (Refer to Chapter Four on Assessments in regards to additional details on TVA breathing). The key is teaching the client to inhale through the nose and allow his/her abdomen to swell as he/she fill the lungs. Then, he/she should exhale through the mouth with the teeth closed but not clenched and the tongue on the roof of the mouth. As your client breathes—or, if preferred, another type of stretch or slow-moving exercise—have him/her clear the mind as part of the meditation process. Have your client wash out the rest of the day and focus on the "here and now" in full preparation for the excellent session you have planned.

The next step is to have your client say *affirmations*, which are simple, powerful statements that imprint or make firm these thoughts in the sub-conscious mind. Sports psychologist use affirmations to help athletes develop a strong attitude about certain aspects of their performance. It is great to have your clients make their own affirmations, but here are a few basic examples:

- I feel good; I feel great; and I feel terrific.
- I have a super strong body.
- I have a super strong mind.
- I have confidence in all situations.
- I am calm in all situations.

The third technique is *visualization*, which is another amazing mental exercise for peak performance, and can be easily taught to your clients. As you progress through the workout with your client, instruct your client to picture in his/her mind themselves performing the exercise, activity, or sport. He/she should create a mental movie and attempt to have as much detail as possible including specific sights, sounds, odors, feelings, sensations and emotions. The visualization should be positive and your client should be successfully accomplishing the task. For example, a tennis player might envision hitting the perfect ace while a businessperson might visualize leaving a flawless board presentation meeting. If he/she has never done it before, have your client attempt to "see" himself/herself doing it and imagine what it would be like (i.e., the roar of the crowd, or the high fives from your colleagues). This technique can be very effective in helping people accomplish something that they struggle at or want to perform better in.

The final technique is called *anchoring*, or basically controlling your successful emotional and mental state. This is often the favorite of clients, and is used by every professional athlete in every sport. When a person achieves success and is filled with strong, positive emotions and a mental state of confidence, he/she can make a simple physical gesture and say a power word or phrase. This will connect the emotions and mindset of success to the gesture and power phrase. For example, a tennis player may pump his/her first after winning a big point, yelling "let's go!" or an NFL player may perform a handshake and a scream with a teammate in celebration of a touchdown. Athletes often associate these physical actions and verbal phrases with being "in the zone." When your client repeats this regularly, he/she will eventually conjure the positive emotional and mental state of being by using the familiar anchor. As a trainer, using an anchoring technique is an excellent way to build repertoire with your client; every time he/she finishes a set, for example, you and your client can perform an anchor together (like a fist bump) that is motivating and unique to your client-trainer relationship.

Yet, how does a trainer work this into a client's program design? After getting a client's permission, you can introduce him/her to the basics of Sports Psychology and explain the techniques of meditation, affirmations, visualizations, and anchoring. If this individual is open to the process, you can help him/her choose some affirmations (and have the client say them at the beginning and end of the session), a power move for his/her personal anchor (everyone will be different), and his/her own power word or phrase.

Creating a Physical *and* Mental Workout

Another effective tool that can be used to incorporate attitude training into a program is to discuss important aspects of success and make one simple component as the theme for the day. These can be themes such as discipline, confidence, teamwork, poise, etc. You pick one for the day and then, during the workout, you and the client can talk about what it means within the context of both the session and his/her daily life.

One of the greatest examples of this strategy is the Pyramid of Success, created by the legendary Coach John Wooden, an 11-time NCAA Champion Men's Basketball Coach at UCLA who is considered the one of the greatest coaches of all time. During Coach Wooden's career, he developed and perfected his Pyramid of Success, as each brick (i.e., theme) builds on top of each other. His program has been utilized by countless sports teams and companies as a way of teaching the finer points of leadership and success in sports, business, and life. As a trainer, you can print out the Wooden Pyramid of Success and include it with your client's program card. (Visit www.coachwooden.com/pyramid-of-success) Then, during each workout, you can choose one of the bricks and discuss it with your client throughout the session. If you were to teach the whole Pyramid at once, it would be overwhelming, but, discussing one a day can be immensely powerful! For example, one day the theme could be "poise," where you discuss what it means to be poised both during this session and the client's life. This inclusion of attitude training—or working to improve your client's mental state—is something that can elevate the quality of your training sessions in unique ways. The best trainers provide both a physical and mental workout, and tools such as this work well to intertwine the mind and the body.

Furthermore, these techniques are not exclusive to modern psychology and have been utilized for thousands of years. Many martial art systems use "school principles" to teach their students mental strength, discipline, and creative thinking. For example, in Rainbow Warrior Martial Arts, there are five principles of the Rainbow Warrior:

- ◊ *To always have a positive mental attitude in everything we say and do*
- ◊ *To always maintain proper conduct, good manners, dignity, humility and honesty towards others*
- ◊ *To seek self-awareness, aiming towards self-perfection of the mind, body, and spirit*
- ◊ *To always maintain strong will power, strength, courage and self-confidence*
- ◊ *To always have unwavering faith in ourselves*

The students of the school must learn, memorize, recite and most importantly live by these principles. As a trainer, you can teach your clients these principles and work with them on these mind power skills.

Ultimately, we at the National College of Exercise Professionals believe in an "Attitude of Gratitude" and our slogan, "teach it forward." As you become more experienced, you will develop your own attitude training "tools" and strategies to motivate your clients in their workout while also improving their mental fortitude in ways that can benefit both their training sessions and their life activities. The tips and suggestions here are only examples that have worked for us, and we encourage you to incorporate your strategies for attitude training into your repertoire of skills.

CHAPTER NINE

Fascia Fundamentals

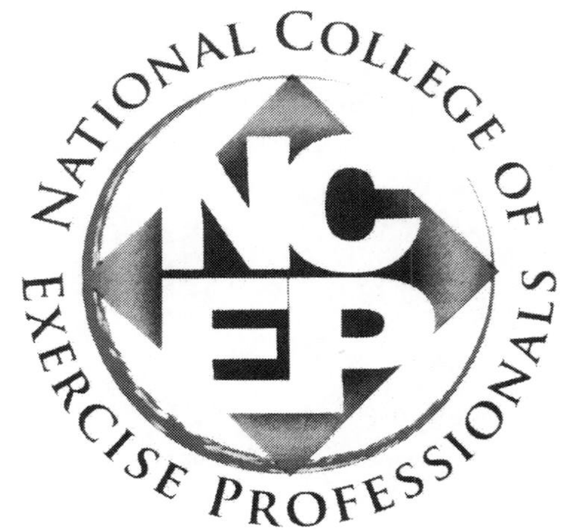

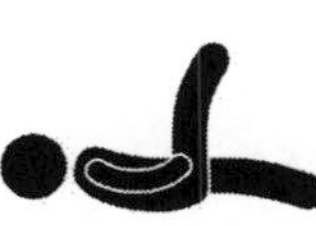
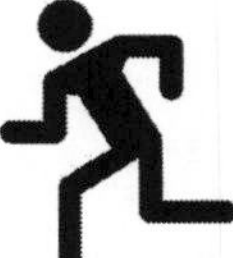
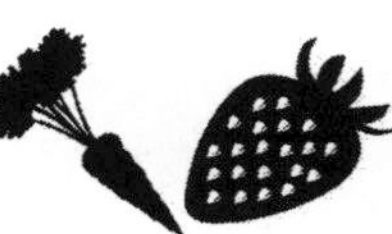
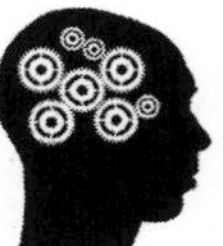

FASCIA FUNDAMENTALS

COURTESY OF MICHELE BOND

What is Fascia and Why Study It?

If we did not have the fascial system, the 70% of our body that is made up of water would be a big puddle around us at our feet. In terms of form, our trillions of cells would be a pile of mush and incapable of organizing much of anything inside our body.

Fascia is the soft tissue component of the connective tissue system that permeates, surrounds, and connects every muscle, bone, organ and nerve from head to toe. It is a three dimensional matrix of structural support, among other things. This fascial system is a continuous network through the entire body. It plays an important role in transmitting mechanical forces between muscles and other structures as well as movement perception and coordination. With this information alone, it is very apparent that some knowledge about the fascial system is important for a deeper understanding of human movement as well as evaluating postures and exercise programming.

Muscle's Partner

Muscles do not work in isolation. One muscle does not work alone to perform movement and communicate with other structures. Muscles work together to accomplish this. However, the fascia (fascial system) is highly responsible for assisting with this as well as providing a communication along a pathway in the body. Did you know that this pathway is how the big toe on your right foot is connected to the left shoulder? We know that one bone is connected to the next bone by a joint (the kinetic chain), but there is more to it than that. There are traceable lines of connective tissue that connect various points of the body to another point. An injury or "snag" in this line can have effects beyond the point at which the injury occurred. With the research we have now, you have the opportunity to take advantage of this information and be one of the first trainers to study these concepts and apply them to your practice. You will understand the lines of communication that flow throughout the body and how that can help further your expertise with the assessment process and exercise programming for a client.

Total Body Connection

In addition to these lines of communication, there is also the three dimensional aspect of this tissue. This 3-D web fills the volume of the body in every direction. Here is why this is important to understand. If you lift a weight, kick a soccer ball, sprint, or clean a house, you are activating this body-wide web in all its glory. Everything has to push and pull and create the right tension in the right places to get these tasks done as efficiently as possible while minimizing risk of injury. This information is vital to how we will evaluate a client's movement and program accordingly. You will be taking into consideration an important aspect of the human body that is integrated into everything we do. It will take you beyond just the muscle.

Energy Storage Capacity

The fascial system can explain how movement is really created, beyond the "only" traditional muscle and bone system. For example, the calf muscle is not nearly as important as the tendon and other connective tissues in propelling the body. The fascia, in this case, has a major capacity to store energy and that is what is allowing the repetitive patterns such as in walking or running. This energy storage can be applied to the wind up in a baseball pitch, the trunk rotation in the backswing of a golf swing, and a powerful jump to dunk a basketball. So, understanding how this system works and how to train it would be a very beneficial addition to a training and conditioning program for athletes and recreational exercisers alike. Understanding how the fascial system works can also be applied to fascial system training in a yoga, Pilates, athletic training, martial arts, dance, and even walking/running regimens.

Sensory and Innervation

The fascial system also has a role as a pain generator. There are free nerve endings in the fascia, and they contain a certain receptor that is nociceptive (pain generating). With respect to exercise, delayed onset muscle soreness (DOMS) can occur because of repetitive eccentric contraction (mentioned in this chapter and throughout the manual). This is the 'sore' in 'sore muscles'.

Proprioception (the sense that tells your body [joints] where it is positioned in space) is aided by the fascial system. The fascial system is equipped with a special type of sensor (mechanoreceptor: a sense cell that responds to mechanical stimuli such as touch or sound) that assists with this ability. Understanding how to properly recruit these mechanoreceptors will assist with a client's ability to become better aware of their body orientation and movement. When you understand the 'why' or the theory, it makes the practice of everything you do as a trainer more valid and productive.

Since the fascial system is innervated by about six times more sensory nerves than muscle spindles (defined in the next chapter), your brain is actually more in tune with the fasica rather than the red muscle tissue. Fascia is indeed muscles' helper!

The Remodel Response

This research about fascia is allowing people, like personal trainers, to understand how to affect this tissue so that the health of the fascial system can be addressed in conjunction with building a strong, balanced, and coordinated muscular system. They are not separate, so adding this information about fascia onto the trainer tool belt just makes sense. Understanding this tissue system is a must for serious trainers who wish to avoid injury. Most injuries are connective tissue injuries, even if muscles are involved. Essentially, fascia responds to training, just like red muscle tissue, but in a different way. You are changing this matrix of fibers during exercise, or lack there of, whether you are aware of it or not. These interconnected fibers direct a multitude of directional forces around the body and are capable of responding to forces by remodeling itself accordingly. For example, if a person sits for the better part of the day, the fascial system will respond to the force accordingly by shortening the hip flexor muscles, lengthening the hamstrings, and if there is poor spinal support, perhaps tightening the chest due to rounded shoulders. This connective tissue system is *the* living biological matrix that causes this remodeling. It is *always* responding!

TRAINER APPLICATION: The relevance here is that after you are more educated in this subject matter, you can approach potential clients from a more complete standpoint. You can explain your reasons for your exercise programming with even more knowledge about another system in the body that affects form and function. You will also be able to correct someone on the gym floor with more conviction because you will better understand how the fascial system contributes to form and function. An exercise done incorrectly or in an inappropriately advanced way can have negative effects on the fascial system and thus cause injury or impede fitness/wellness goals. To be able to communicate that knowledge to someone will be invaluable.

Fascia and Fitness/Sport

The discussion about fascia has reached the fitness/sport community already. Major personal training conferences are featuring workshops about fascia and how to affect it so that movement can be more productive. However, most of these workshops are focused very little on the theory and background about fascia and more on the practical applications. NCEP strives to provide both theory *and* practice. This is so that the personal trainer will understand the mechanisms that make the fascial system work the way it does and be able to speak about it intelligently.

The sport science world is also coming around to this information. There have been several conferences regarding this. One conference is called Connective Tissue in Sports Medicine. This is hosted by one of the main researchers in Germany, Dr. Robert Schleip. Also, the first fascia research conference was in 2007 at Harvard Medical School. If Harvard hosts something, you can bet it's something well validated. Any trainer who invests some time and energy on this subject matter starting here and continuing on, will be ahead of the curve. Fascia research and application has already permeated the therapeutic and movement science arenas. Being able to discuss this tissue and system at a basic level and apply several of fascia's conditioning principles to your client's programming will be very rewarding. Not only will you set yourself apart both as an exercise professional and a business professional, but you will open doors for conversations with personnel in those various arenas that will begin to trust you and refer clients to you.

Why Now?

Why has this material not been presented in an exercise certification setting until now? Historically, fascia research has not really been at the forefront of personal training. One researcher noted that the traditional method of studying muscle as independent units has been a barrier to examining the larger picture and overlooking the function of the fascial system. Even in traditional medical school, the fascia is stripped away (thought of as just packaging) to get to the study of other structures. This is all about to change with the surge of prominent research since the turn of the millennium. For our chapter about muscle physiology, we will focus on how the discovery of this entity in the body, that has always been there, is now illuminating some of the mechanisms behind why muscle functions the way it does. Again, the fascial system is not a new structure in the body. It has always been there. It is just that the brilliant anatomists, clinicians, and researchers that kept digging and asking questions have paved a way to reveal the true function of this magnificent tissue and system.

In this case, we are talking about the fascial system of the body, and in the case of this chapter, the deep fasciae (plural) that relates to the muscle. This can be thought of as the myofascia. The myofascia is found on the surface of the muscle, around a muscle group (e.g. quadriceps muscle group), and in the various layers within a muscle (epimysium, perimysium, endomysium).

Fascia Research

The first fascial research conference was held at the aforementioned Harvard School of Medicine in 2007. The Fascia Research Society was born from this success to facilitate, encourage, and support the dialogue and collaboration between clinicians, researchers, and academicians, in order to further the understanding of the properties and functions of fasciae. From this effort, we can now review various research studies on an array of topics—biomechanics, sensory aspects, anatomical structures, pathology and several others. So, the take away here is this topic of fascia is not some kind of fad. It is a topic that is heavily embedded in the medical, therapeutic, exercise/sports science, and pain management arenas. As an exercise professional, you need to be aware of it.

Bottom line: the fascial system research now blows away once thought of modalities of the connections in the body and how they work. This research will continue to change textbooks and applications to sport, exercise, and therapy.

Training the Fascial System

It's more than about stretching or foam rolling. Training the fascial system is really more about a stand-alone training and conditioning program for this specific system. The fascial components of this system respond to specific types of stimulus because of mechanoreceptors that were discussed earlier. There have been movement programs developed based on specific principles to illicit changes in the fascial system. These changes could allow corrective exercise to be more productive to address the postural deviations mentioned in Chapter 4. Further study with NCEP in this subject matter is highly recommended.

Concluding Remarks

This information is also keeping in alignment with NCEP's dedication to a holistic approach to personal training. The function of the layers of fascia as they relate to muscle could not be more holistic in nature. This component of the body as it relates to muscle needs to be touched upon to really appreciate the work that both tissues do. What is important now, is to help you understand the foundations of fascia and fascial research so that further study and application will be motivating and rewarding for both you and your client.

We are first generation users of this modern research. We are the pioneers. Today. Right now. You will be able to say you are a facial research applications pioneer. This will, no doubt, set you apart at another level. This information is heavily applicable to personal training and exercise therapy due to fascia's intimate involvement with muscle anatomy and function. Welcome to the wondrous world of fascia!

Note: The NCEP would like to thank Michele Bond for writing this chapter and generously allowing us to include this important introduction to fascia-related research in our manual.

CHAPTER TEN

Physiology

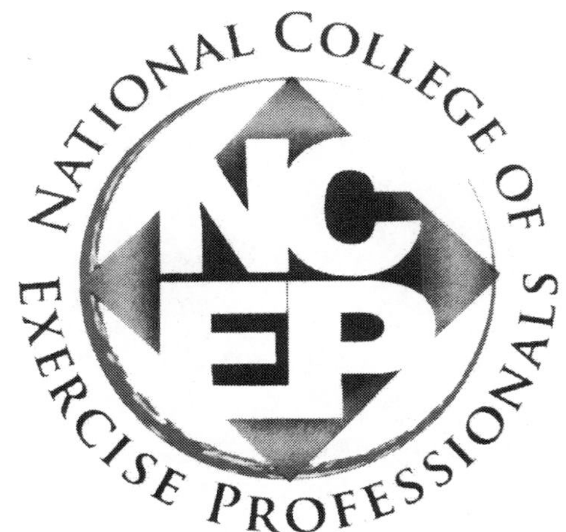

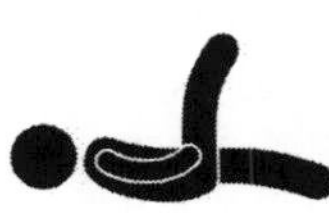
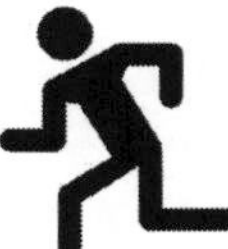
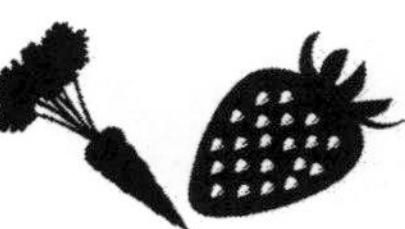
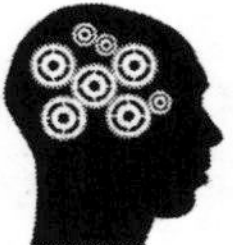

PHYSIOLOGY

How Does a Muscle Work?

Since understanding the details of muscle movement is complicated and nuanced, this chapter provides only the basic, foundational principles central to muscle physiology, starting with the terms on this page. Essentially, the nerve and all the muscle fibers that it connects with, or innervates, are referred to as a ***motor unit***. An ***action potential,*** or electric impulse, travels along the nerve or ***neuron*** but is not directly capable of stimulating the muscle fiber. It is the release of a chemical called ***acetylcholine*** which crosses into the muscle fiber causing a release of calcium to stimulate a contraction. This neural signal causes a momentary twitch of all the fibers in the motor unit. This is referred to as the ***all or none principle***. Either the action potential is great enough to contract all the muscle fibers or it is not strong enough to contract any. If the contraction is needed for longer than a moment, a second twitch takes place, and then a third and so on. The twitches add up or ***summate*** and the force becomes greater. With training, the frequency of twitches can increase and also the number of motor units activated or ***recruited*** will increase. This frequency and recruitment increase is the development of neural pathways associated with new levels of exercise.

It is important to understand that some muscle fibers are more suited for slower twitches and are not capable of high intensity contractions. These muscle fibers are called ***slow twitch type I*** and are associated more with endurance or postural muscles. There are other muscle fibers that are capable of producing high intensity high velocity twitches and they are referred to as ***fast twitch type II*** muscle fibers. There are also many different fibers that fall somewhere in between fast and slow twitch. These are called ***intermediate fibers*** and they have the uncanny ability to take on the characteristics of either fast or slow twitch fibers depending upon how they are trained. This is the logic behind training in a speed environment if you want to improve power or absolute strength as well as the purpose of training in a slow and controlled environment if you want to get better at endurance activities.

In and around the muscle fiber there are a number of ***neural receptors*** that can also control the contraction. ***Muscle spindles*** sense stretch and/or rate of length change in a muscle and cause a contraction. Conversely, ***golgi tendon organs*** respond to high levels of tension which will cause the muscle to relax—thus, the reason why we hold static stretches at least 20 seconds. When the muscle spindles sense a rate of change in the muscles' length it will cause the muscle to first fight the change and contract. Finally, when consistent tension is placed on the muscle for a length of time, the golgi tendon organ will override the message from the muscle spindle thus causing the muscle to relax.

The content that follows in this brief chapter only touch the surface of muscle movement, but provide a basic overview for what you, as an exercise professional, should be familiar with and that you can apply in practice.

SLIDING FILAMENT THEORY

4 components
Electrical impulse stimulates calcium w/ Tropomysin, Actin, Myosin to form cross bridge
4 pts

Active Components

- Actin
- Myosin
- Tropomyosin (troponin and myosin)

Reaction

1. Electric impulse from brain
2. Calcium ++ ions
3. Troponin is pulled away
4. Crossbridging occurs

SKELETAL MUSCLE CONTRACTION (WITH CROSSBRIDGE)

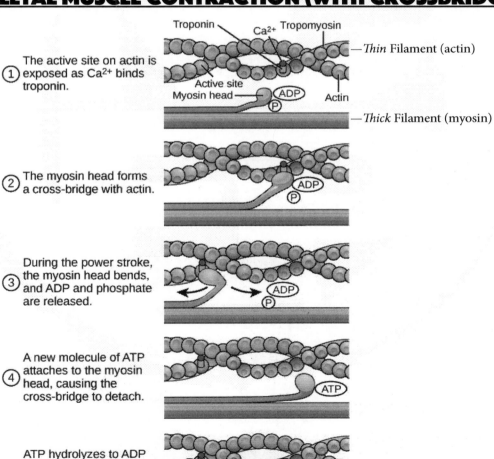

(1) The active site on actin is exposed as Ca^{2+} binds troponin.

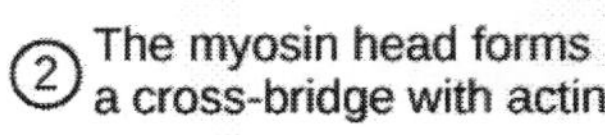
(2) The myosin head forms a cross-bridge with actin.

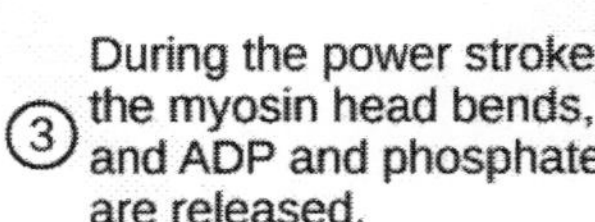
(3) During the power stroke, the myosin head bends, and ADP and phosphate are released.

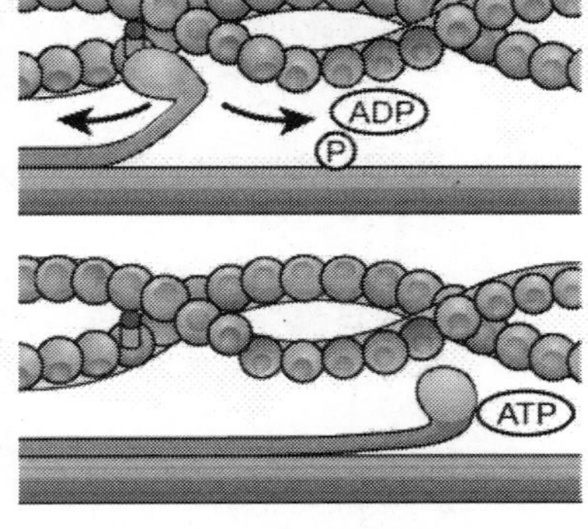

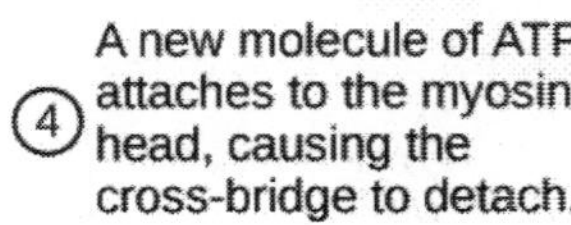
(4) A new molecule of ATP attaches to the myosin head, causing the cross-bridge to detach.

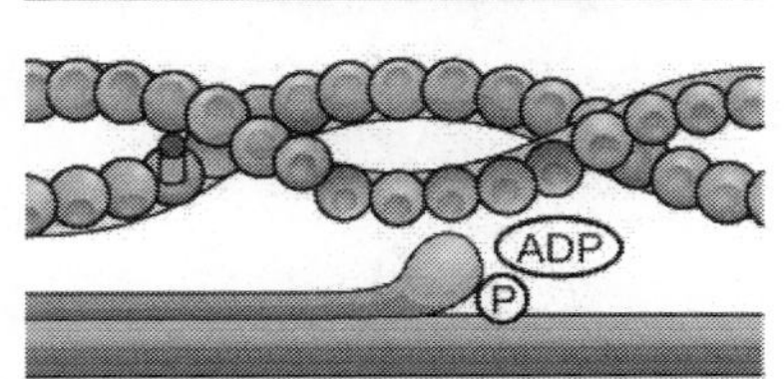

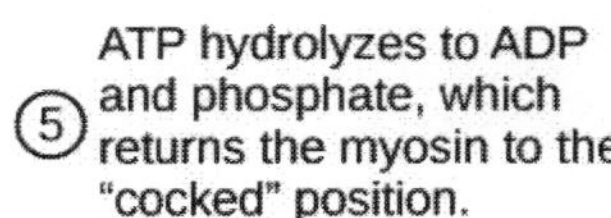
(5) ATP hydrolyzes to ADP and phosphate, which returns the myosin to the "cocked" position.

STRENGTH CURVE

A. **What is the Strength Curve?**
The strength curve basically states that in every movement there are times when the muscle has a greater capacity for work and a lesser capacity for work. The work capacity is determined by the number of crossbridges that have been formed at any given moment. The most amount of crossbridges occur in the middle of the motion.

B. **Number of Crossbridges**
1. Least amount = *smallest capacity for work*
2. Most amount = *greatest capacity for work*
3. H-zone = *no ability to crossbridge*

MUSCLE FIBERS

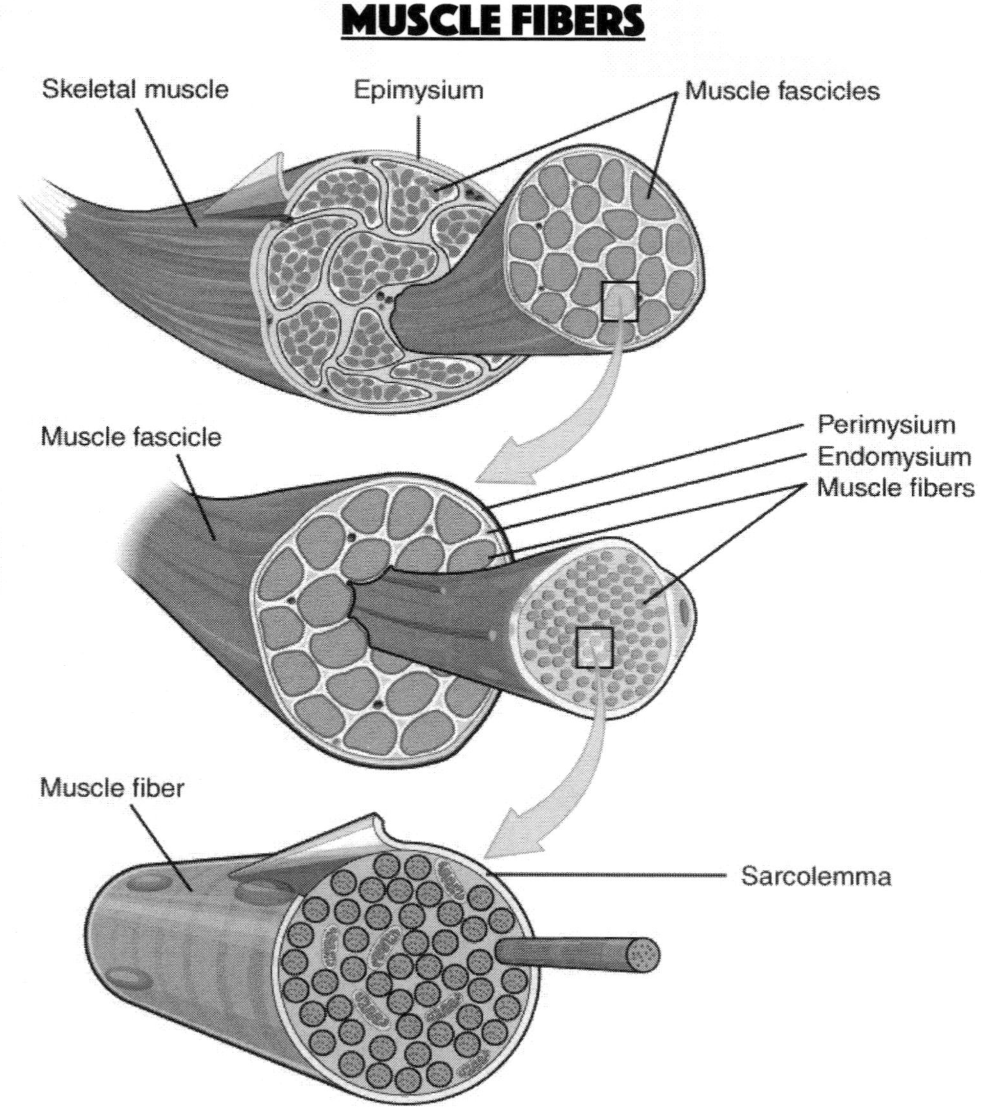

MUSCLE FIBERS (DETAILED)

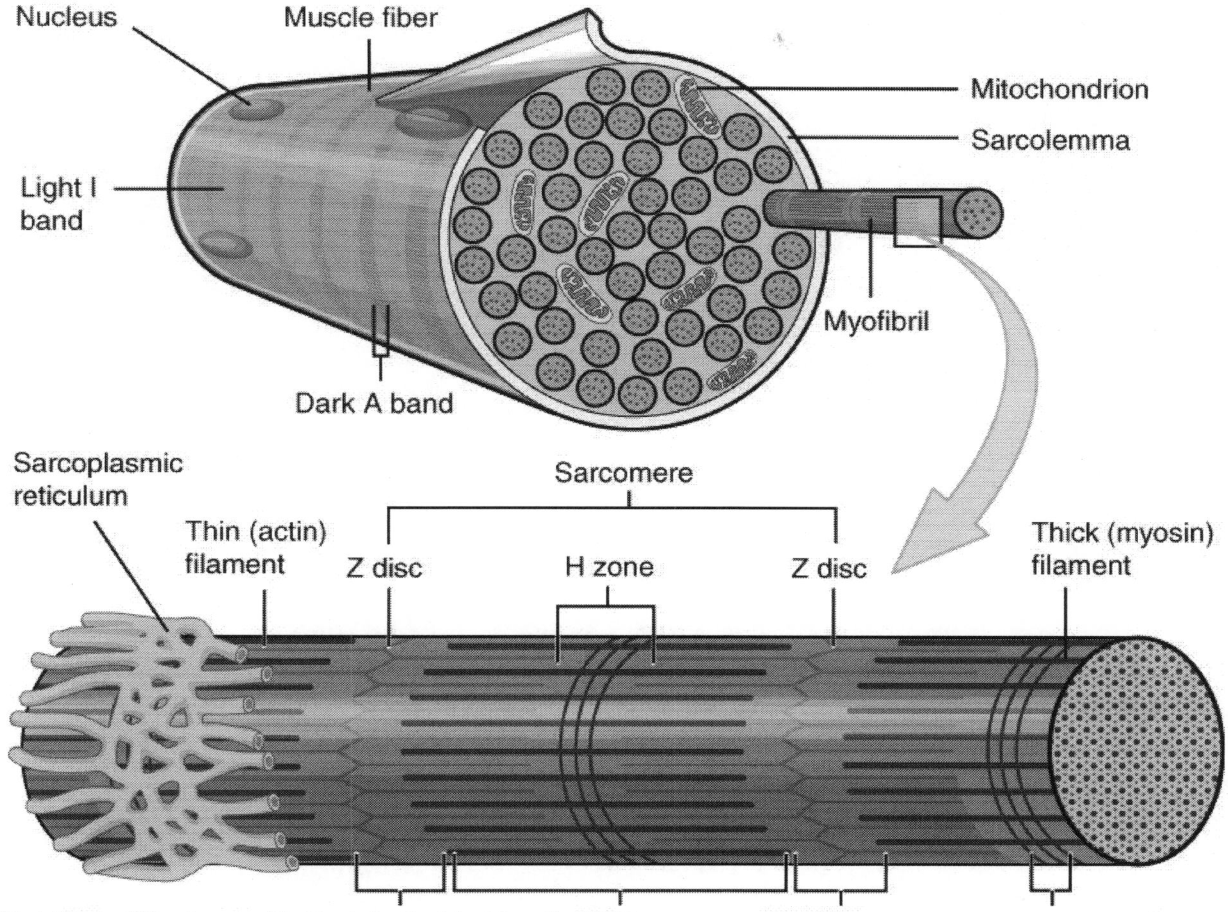

"Muscle Fibers (small)" from Anatomy and Physiology by OpenStax College is licensed by CC BY 3.0

NOTE: *The diagram above is a continuation of the previous diagram (page 108), with a more detailed look at the muscle fiber by going "deeper" and viewing a closer look at the sarcomere inside the myofibril. Remember, this is where muscle contractions happen, as you will see on the next page via the diagram illustrating the shortening of the sarcomere.*

SHORTENING OF THE SARCOMERE

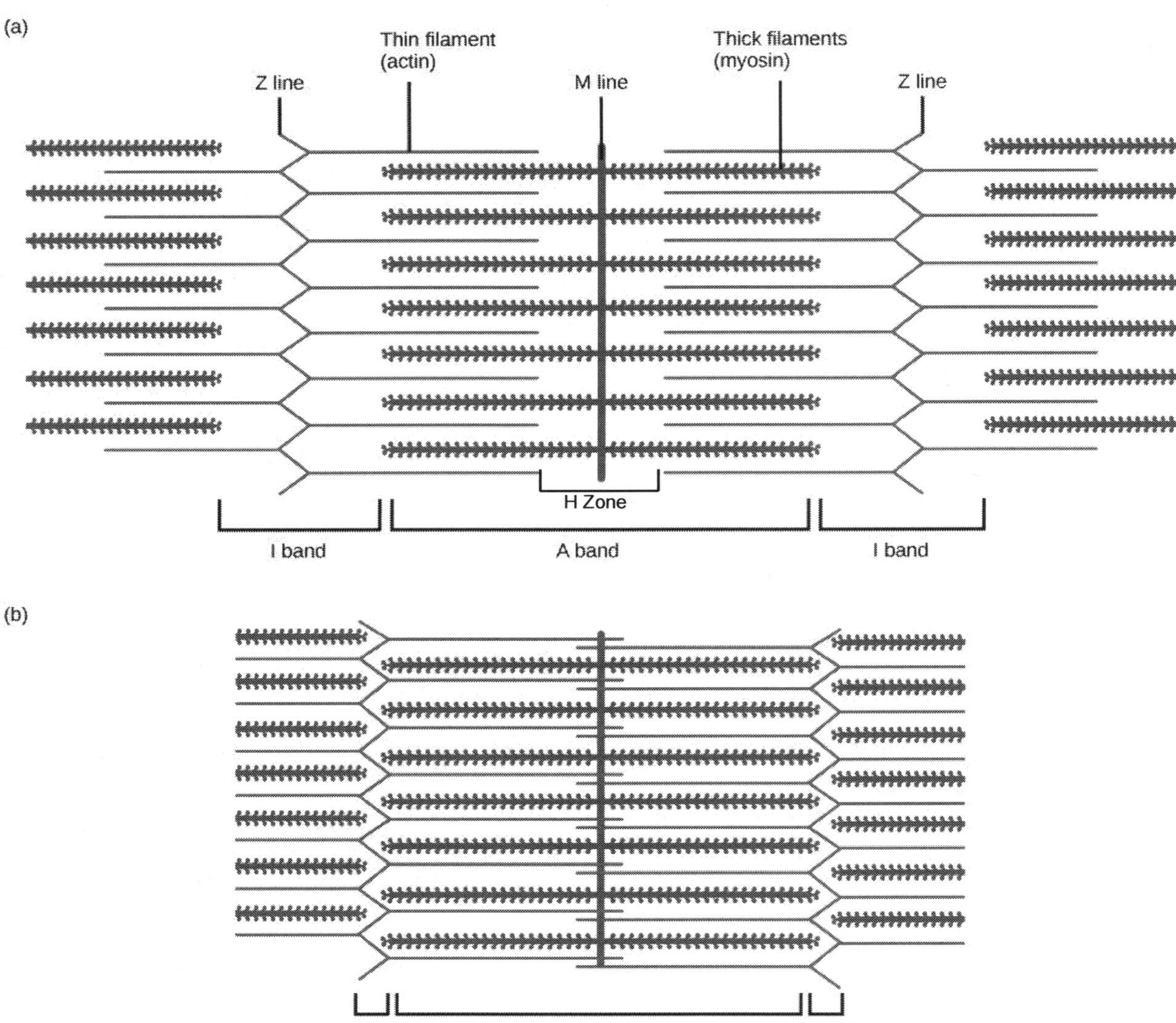

"Sliding Filament Model of Contraction" from Muscle Contraction and Locomotion by OpenStax College is licensed by CC BY 3.0

In a relaxed muscle, actin and myosin myofilaments lie side-by-side and the H zones and I band are at maximum width (figure a). During contraction, the actin and myosin myofilaments interact. The actins slide toward the center of each myosin myofilaments and as a result, the sarcomeres shorten. In the fully contracted muscle, the ends of the actin myofilaments overlap, the H zones disappear and the I band becomes very narrow (figure b).

THREE TYPES OF CONTRACTIONS

Concentric Action - *when the force within the muscle overcomes the resistance against it and the muscle shortens* **(FORCE PRODUCTION)**

Isometric Action - *when the force within the muscle is equal to the resistance placed upon it and there is no movement* **(STABILIZATION OF FORCE)**

Eccentric Action - *when the resistance overcomes the force being generated by the muscle; although the muscle is contracting, it is forced to lengthen with control (also called a "negative")* **(FORCE REDUCTION)**

Conclusion: What Do I Need to Know About Physiology?

For many beginning trainers, learning the physiology of a person and the dynamics of muscle movement can often be overwhelming, and understandably so. While we believe that it is important to know some of the basic components of this section—for example, how training in different speeds affects different muscle fibers relevant to certain activities—by and large, understanding the minutiae of muscle contractions will not make you become a quality trainer. In fact, some of the most knowledgeable exercise physiologists may not know how to create an appropriate resistance program for a client. Thus, staying true to our philosophy, we believe that program design is most critical to success.

However, knowing the basic knowledge of how a muscle contracts can still be highly relevant and we do believe that, as an exercise professional, this information is worth learning. *Ultimately, the best trainers are those who can use this knowledge and incorporate it into program design.* For example, understanding the three different types of contractions (above) can then allow you to have your client engage in these different contractions in ways that help them move better and more efficiently—and create a unique program that is different than trainers who lack this knowledge (for example, only training their clients concentrically). As you continue your education and career in the industry, there will be many opportunities to go deeper into exercise physiology and we wholeheartedly encourage you to do so.

CHAPTER ELEVEN

Energy Systems

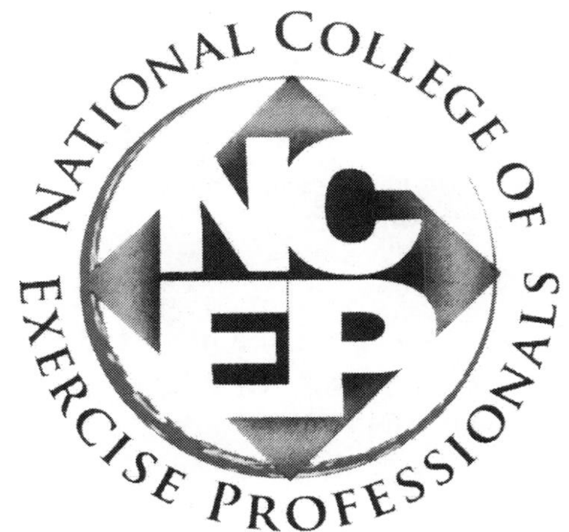

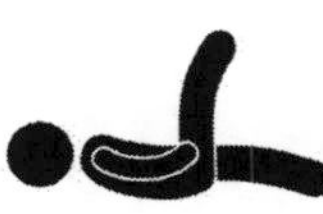
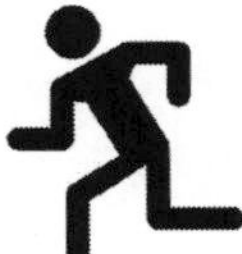
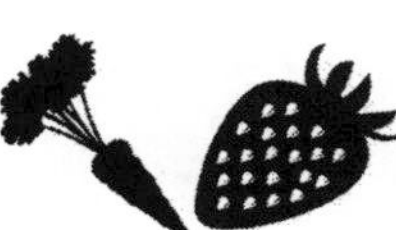
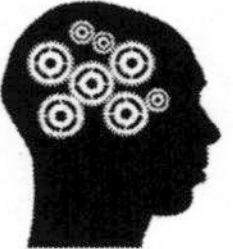

ENERGY SYSTEMS
(OR METABOLIC PATHWAYS)

This chapter briefly discusses how the body creates energy via the three main "metabolic pathways," or what we like to refer to more simply as "energy systems." While there are many specific forms of knowledge around substrate utilization (i.e., how the body uses different types of fuel, such as carbohydrates or fats) that are beyond the scope of this manual, it is important to know that the body has three main energy systems. These energy systems are outlined in this chapter. The reasons for knowing how the body's energy systems function is simple: certain activities rely on different energy systems, which align to the type of exercises you will design for a client as well as help him/her prepare for specific activities. The ability to understand these congruences—such as the fact that the ATP-CP system takes the same time to replenish as the "rest time" for "strength training" (see Chapter Six)—will only add to your skill set as an exercise professional.

"THE QUEST FOR ADENOSINE TRI - PHOSPHATE"

A. The ATP-CP System -

This metabolic pathway uses the **ATP** that is stored in the muscle and the use of **creatine phosphate** to rephosphorylate **ADP**. The **ATP-CP System** is engaged at the onset of exercise and when an individual is participating in short duration, high intensity exercises (i.e., sprinting, weight lifting, etc.). This pathway is considered an **anaerobic pathway**.

B. Glycolysis -

This second metabolic pathway is capable of rapidly producing **ATP** without oxygen. **Glycolysis** is a metabolic pathway in the cytoplasm of the cell that results in the degradation of glucose into pyruvate or lactate. Oxygen is not directly involved in the process of glycolysis, therefore the pathway is considered anaerobic. In the presence of oxygen in the mitochondria, pyruvate can participate in the aerobic production of ATP. Thus, glycolysis is an **anaerobic pathway** capable of producing ATP without oxygen, as well as the first step in the aerobic degradation of carbohydrates (i.e., playing soccer).

C. Oxidative Phosphorylation -

The interaction of two cooperating metabolic pathways are involved in the aerobic production of **ATP** inside the mitochondria: (1) **the Krebs Cycle;** and (2) **electron transport chain**. The Krebs Cycle is the metabolic pathway in the mitochondria in which energy is transferred from carbohydrates, fats, and amino acids through the electron transport chain for the production of ATP. The electron transport chain is a series of oxidation reductions that occur in the mitochondria and are responsible for oxidative phosphorylation (i.e., running).

ENERGY SYSTEMS/METABOLIC PATHWAYS

Energy System	Substance Used	Limitations	Primary Use	
1. ATP-CP anaerobic	Creatine Phosphate (CP) stored ATP	Muscle can store very little CP and ATP	High intensity activities, less than 10 seconds	HIIT tabata
2. Glycolysis anaerobic	Glucose & Glycogen	Lactic acid (the burn)	High intensity activities, lasting 1- 3 minutes	most sports
3. Oxidative Phosphorylation	Fatty acids, Glucose and Gly-cogen	Depletion of Glycogen and sugar	Long duration sub-anaerobic threshold activities lasting more than 3 minutes	long distance running

Examples of Exercises Using Specific Metabolic Pathways

1. ATP-CP

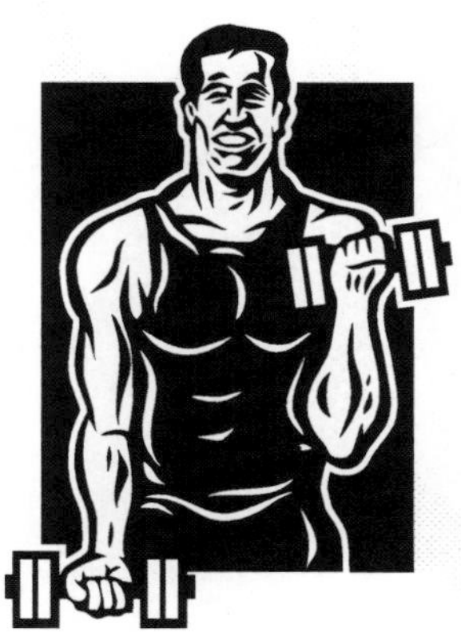

2. Glycolysis

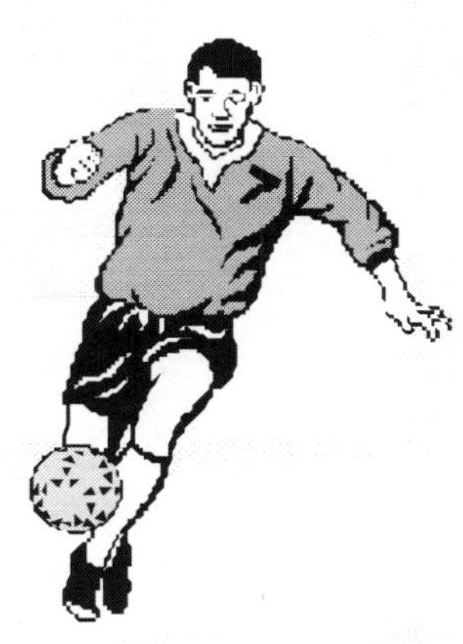

3. Oxidative Phosphorylation

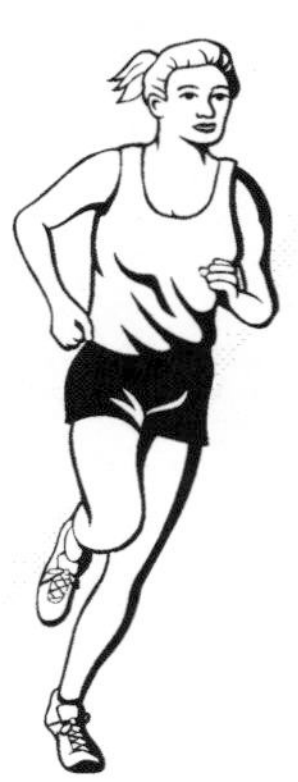

NOTE: *All three energy systems are always "on" and just because one energy system becomes more predominant based on the specific activity does not mean thae others stop functioning (i.e., no system shuts "off"). Essentially, your body just "shifts" from system to system (or pathway to pathway) depending on the exercise and/or activity.*

BREAKDOWN OF MACRONUTRIENTS

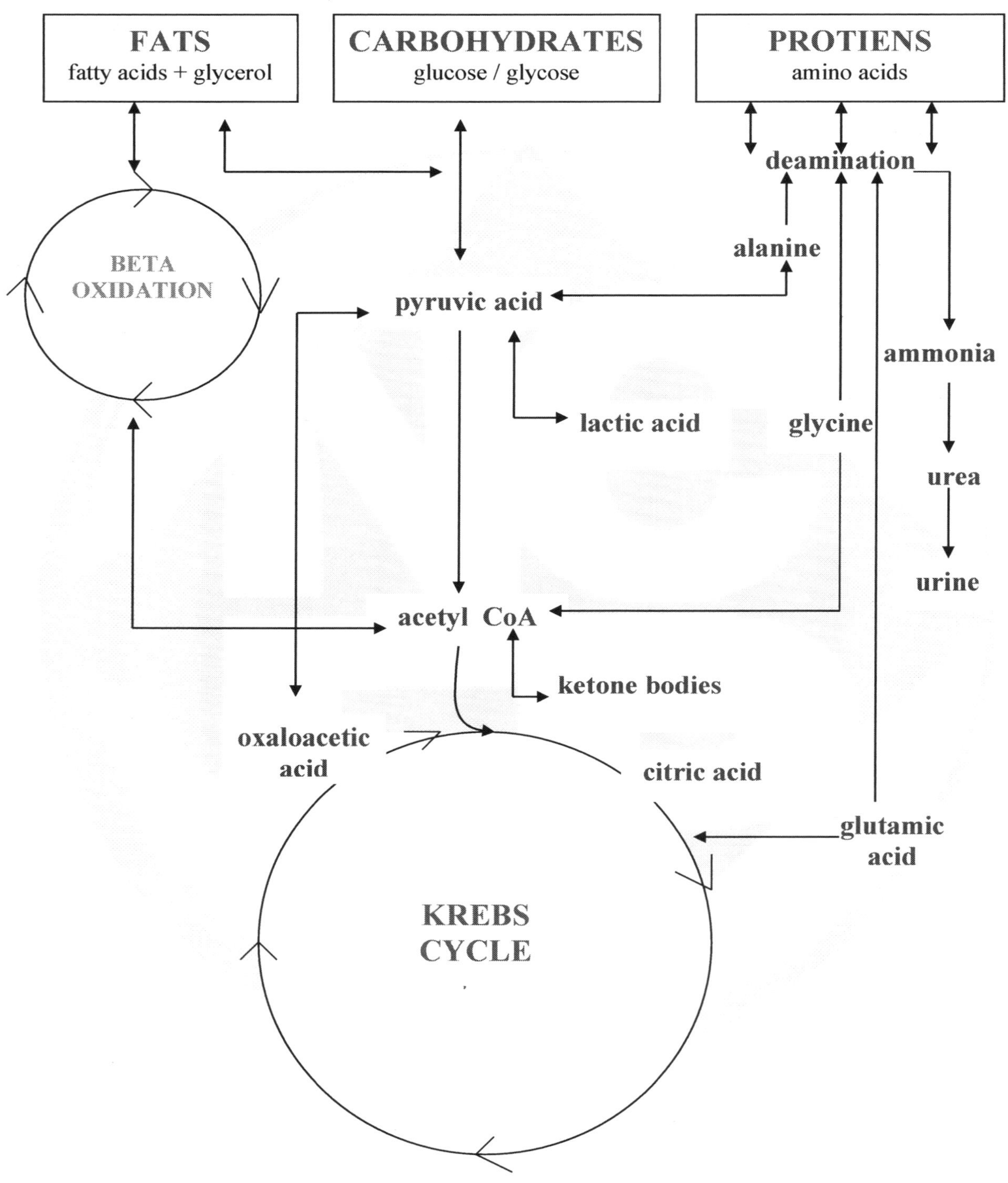

CHAPTER TWELVE

Anatomy

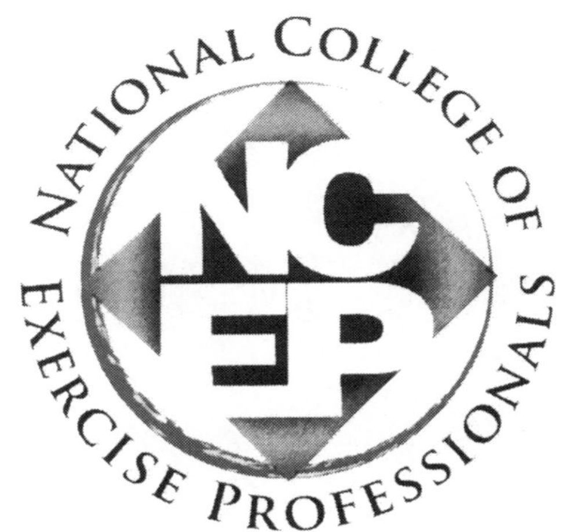

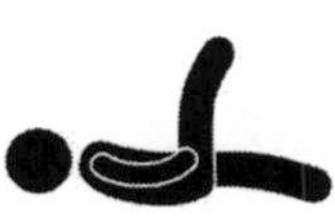

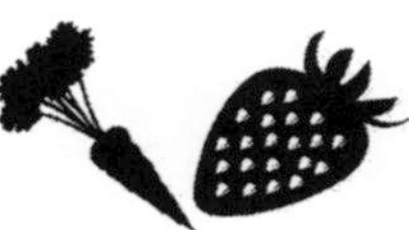

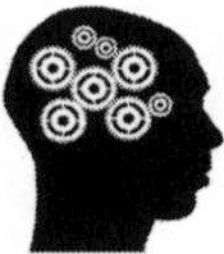

SKELETAL SYSTEM
(ANTERIOR)

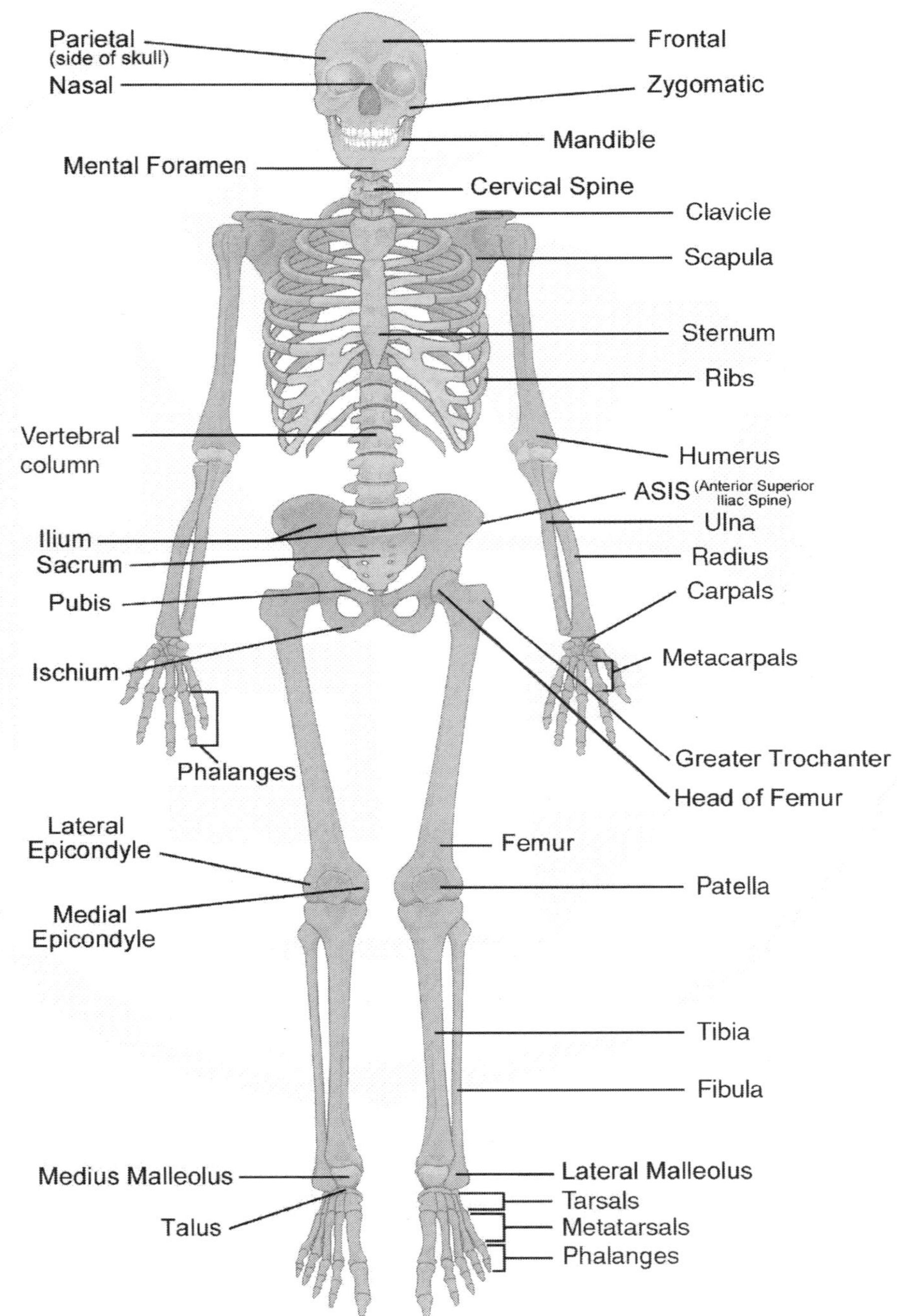
Parietal
(side of skull)
Nasal
Frontal
Zygomatic
Mandible
Mental Foramen
Cervical Spine
Clavicle
Scapula
Sternum
Ribs
Vertebral column
Humerus
ASIS (Anterior Superior Iliac Spine)
Ulna
Ilium
Sacrum
Radius
Carpals
Pubis
Metacarpals
Ischium
Phalanges
Greater Trochanter
Head of Femur
Lateral Epicondyle
Femur
Patella
Medial Epicondyle
Tibia
Fibula
Medius Malleolus
Lateral Malleolus
Tarsals
Talus
Metatarsals
Phalanges

SKELETAL SYSTEM
(POSTERIOR)

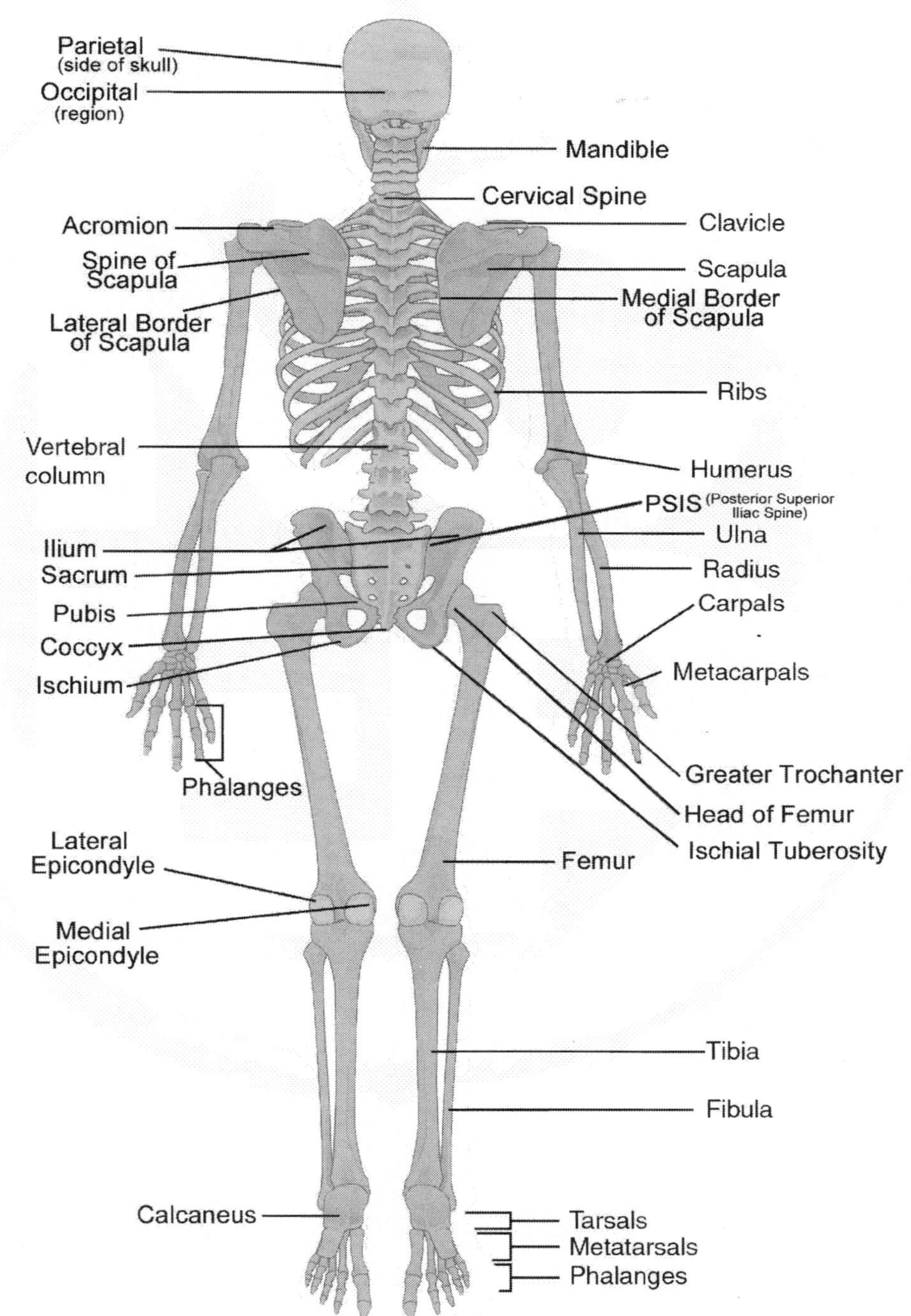
Parietal
(side of skull)
Occipital
(region)
Mandible
Cervical Spine
Acromion
Clavicle
Spine of Scapula
Scapula
Lateral Border of Scapula
Medial Border of Scapula
Ribs
Vertebral column
Humerus
PSIS (Posterior Superior Iliac Spine)
Ulna
Ilium
Sacrum
Radius
Pubis
Carpals
Coccyx
Ischium
Metacarpals
Phalanges
Greater Trochanter
Head of Femur
Ischial Tuberosity
Lateral Epicondyle
Femur
Medial Epicondyle
Tibia
Fibula
Calcaneus
Tarsals
Metatarsals
Phalanges

SKELETAL SYSTEM
(LATERAL)

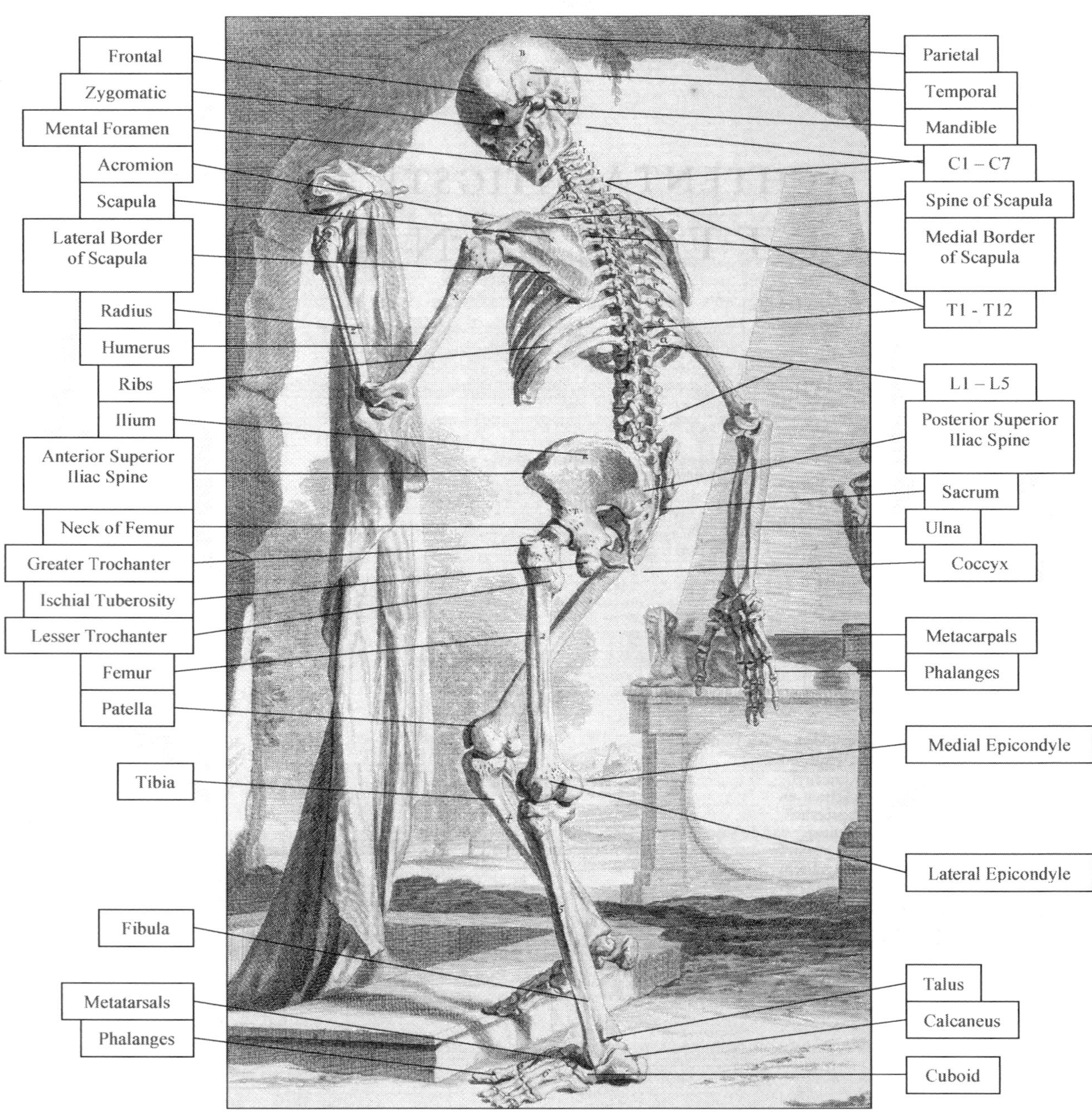
Frontal
Zygomatic
Mental Foramen
Acromion
Scapula
Lateral Border of Scapula
Radius
Humerus
Ribs
Ilium
Anterior Superior Iliac Spine
Neck of Femur
Greater Trochanter
Ischial Tuberosity
Lesser Trochanter
Femur
Patella
Tibia
Fibula
Metatarsals
Phalanges
Parietal
Temporal
Mandible
C1 – C7
Spine of Scapula
Medial Border of Scapula
T1 - T12
L1 – L5
Posterior Superior Iliac Spine
Sacrum
Ulna
Coccyx
Metacarpals
Phalanges
Medial Epicondyle
Lateral Epicondyle
Talus
Calcaneus
Cuboid

MAJOR MUSCLES
(LATERAL)

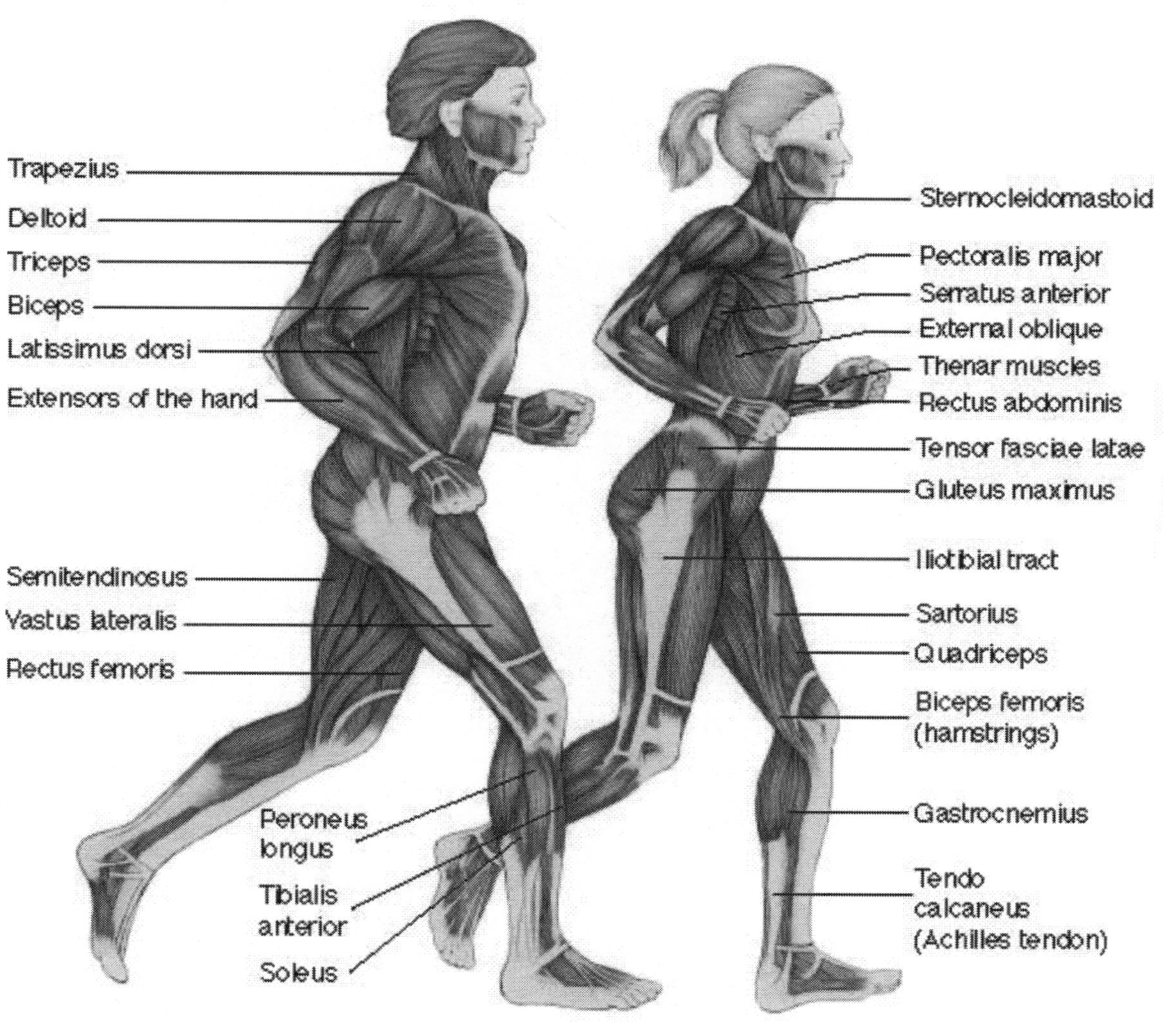
Trapezius
Deltoid
Triceps
Biceps
Latissimus dorsi
Extensors of the hand
Semitendinosus
Vastus lateralis
Rectus femoris
Peroneus longus
Tibialis anterior
Soleus
Sternocleidomastoid
Pectoralis major
Serratus anterior
External oblique
Thenar muscles
Rectus abdominis
Tensor fasciae latae
Gluteus maximus
Iliotibial tract
Sartorius
Quadriceps
Biceps femoris (hamstrings)
Gastrocnemius
Tendo calcaneus (Achilles tendon)

MAJOR MUSCLES
(ANTERIOR)

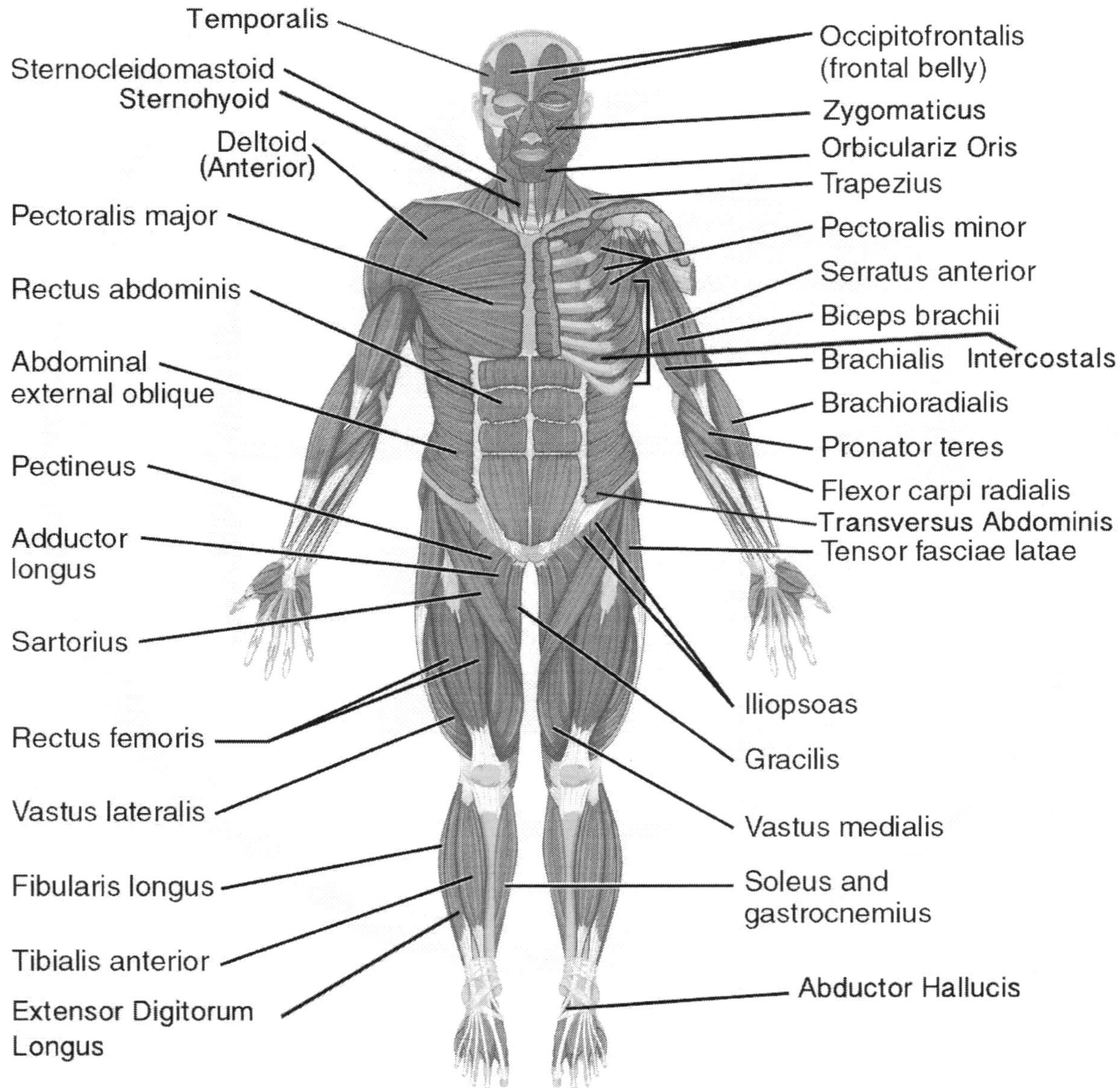

Left side: *superficial muscles* **Right side:** *deep muscles*

MAJOR MUSCLES
(POSTERIOR)

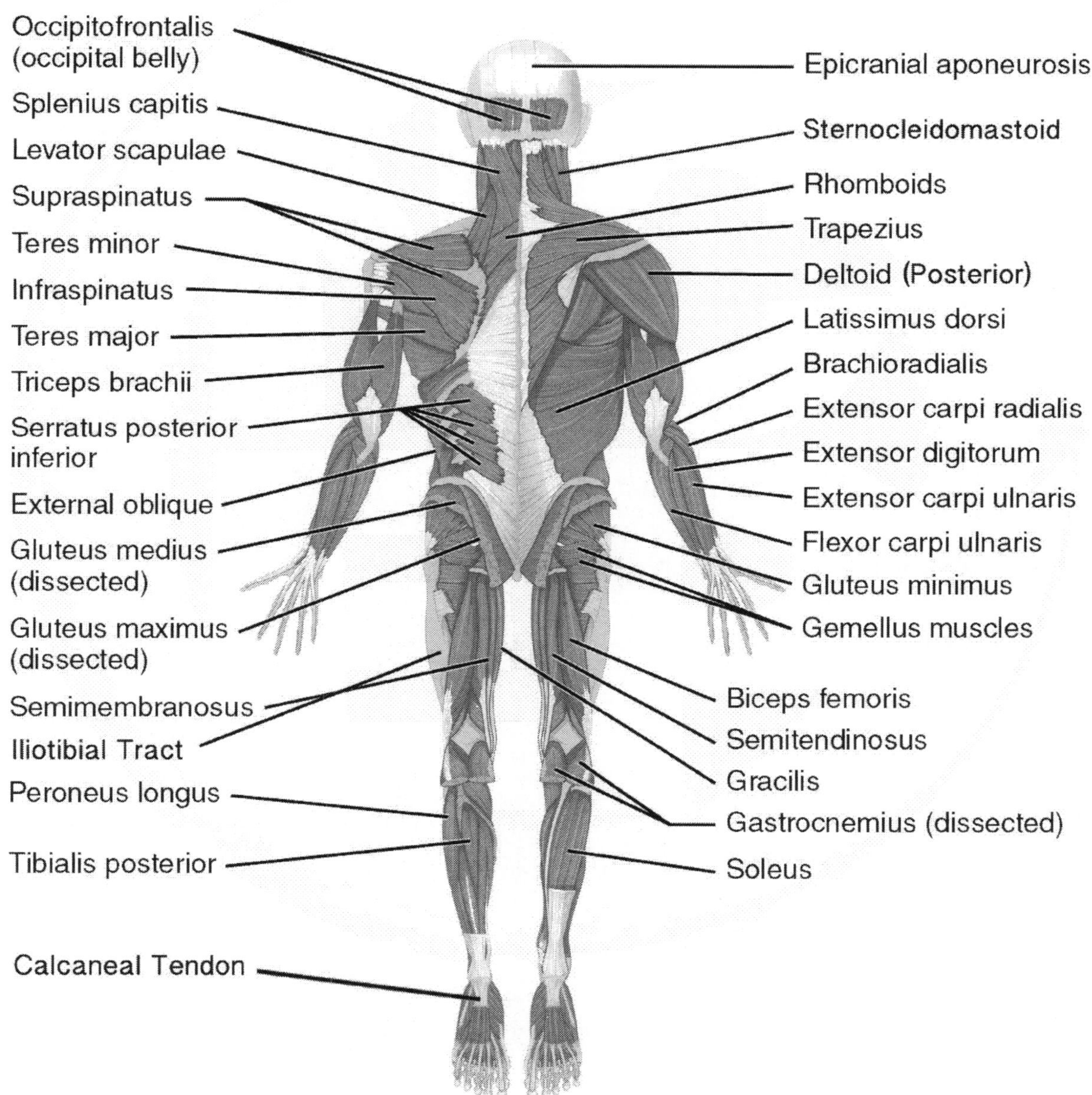

Left side: *deep muscles*

Right side: *superficial muscles*

ANATOMY

Vocabulary

- ***Joint*** – where two bones articulate or come together
- ***Ligament*** – attaches bone to bone, does not stretch
- ***Tendon*** – attaches muscle to bone, does not stretch
- ***Disc*** – cushion between each vertebra
- ***Meniscus*** – cushion between the tibia and femur
- ***Fossa*** – hole or depression in bone
- ***Process*** – protrusion on a bone
- ***Kyphotic Curve*** – concave curve of upper back, thoracic region
- ***Lordotic Curve*** – convex curve of lower back, lumbar region

Four Components of Movement

1. ***Osteokinematics*** – study of the movement of the bones
2. ***Arthrokinematics*** – study of the way the joints move
3. ***Ligamentous and Articulating Structures*** - look at the ligaments and surrounding structures affected by the movement
4. ***Musculature*** – examine muscles involved in each joint action

MECHANICS OF MUSCLE MOVEMENT

To have movement occur, the muscles pull on the bones in which one bone acts as an anchor. The end of the anchor creates an **axis point**, or joint which the other bone can rotate around. The force that is felt around the joint is referred to as **torque**. The torque can be increased as the center of gravity of free weight falls further away from the axis of rotation. The distance between where the center of the weight falls and where the center of the axis falls is called a **moment arm**. Take a bicep curl for example. When the weight is hanging straight down the moment arm is quite small. However, as the weight goes up and reaches the halfway point, it is the furthest away from the axis and the torque is essentially the greatest. As the weight continues to rise, the moment arm again decreases and the torque decreases proportionately.

TERMS OF MOVEMENT

***Flexion*:** decreasing the angle between two bones

***Extension*:** increasing the angle between two bones

***Hyperextension*:** movement beyond normal extension

***Abduction*:** moving away from midline

***Adduction*:** moving towards midline

***Horizontal abduction*:** moving upper arm away from midline in horizontal plane

***Horizontal adduction*:** moving upper arms towards midline in horizontal plane

***Pronation*:** rotating palms up to palms down

***Supination*:** rotating palms down to palms up

***Dorsiflexion*:** bringing the toes and foot up as a unit to decrease the angle between the foot and anterior tibialis

***Plantar Flexion*:** pushing the foot and toes down as a unit to increase the angle between the foot and the anterior tibialis

***Inversion*:** turning the sole of the foot towards the midline

***Eversion*:** turning the sole of the foot away from the midline

***Rotation*:** movement of the long bone around its axis

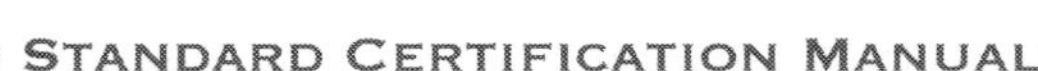

JOINT RANGES OF MOTION

(For quick reference only)

Shoulder	Degrees From Neutral
▪ Flexion	180
▪ Hyper-Extension	60
▪ Abduction	180
▪ Adduction	75
▪ External Rotation (Sag. Plane)	90
▪ Internal Rotation (Sag. Plane)	70
▪ External Rot. (Trans. Plane)	60
▪ Internal Rot. (Trans. Plane)	60
▪ Horizontal Adduction	120
▪ Horizontal Abduction	30
▪ Scapular Elevation	30
▪ Scapular Depression	10
▪ Scapular Abduction/Protraction	30
▪ Scapular Adduction/Retraction	30

Elbow

▪ Flexion	175
▪ Extension	0
▪ Pronation (Radial/Ulnar)	80
▪ Supination (Radial/Ulnar)	80

Wrist

▪ Flexion	80
▪ Hyper-Extension	70
▪ Radial Deviation	20
▪ Ulnar Deviation	30
▪ Supination (Radial/Ulnar)	80
▪ Pronation (Radial/Ulnar)	80

JOINT RANGES OF MOTION (CONTINUED)

Foot/Ankle	Degrees From Neutral
▪ Plantar Flexion	50
▪ Dorsiflexion	20
▪ Eversion	5
▪ Inversion	5
▪ Supination	35
▪ Pronation	15
▪ Adduction	40
▪ Abduction	30
Neck (cervical)	
▪ Flexion	45
▪ Hyper-Extension	45
▪ Lateral Flexion	45
▪ Rotation	60
Spine (thoracic & lumbar)	
▪ Flexion	90
▪ Hyper-Extension	40
▪ Lateral Flexion	30
▪ Rotation	45
Hip	
▪ Flexion	120
▪ Hyper-Extension	10
▪ Abduction	45
▪ Adduction	30
▪ External Rotation	45
▪ Internal Rotation	45
Knee	
▪ Flexion	135
▪ Extension	0

A Note about Our Anatomy Section

Fulling learning all aspects of the human body is a complicated task. While other certifications may dedicate more time on the anatomy of the body, we believe that at first knowing the major muscles groups, bones, joint actions, and a few other important details generally can suffice for most trainers—it is more about applying this knowledge in a way that helps your clients live healthier lives that will determine your success. Thus, we believe the pages prior to this note broadly encompasses the standard information that you should know.

Again, knowing every aspect of the human body, such as all 206 bones in the body and every biomechnic joint movement, is beyond the scope of this manual and this introductory course, at least at the start. Yet, the body is important, and for this reason, the following pages in this chapter are included for your reference. We hope these pages are useful as you further your education and begin to master the extraordinary miracle that is the human body.

SPINE

> Bones

* Cervical Vertebrae **1-7**
* Thoracic Vertebrae **8-19**
* Lumbar Vertebrae **20-24**
* Sacrum (fused vertebrae **25-29**)
* Coccyx (fused vertebrae **30-33**)

> Joints

* Spine (each vertebral complex is a joint)
* SI (sacroiliac)

> Muscles of the Trunk

* **Flexion** – Rectus Abdominus
* **Extension** – Erector Spinae
* **Rotation** – External and Internal Obliques
* **Stabilization** – TVA (Transverse Abdominus)

CENTRAL NERVOUS SYSTEM

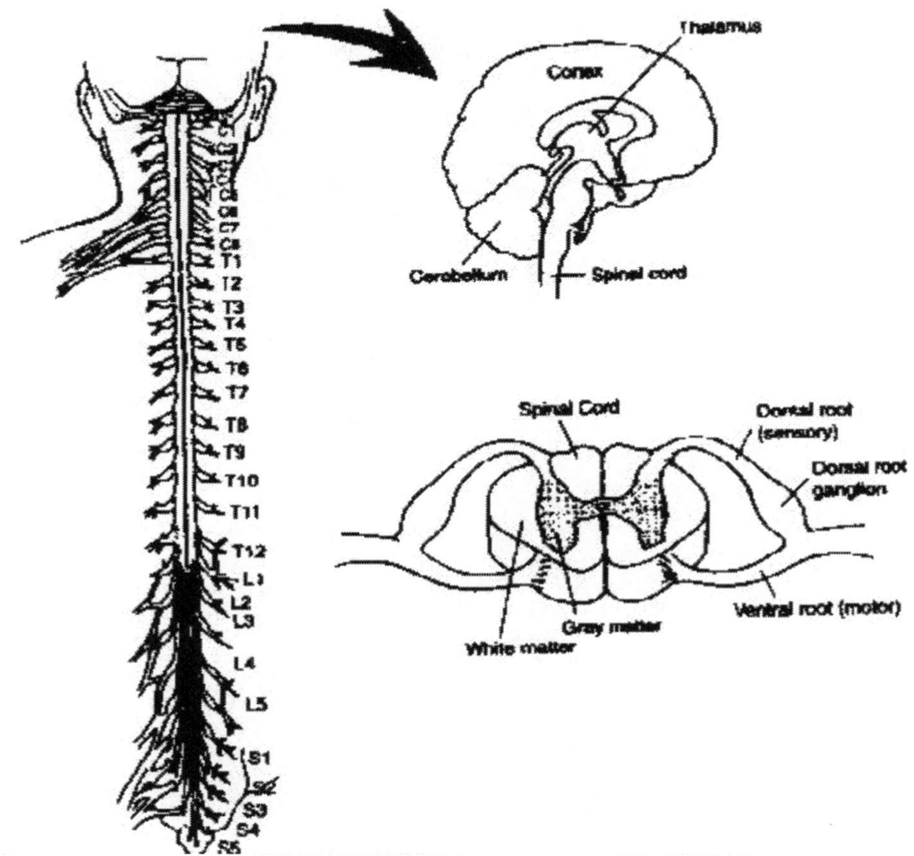

Postural Feed Forward Response Mechanism - the body's ability to contract the muscles that support and protect the spine several milliseconds before the body begins to move

SPINE

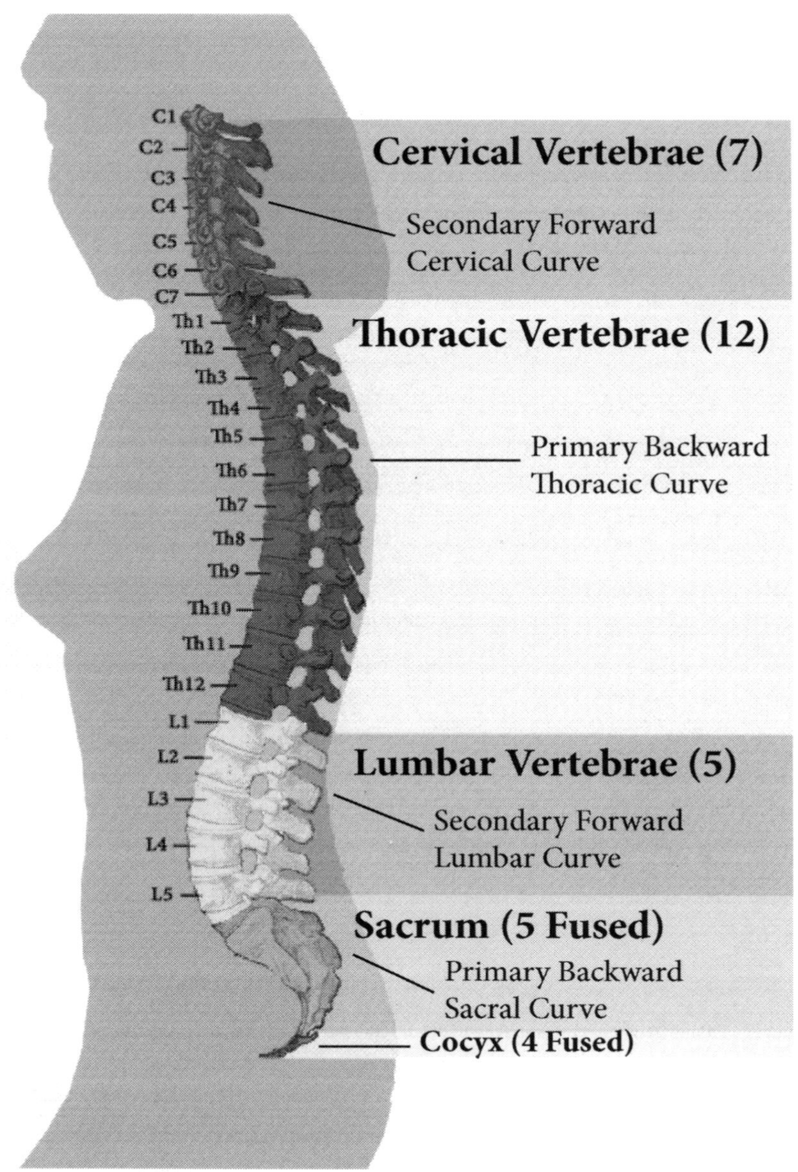

- In the spine there are **33 vertebrae**
- 24 are moveable and 9 are fused
- The five segments form four curves
- The thoracic curve is also known as the **kyphotic curve**
- The lumbar region has a **lordotic curve**

Neutral Alignment means there is the least amount of stress on the structures.

There are two parts within each disc. The outer part is called the **annulus fibrosa** while the center is called the **nucleus pulposus**.

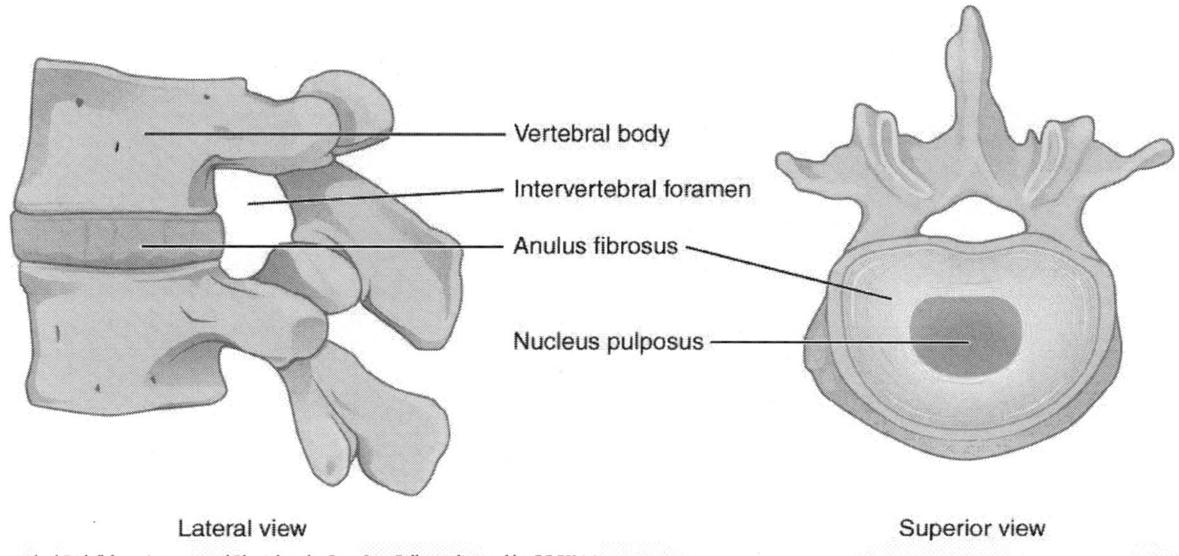

"Inteverbral Disks" from Anatomy and Physiology by OpenStax College is licensed by CC BY 3.0

Common Facts About Back Pain and Spinal Alignment

- One of the most vulnerable positions for the disc appears to be during flexion, while under compression.
- More than 80% of all Americans will experience back pain. People who are seated at their jobs every day have 30 - 40% more intra-disc pressure compared to those who stand.
- This is significant because the #1 job in the world is a sit down job.
- **The number one cause of back pain is being out of the neutral position for longer periods of time.**

Joints -
- Sacroiliac
- Intra-Spinous Joints – Discs

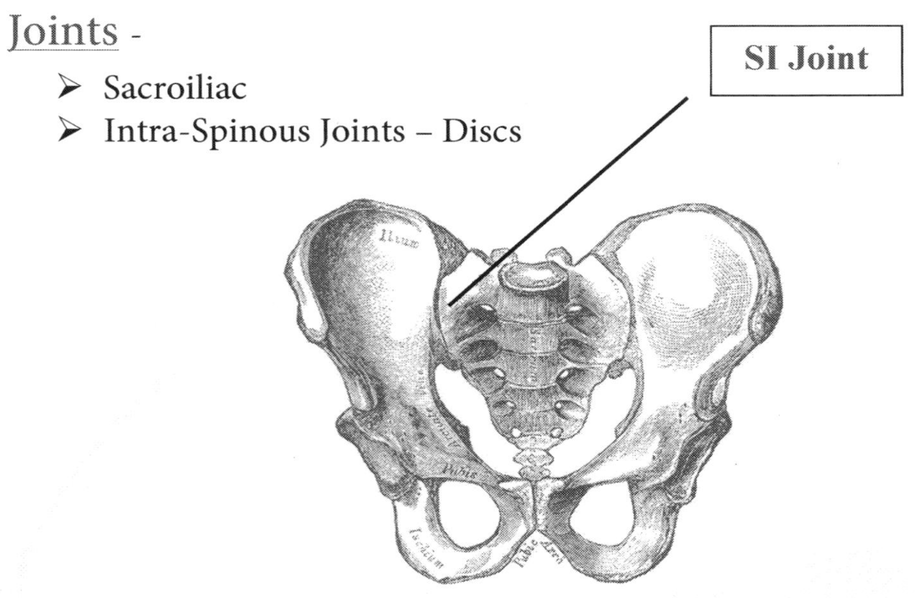

Ligaments - 5 ligaments surround the spine in all directions

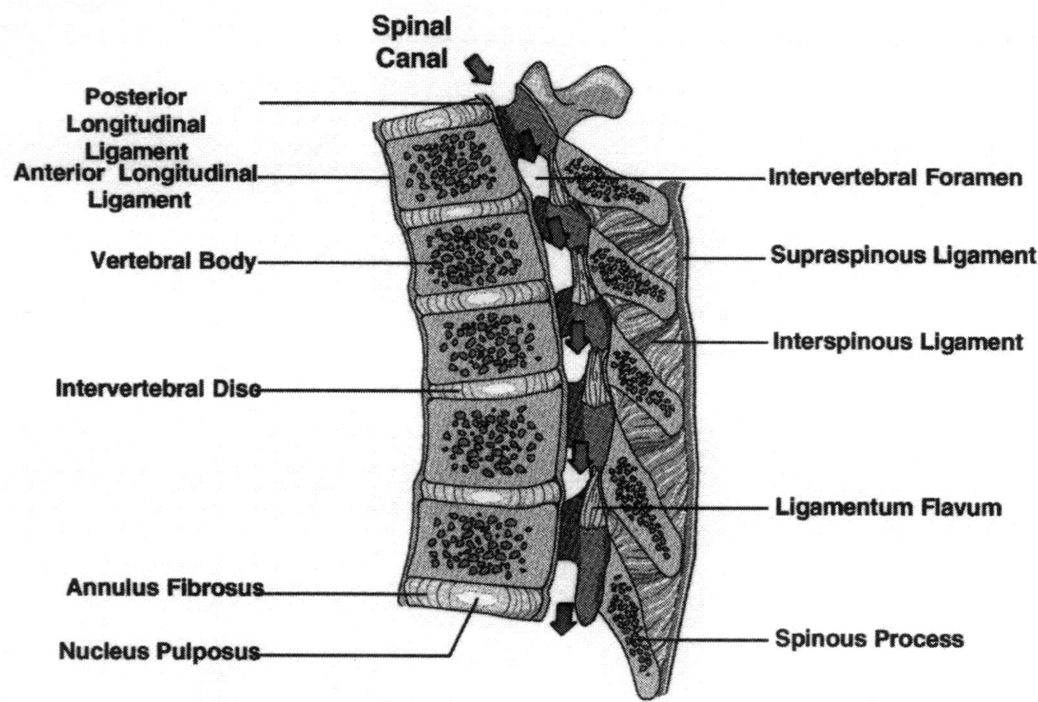

SPINAL MUSCLES/MOTIONS

Muscles & Motions – (Cervical Curvature)

- **Extension** (Backwards Motion)
  - **Levator Scapulae**
  - **Trapezius**
  - **Splenius Capitis**
  - **Semispinalis Capitis**

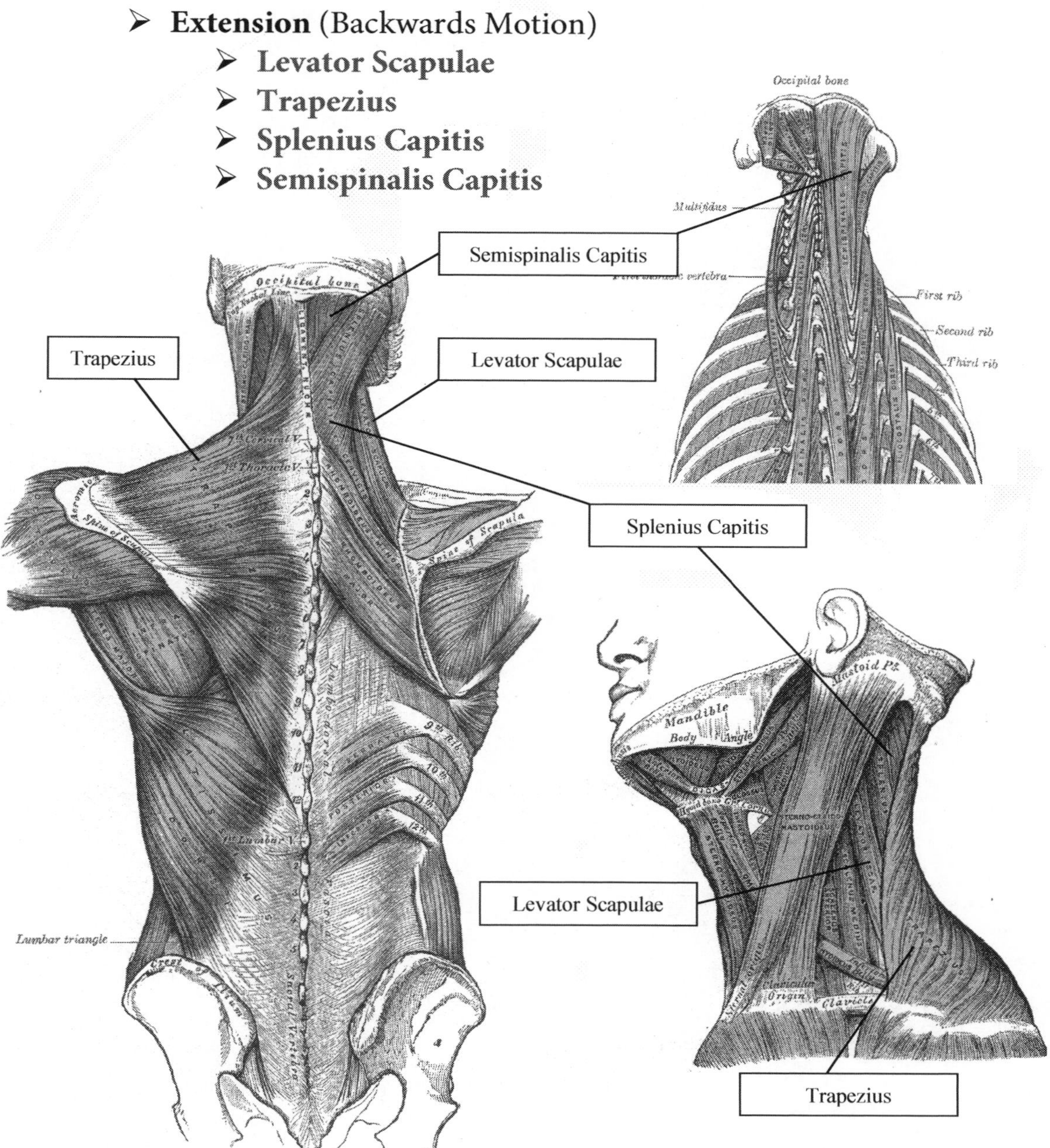

Cervical Extension (Hyper-Extension) (0-45 degrees)

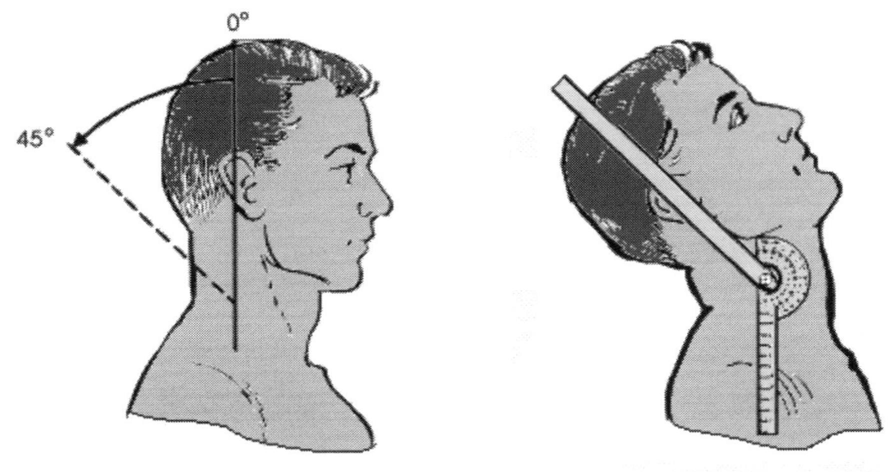

Muscles & Motions – (Cervical Curvature)- cont.

- **Flexion** – (Forward Motion)
  - **Sternocleidomastoid, Scalenes, Infra Hyoids, Longus Colli, Longus Capitis**

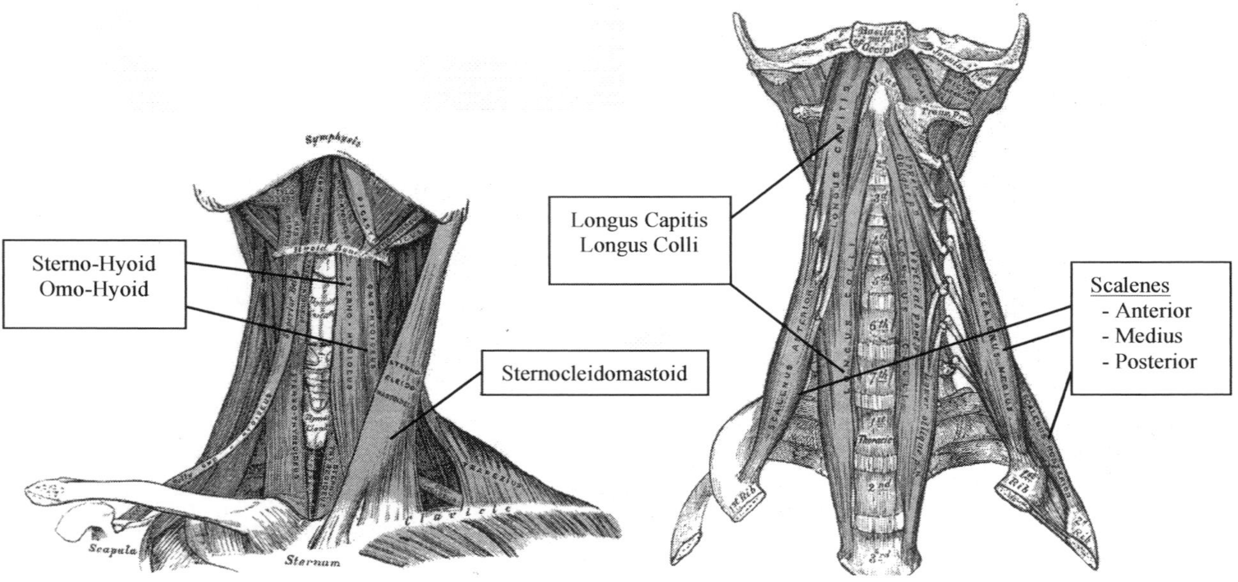

Cervical Flexion (0-45 degrees)

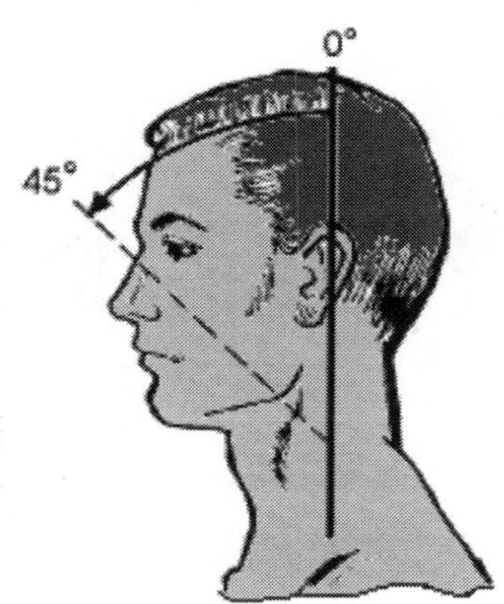

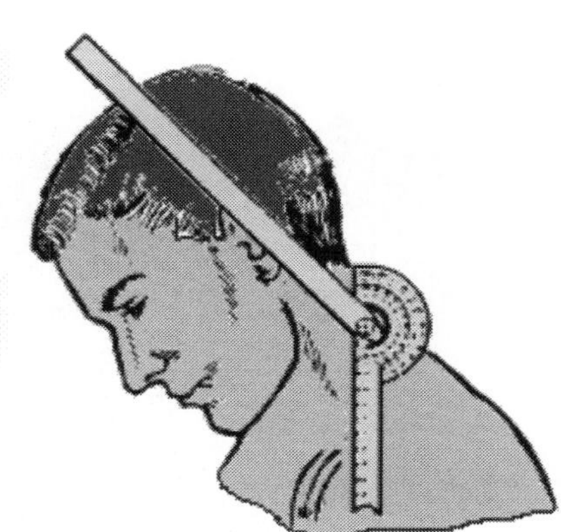

Muscles & Motions – (Cervical Curvature) - cont.

- **Both: Lateral Flexion** (Side to Side) & **Rotation**
- Many of these are deep muscles of the cervical complex.
    - **Longus Colli & Longus Capitis**
    - **Levator Scapulae**
    - **Longissimus Capitis & Longissimus Cervicis**
    - **Sternocleidomastoid**
    - **Splenius Cervicis & Splenius Capitis**
    - **Spinalis Cervicis**
    - **Semispinalis Cervicis & Semispinalis Capitis**
    - **Scalenus Anterior, Scalenus Medius, Scalenus Posterior**

Cervical Rotation (0-60 degrees)

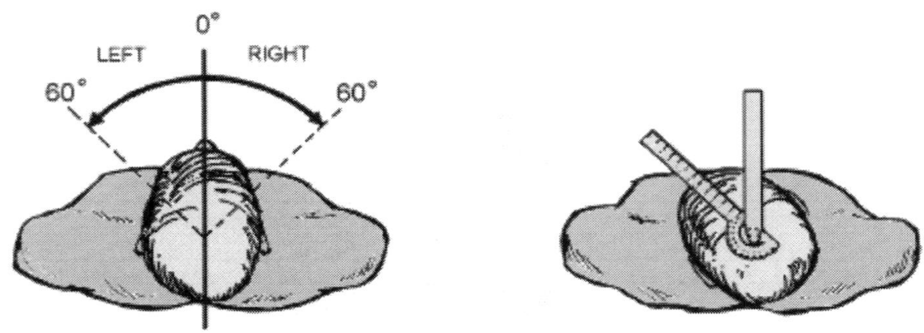

Cervical Lateral Flexion (0-45 degrees)

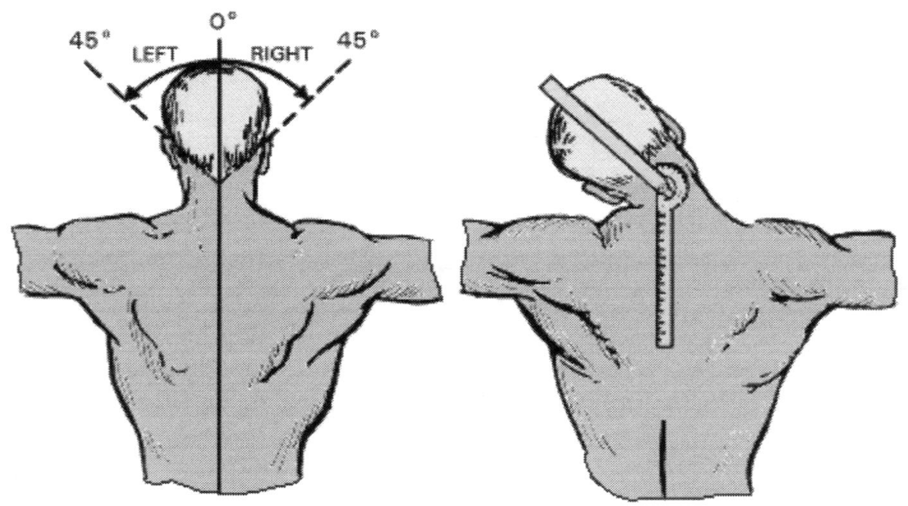

Muscles & Motions - (Lumbar & Thoracic Curvature)

- **Extension** (Backwards Motion) - **Erector Spinae (Group)**

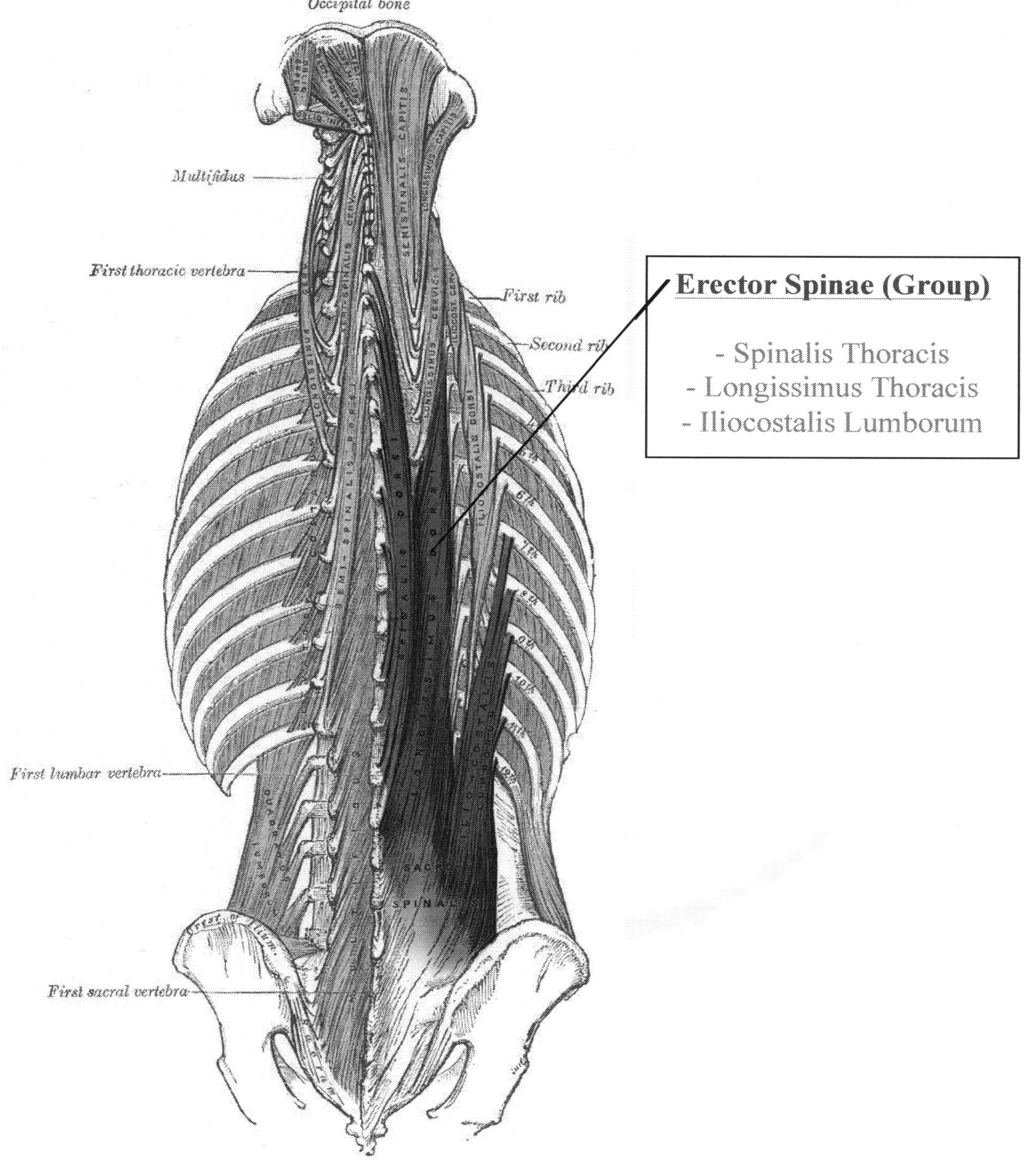

Spinal Extension (Hyper-Extension) (0-40 degrees)

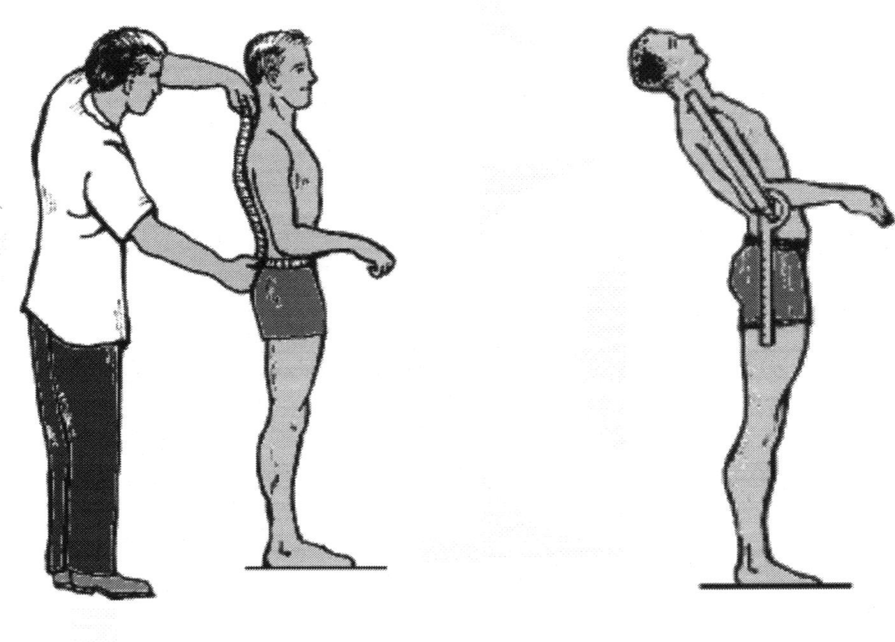

Spinal Flexion (0-90 degrees)

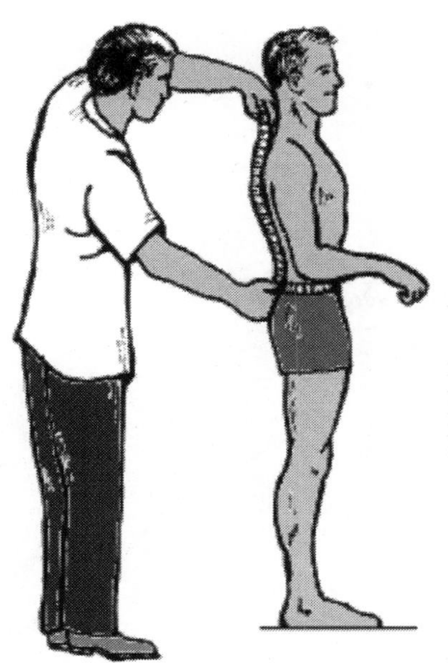

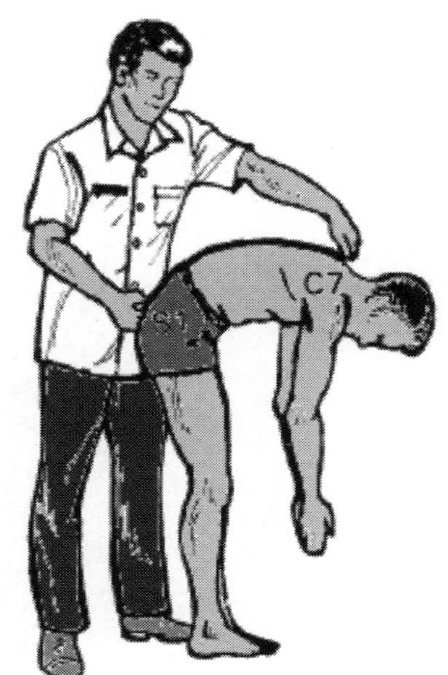

Spinal Rotation (0-45 degrees)

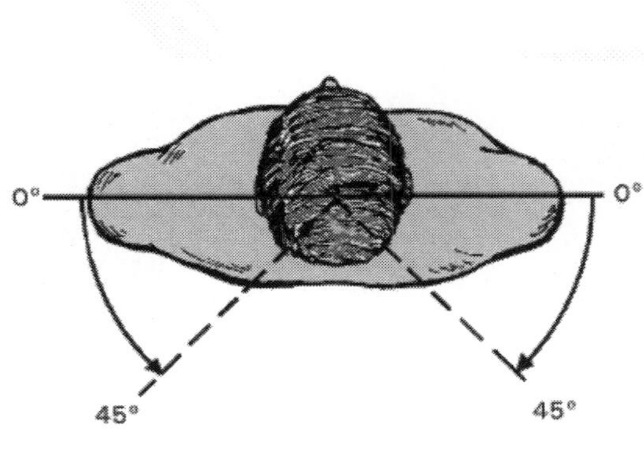

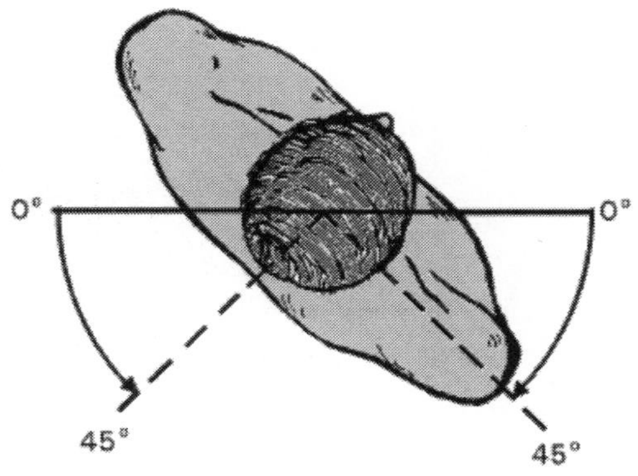

Spinal Lateral Flexion (0-30 degrees)

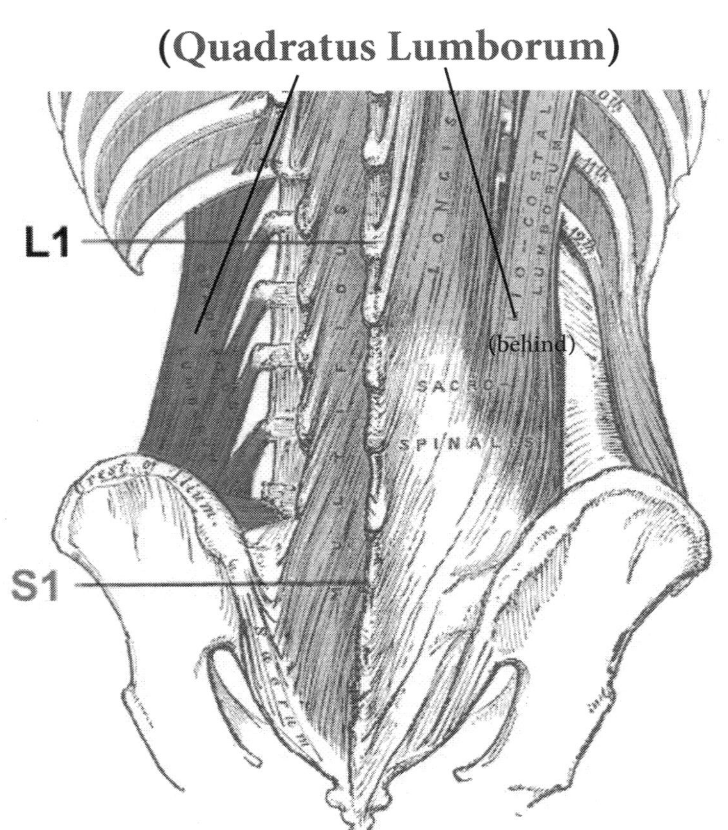

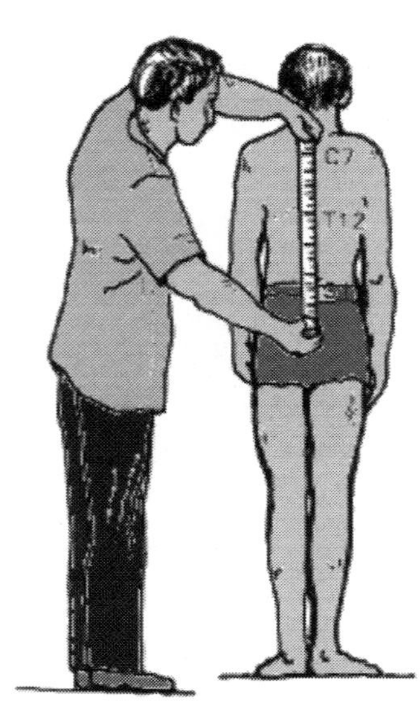

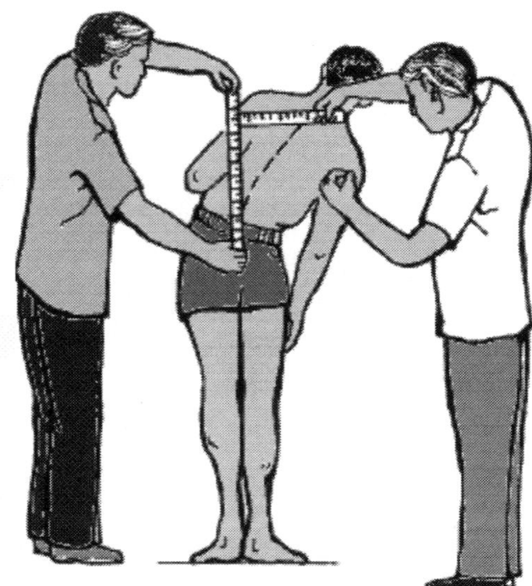

PELVIC TILTING

Anterior Tilt - lumbar extension, hip flexion

Posterior Tilt - lumbar flexion, hip extension

Neutral Lumbo-Pelvis

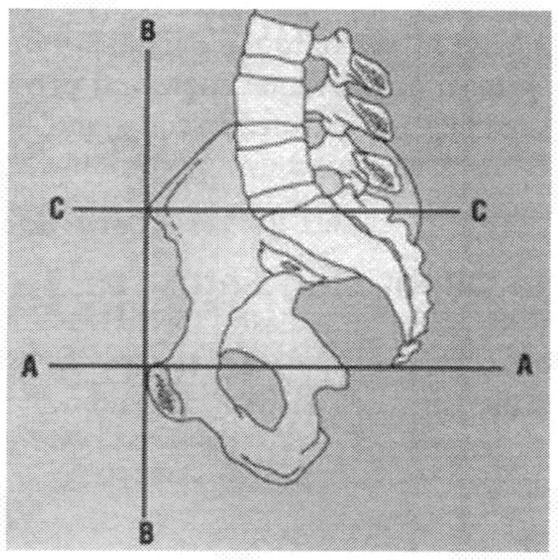

Different Lumbo-Pelvic Tilts

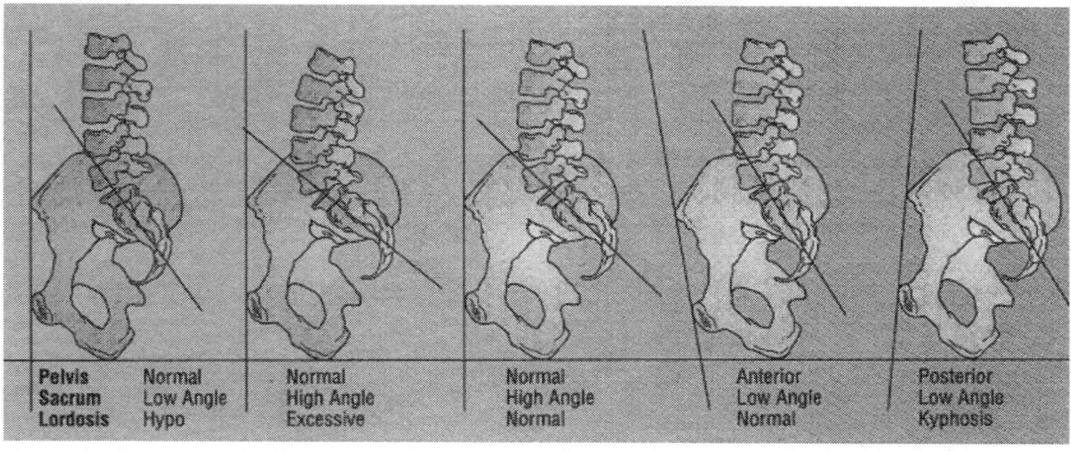

Misleading Body Structures

To

Lumbo-Pelvic Tilts

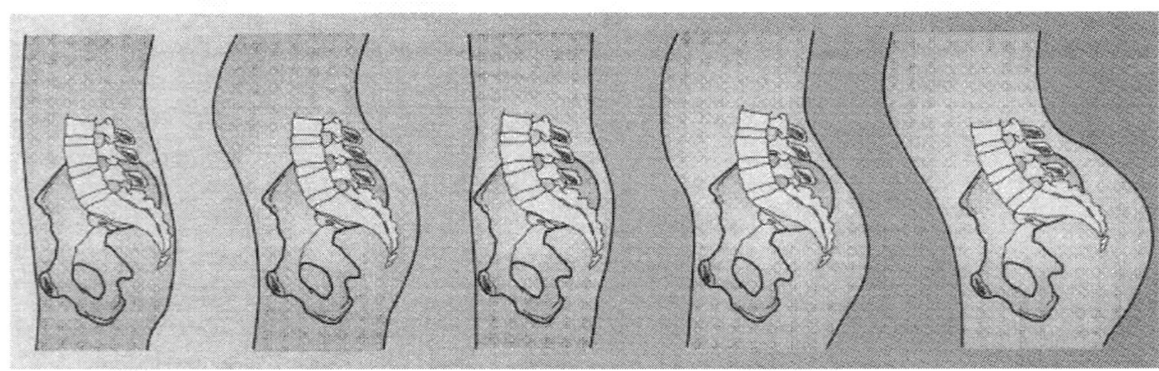

SHOULDER COMPLEX

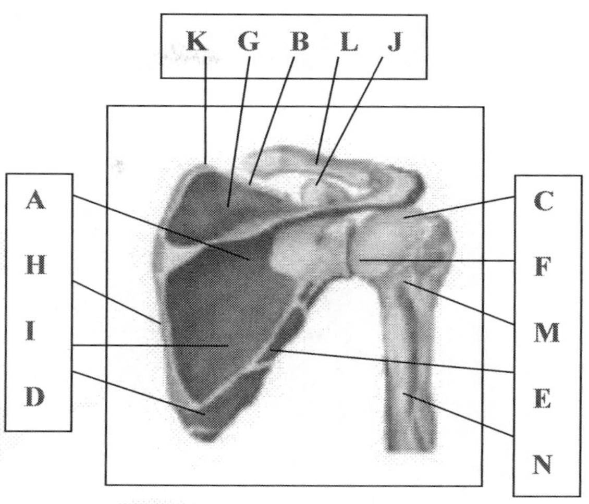

Posterior View

A.) Spine	**B.)** Superior Border
C.) Acromion	**D.)** Inferior Angle
E.) Lateral Border	**F.)** Glenoid Cavity
G.) Supraspinous Fossa	**H.)** Medial Border
I.) Infraspinous Fossa	**J.)** Coracoid Process
K.) Superior Angle	**L.) Clavicle**
M.) Articular Cartilage	**N.) Humerus**

Bones –
- Humerus (N)
- Scapula
- Clavicle (L)

Joints –
- 4 joints of shoulder (2 in this class)
- Gleno-Humeral Jt. (ball and socket)
- Scapulo- Thoracic (gliding)

Ligaments – 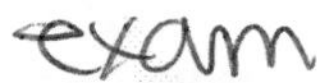

Rotator Cuff - muscles that act as ligaments
- Supraspinatus
- Infraspinatus
- Teres Minor
- Subscapularis

Muscles -

Flexion
- Anterior Deltoid
- Pectorals
- Biceps Brachii
- Coracobrachialis

Extension
- Latissimus Dorsi
- Posterior Deltoid
- Long Head of Triceps

ABduction
- Deltoids
- Supraspinatus

ADduction
- Latissimus Dorsi
- Posterior Deltoid
- Coracobrachialis
- Long Head of Triceps

Horizontal ADduction
- Pectorals
- Anterior Deltoid

Horizontal Abductions
- Posterior Deltoid
- Latissimus Dorsi

SHOULDER COMPLEX
(CONTINUED)

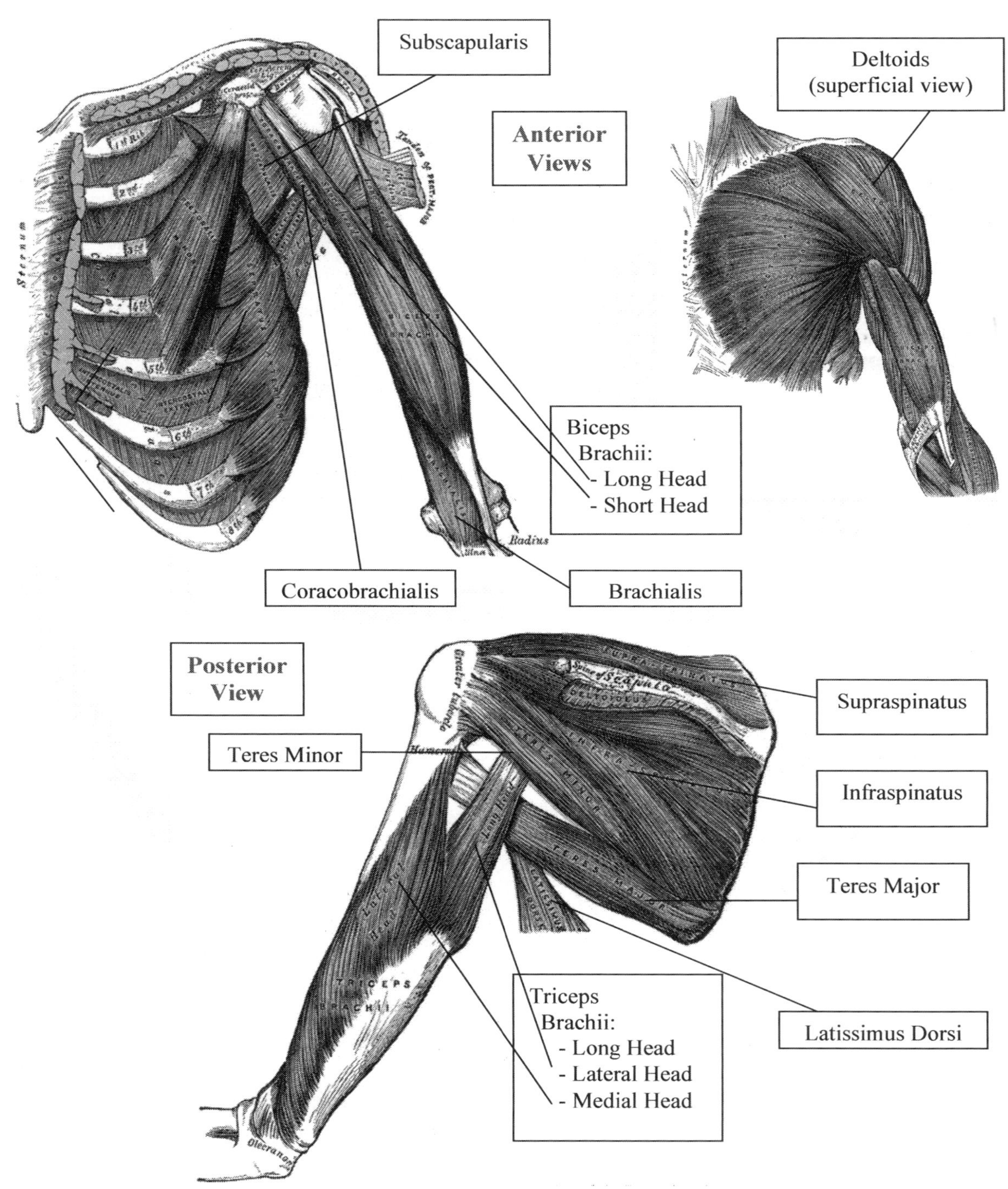
Subscapularis
Anterior Views
Deltoids (superficial view)
Sternum
Biceps Brachii:
- Long Head
- Short Head
Radius
Ulna
Coracobrachialis
Brachialis
Posterior View
Supraspinatus
Teres Minor
Infraspinatus
Teres Major
Triceps Brachii:
- Long Head
- Lateral Head
- Medial Head
Latissimus Dorsi
TRICEPS BRACHII

Shoulder Joint Flexion (0-180 degrees) (Sagittal Plane)

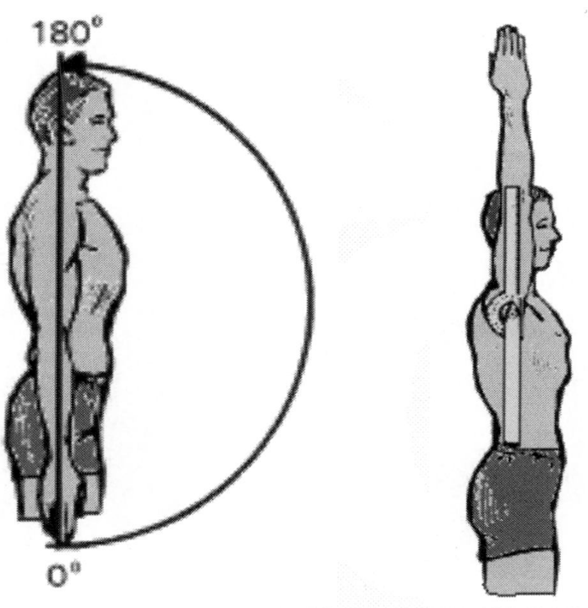

Shoulder Joint Extension (0-60 degrees) (Sagittal Plane)

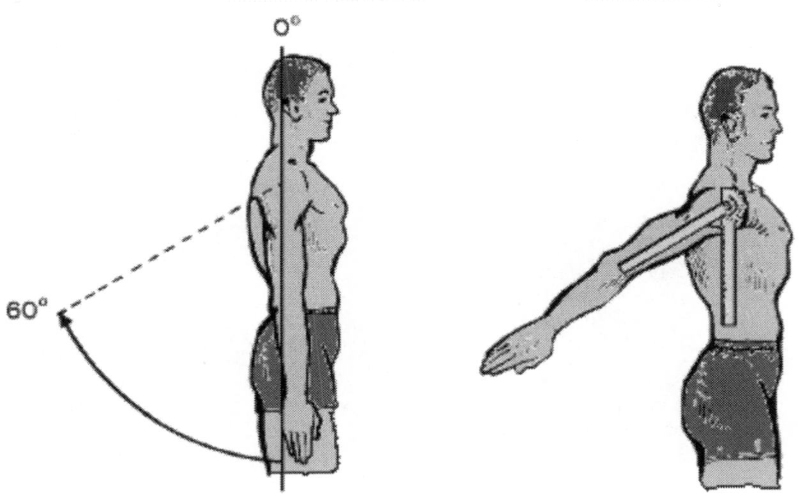

Shoulder Joint Abduction (0-180 degrees) (Lateral/Frontal Plane)

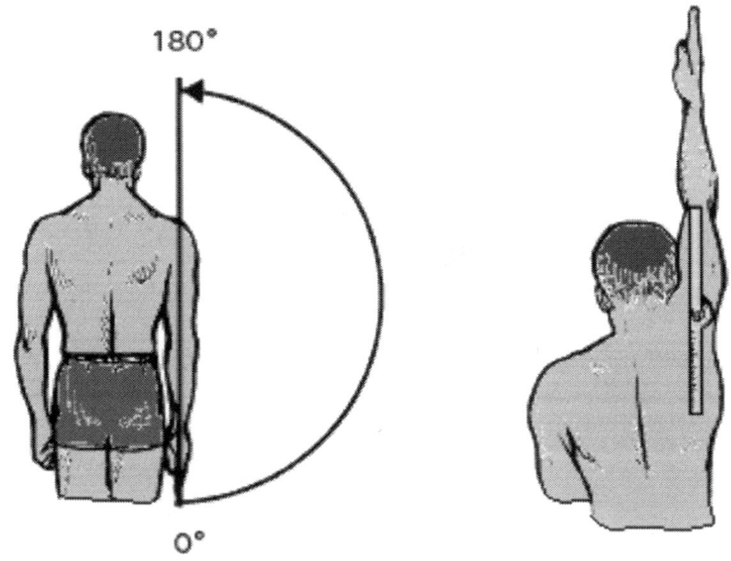

Shoulder Joint Adduction (0-75 degrees) (Lateral/Frontal Plane)

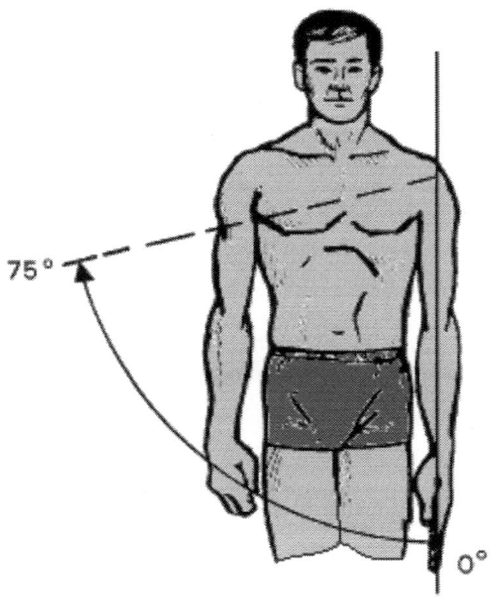

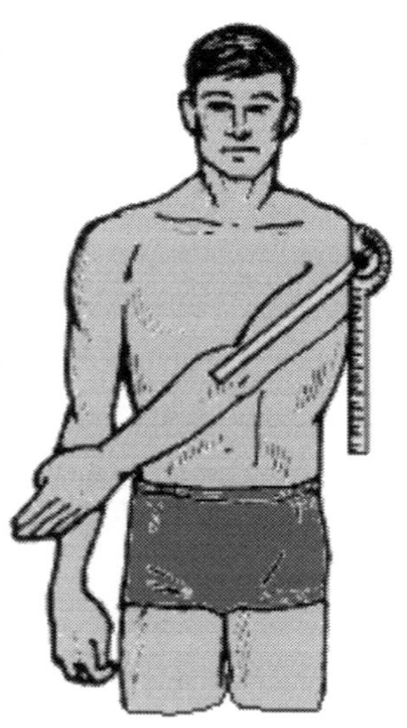

Shoulder Joint
Horizontal/Transverse Plane

Adduction (0-120 degrees)
Abduction (0-30 degrees)

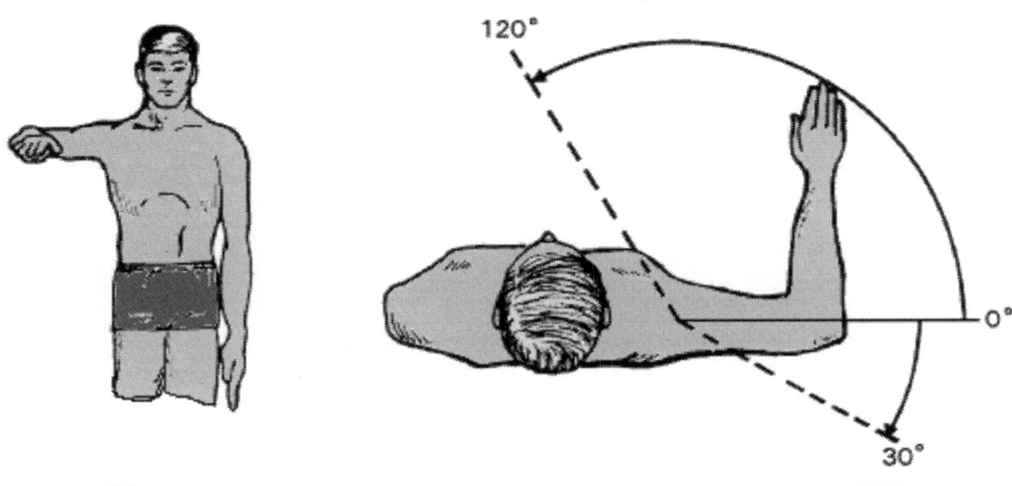

Shoulder Joint
Lying Supine & Shoulder Abducted 90 degrees
Sagittal Plane

Internal Rotation (0-70 degrees)

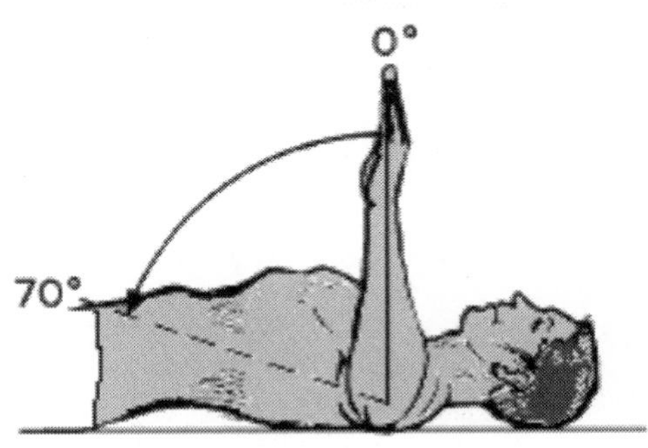

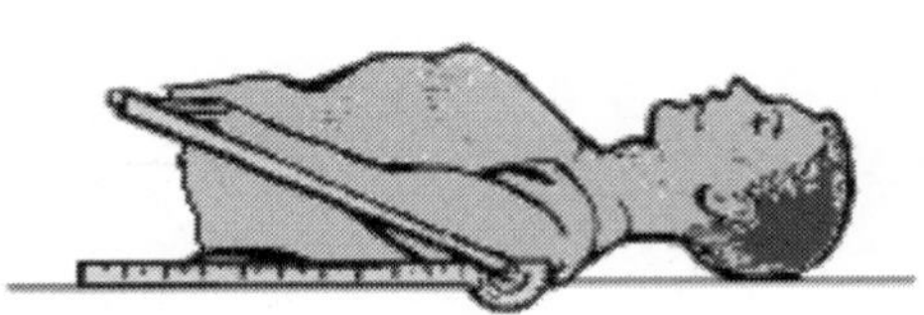

Shoulder Joint
Lying Supine & Shoulder Abducted 90 degrees
Sagittal Plane

External Rotation (0-90 degrees)

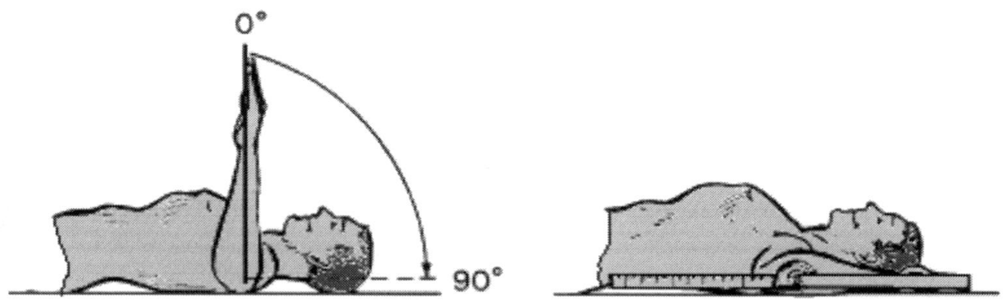

Shoulder Joint Rotation
Horizontal/Transverse Plane

Internal Rotation (0-60 degrees)
External Rotation (0-60 degrees)

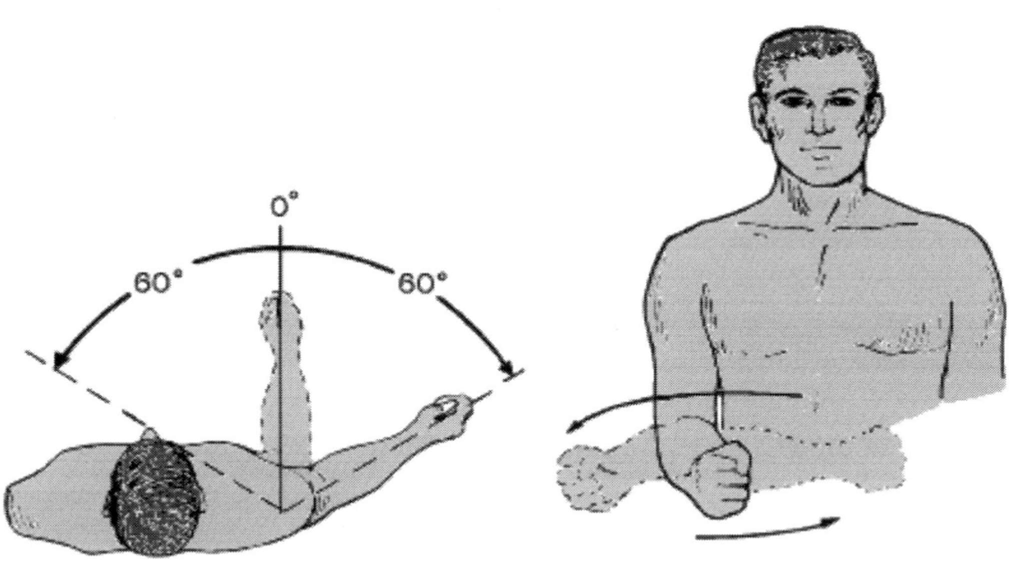

SCAPULO-THORACIC

Elevation > Upper Trapezius	**Depression** > Lower Trapezius & Gravity
Adduction > Medial Trapezius & Rhomboids	**Abduction** > Serratus Anterior

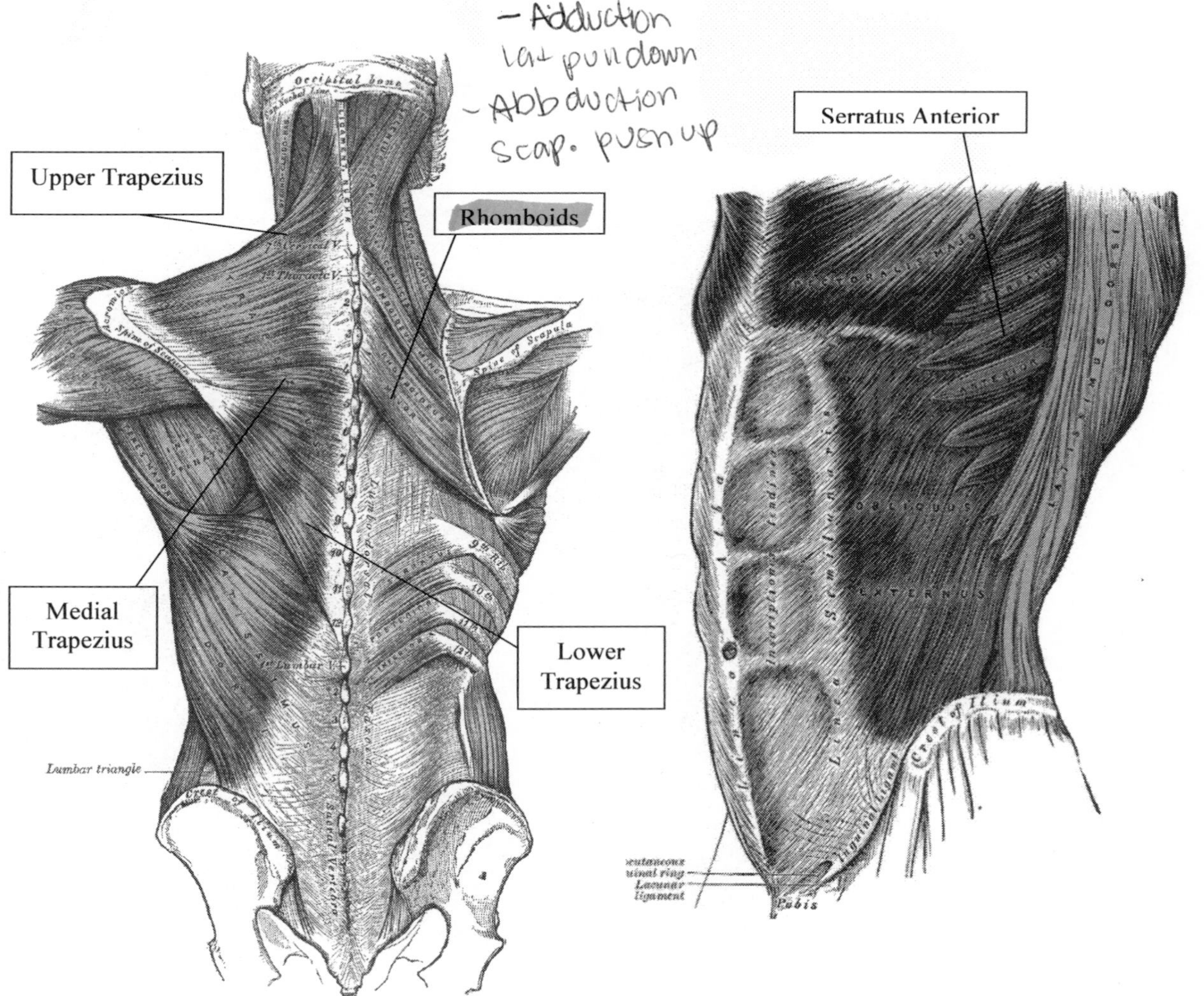

Scapular Elevation (0-30 degrees)

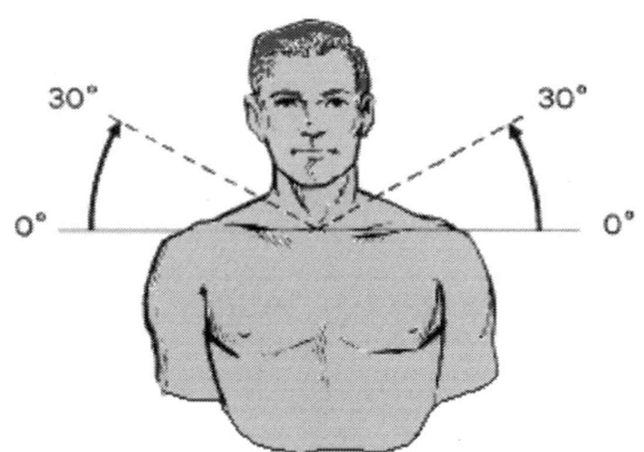

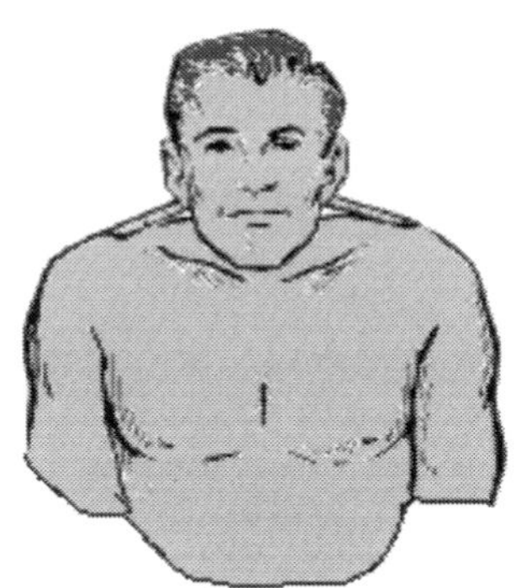

Scapular Depression (0-10 degrees)

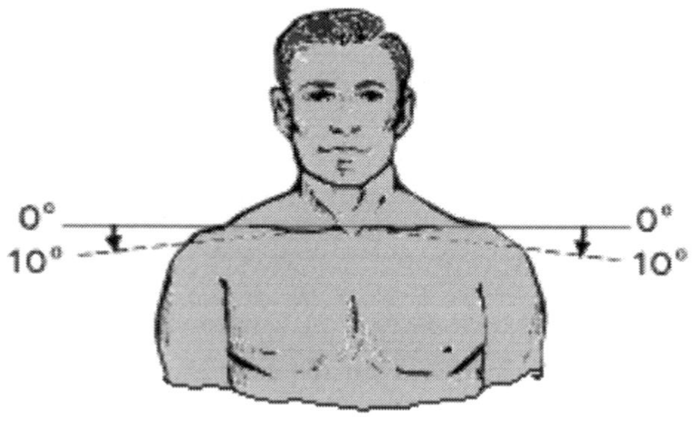

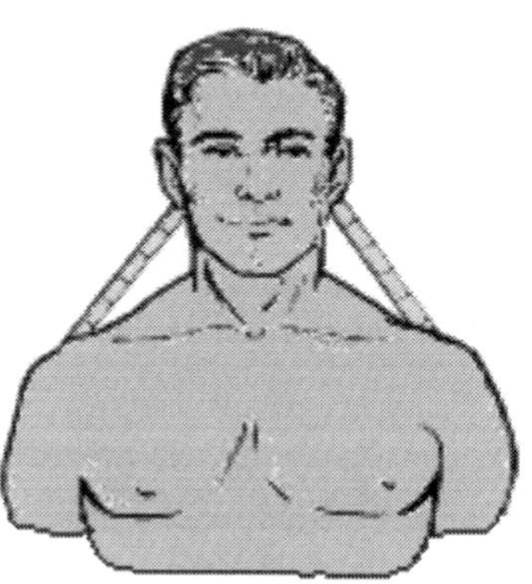

Scapular Abduction/Protraction (0-30 degrees)

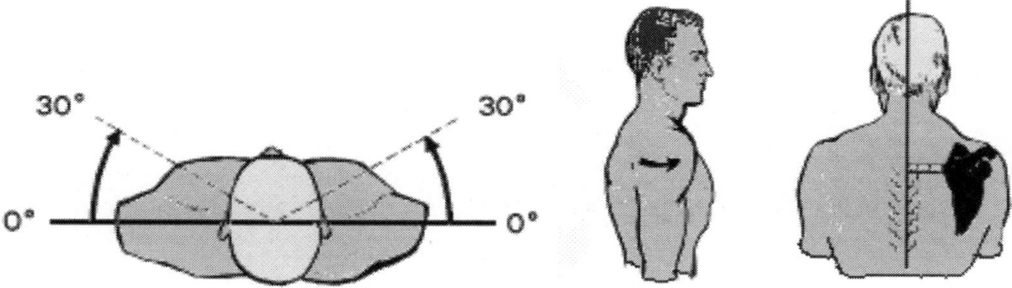

Scapular Adduction/Retraction (0-30 degrees)

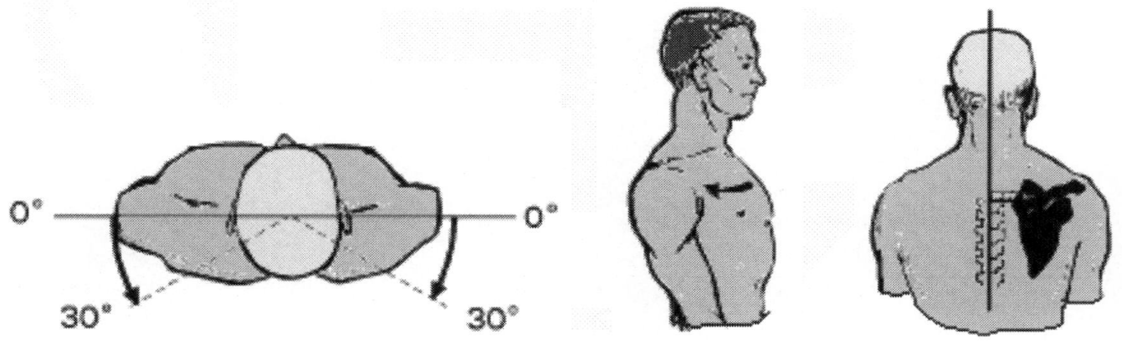

ELBOW

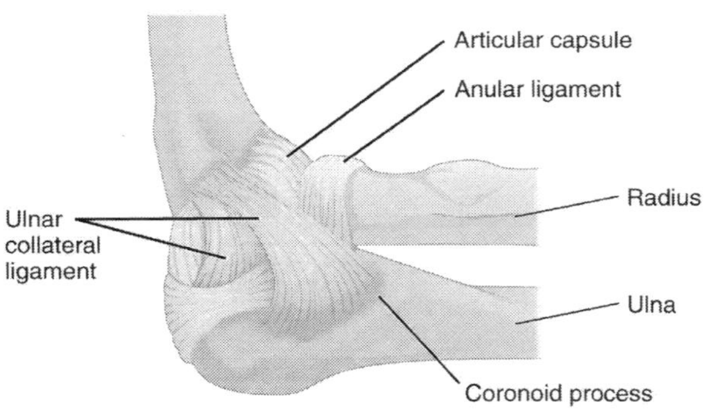

Medial view of right elbow joint

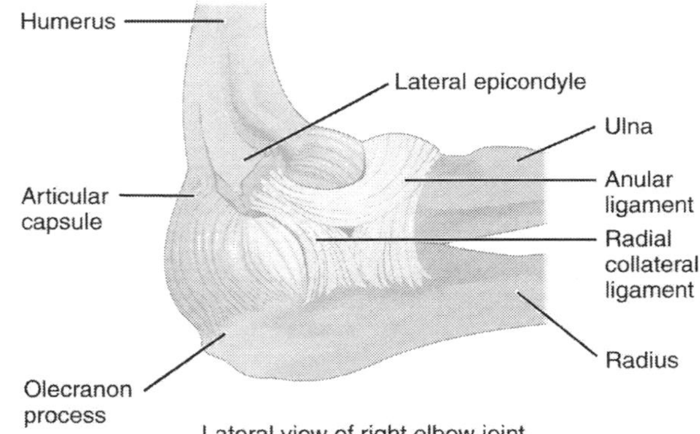

Lateral view of right elbow joint

(Ligaments only for reference)

Bones –

- Humerus
- Radius & Ulna (forearm)

Ligaments –

- Not in this Class

Joint –

- Elbow

Muscles –

- ***Flexion*** **– Biceps Brachii, Brachialis**
- ***Extension*** **– Triceps Brachii**

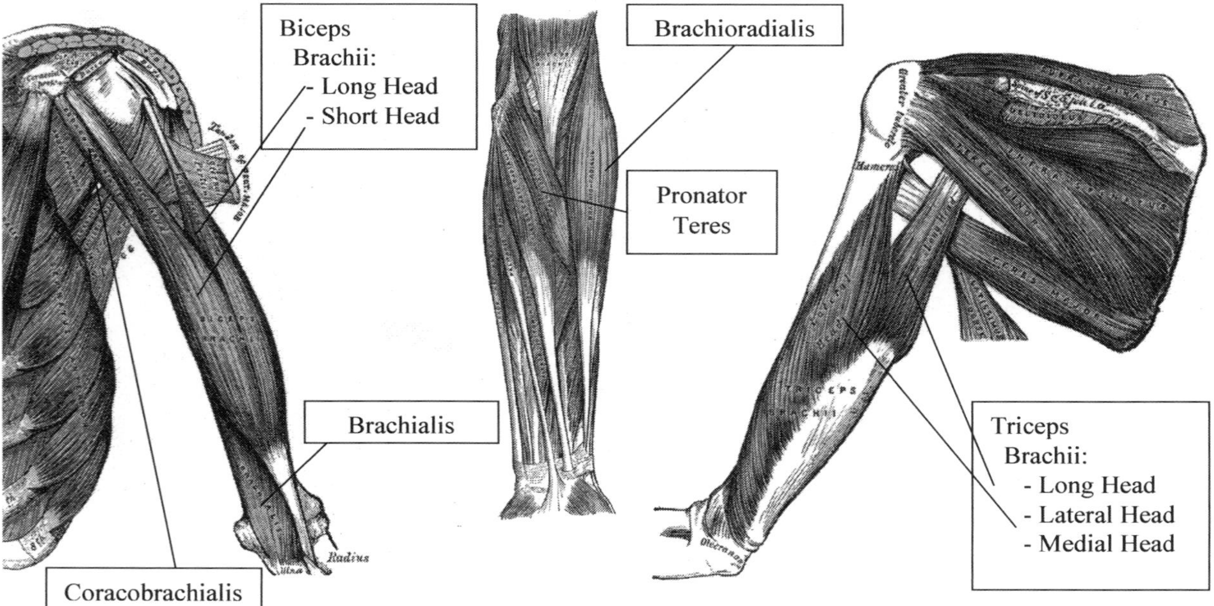

Elbow Flexion (0-175 degrees)

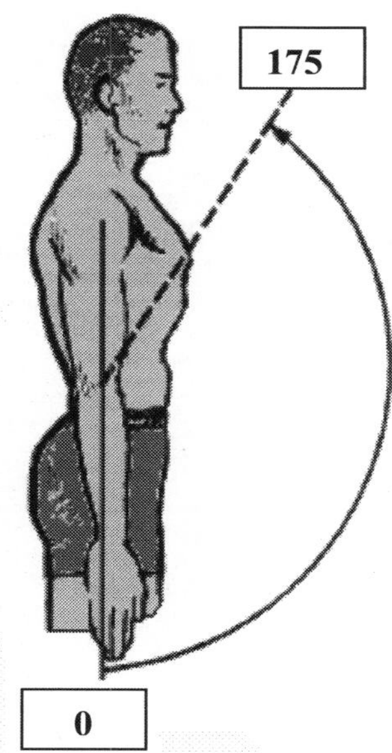

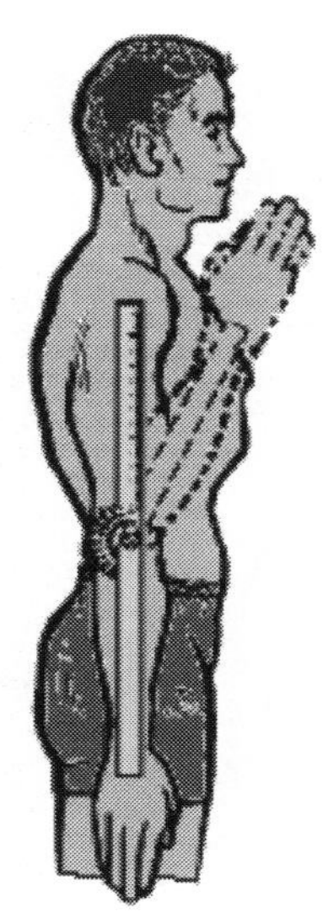

(Elbow Extension is Merely Returning to 0 degrees)

Elbow/Forearm:

Pronation (0-80 degrees) Supination (0-80 degrees)

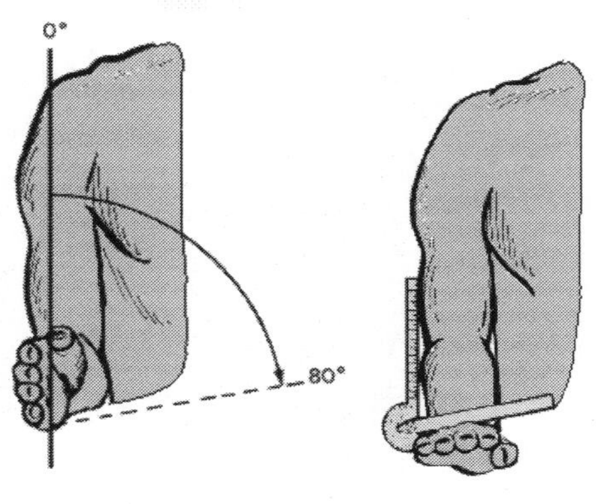

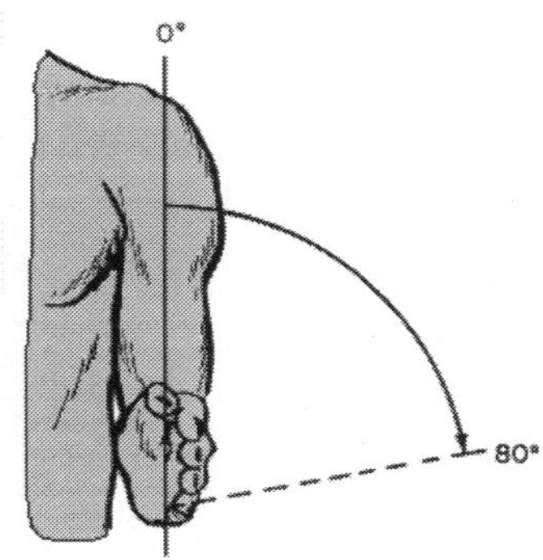

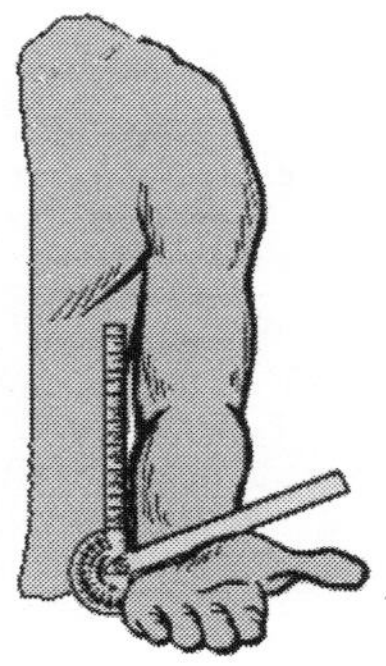

WRIST

Bones –

- Radius & Ulna
- Scaphoid
- Trapezoid
- Capitate
- Hamate
- Lunate
- Pisiform
- Triquetral

Joint –

- Wrist

Ligaments –

- Not in this class

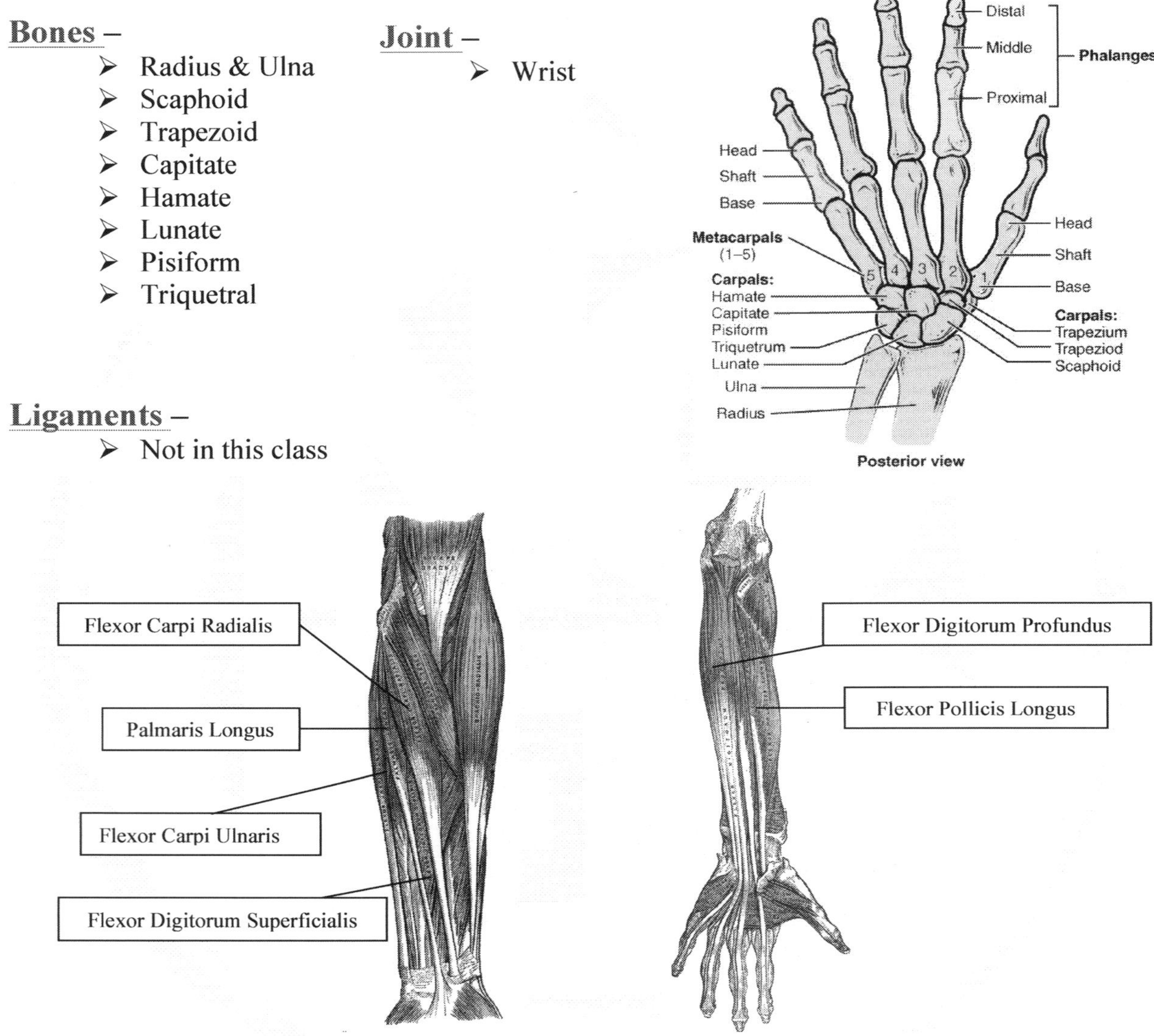

ANTERIOR VIEW

Muscles –

- **Flexor Carpi Radialis**
- **Palmaris Longus**
- **Flexor Digitorum Superficialis**
- **Flexor Carpi Ulnaris**
- **Flexor Pollicis Longus**
- **Flexor Digitorum Profundus**

WRIST
(CONTINUED)

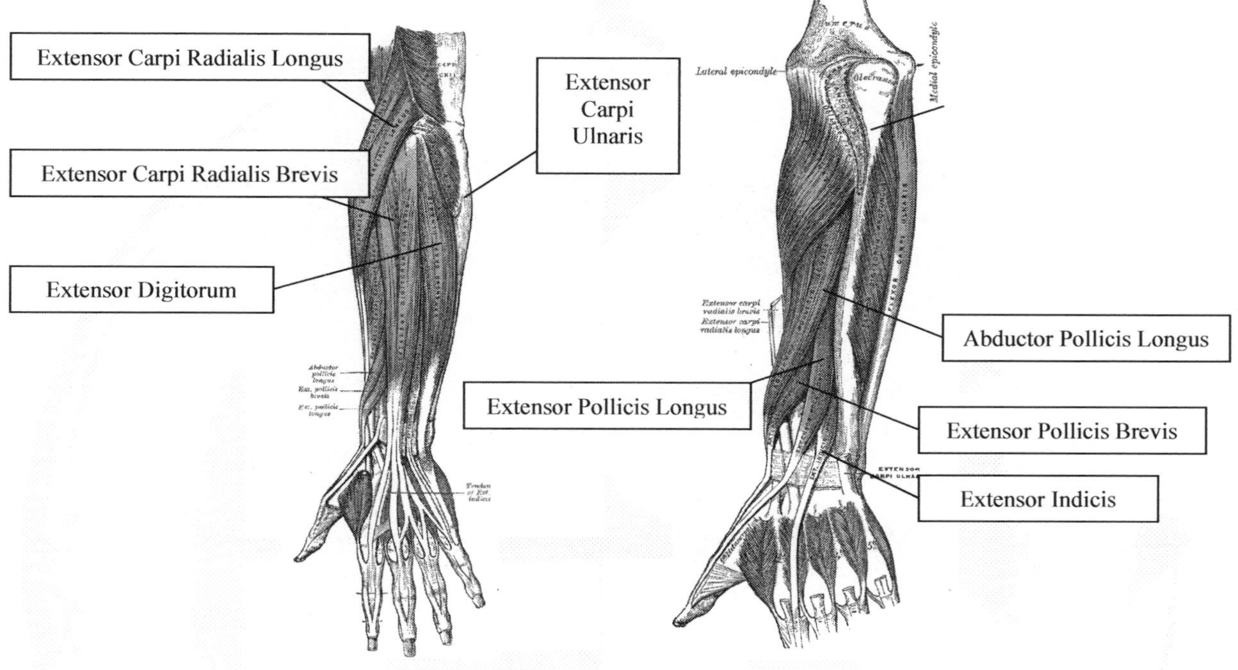

Posterior View

Muscles –

- **Extensor Carpi Radialis Longus**
- **Extensor Carpi Radialis Brevis**
- **Extensor Digitorum**
- **Extensor Carpi Ulnaris**
- **Extensor Pollicis Brevis**
- **Abductor Pollicis Longus**
- **Extensor Pollicis Longus**
- **Extensor Indicis**

Wrist Flexion (0-80 degrees)

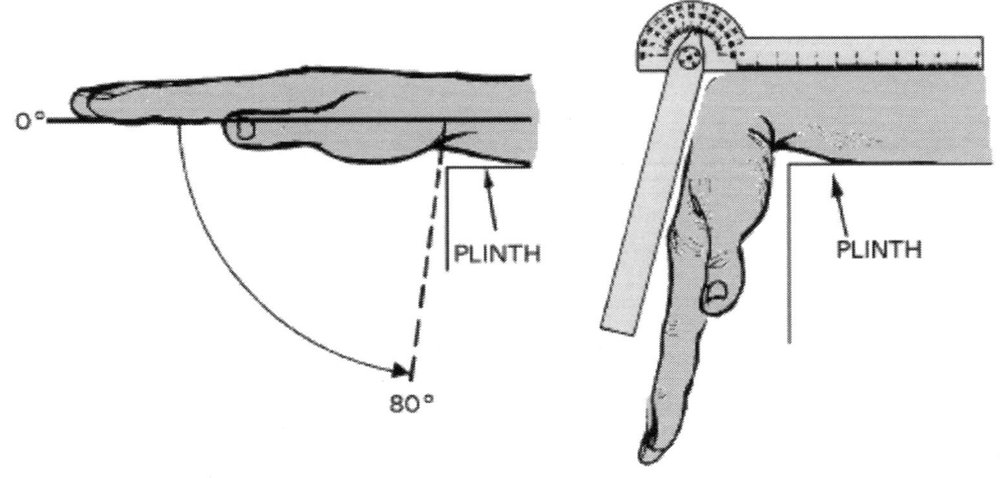

Wrist Extension (0-70 degrees)

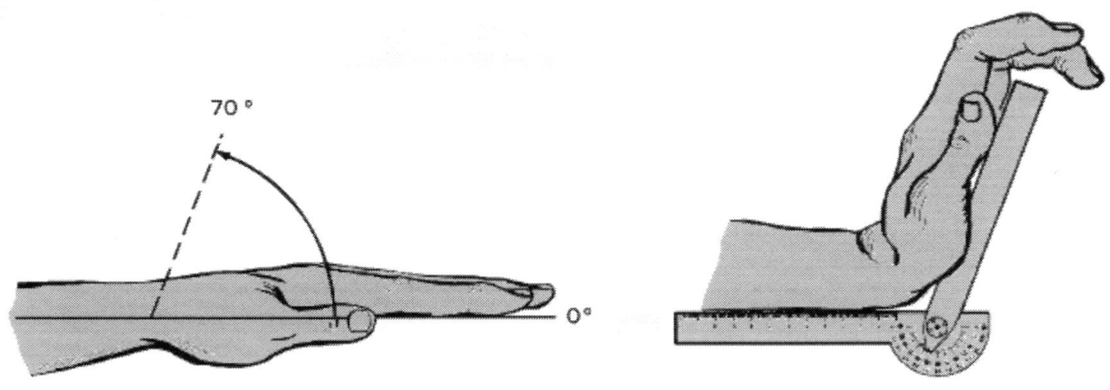

Radial Deviation (0-20 degrees)

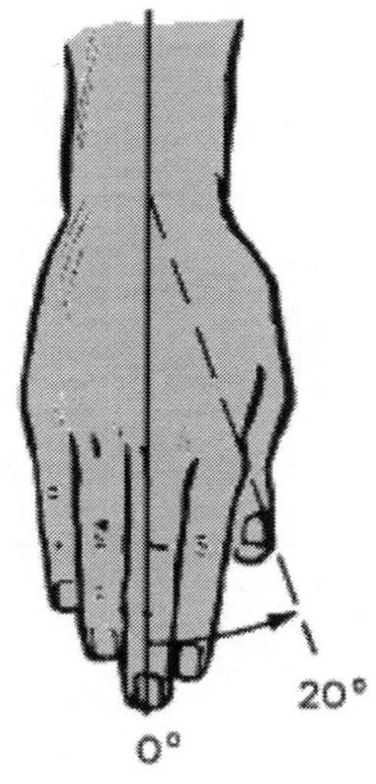

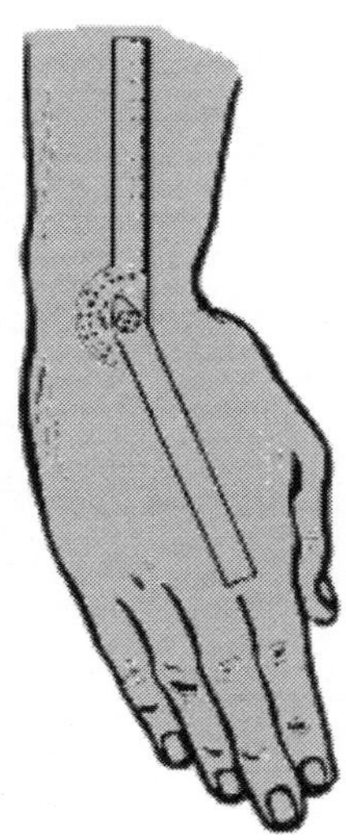

Ulnar Deviation (0-30 degrees)

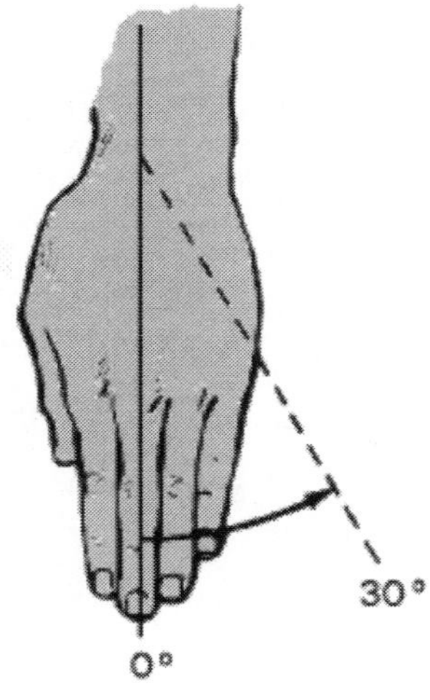

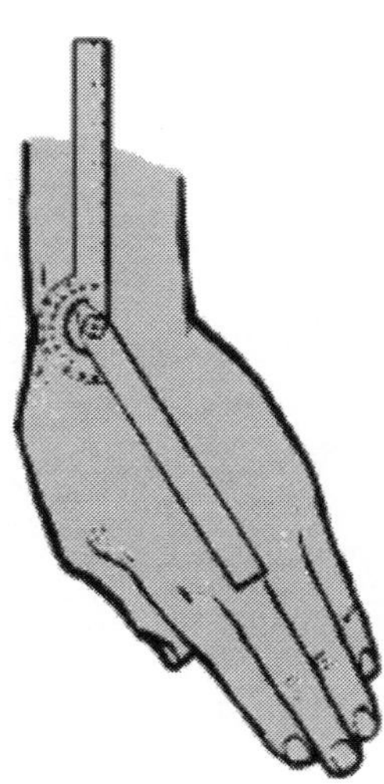

HIP

Bones -
- Pelvis (acetabula fossa)
- Femur

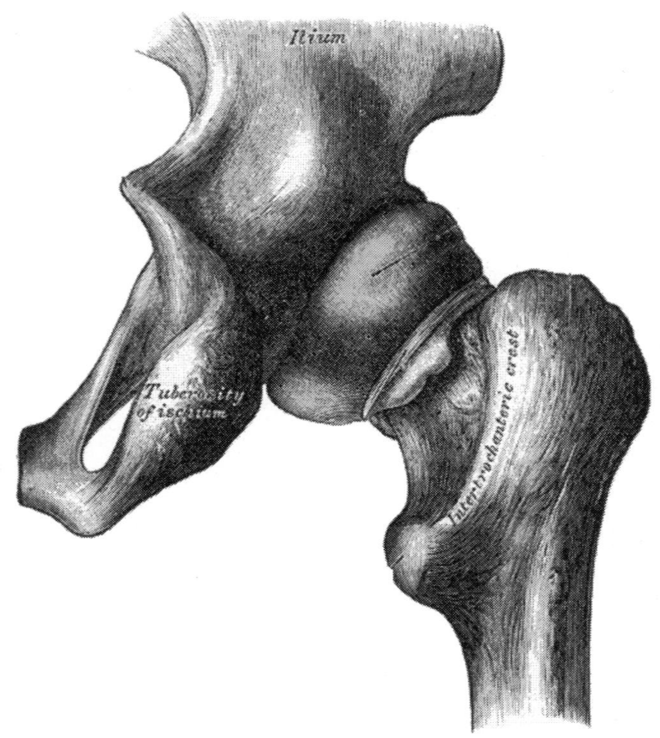

(enlarged for quick reference)

Joint –

Ilio-Femoral Jt.
- Ball and Socket: Three Degrees of Movement

Ligaments –
- Not in this Class

Muscles –
- **ADduction** – Adductor Magnus, Adductor Longus, Adductor Brevis
- **ABduction** - TFL, Gluteus Medius, Gluteus Minimus
- **Flexion** – Iliopsoas, Rectus Femoris
- **Extension** - Gluteus Maximus, Hamstrings (Biceps Femoris, Semimembranosus, Semitendinosus)

HIP
(CONTINUED)

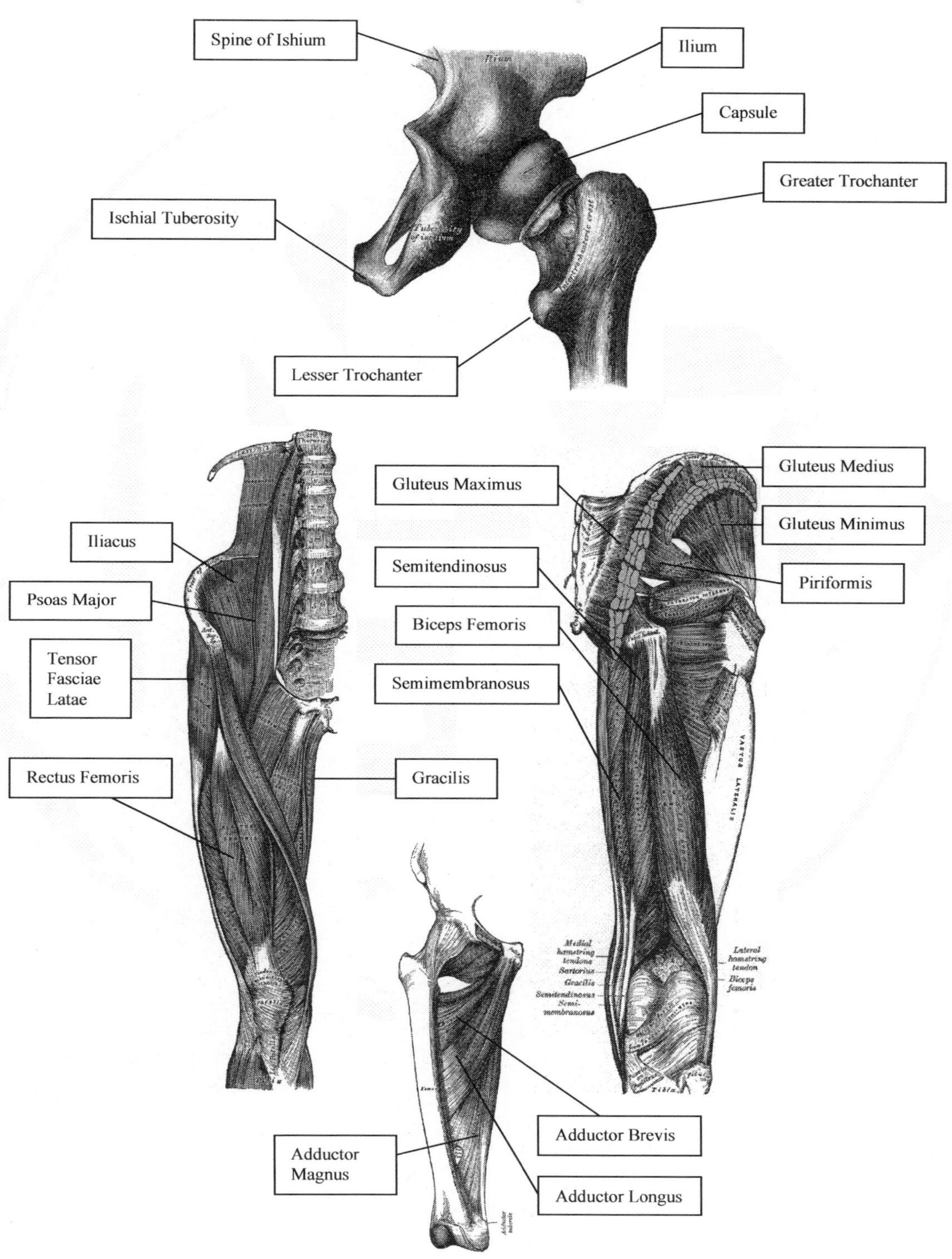

Spine of Ishium
Ilium
Capsule
Greater Trochanter
Ischial Tuberosity
Lesser Trochanter
Gluteus Maximus
Gluteus Medius
Gluteus Minimus
Iliacus
Semitendinosus
Piriformis
Psoas Major
Biceps Femoris
Tensor Fasciae Latae
Semimembranosus
Rectus Femoris
Gracilis
VASTUS LATERALIS
Medial hamstring tendons
Sartorius
Gracilis
Semitendinosus
Semi-membranosus
Lateral hamstring tendon
Biceps femoris
Adductor Brevis
Adductor Magnus
Adductor Longus

Hip Flexion (0-120 degrees)

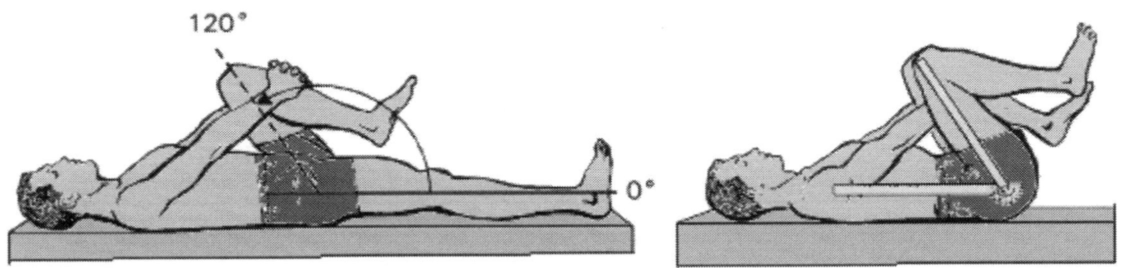

Hip Extension (0-10 degrees)

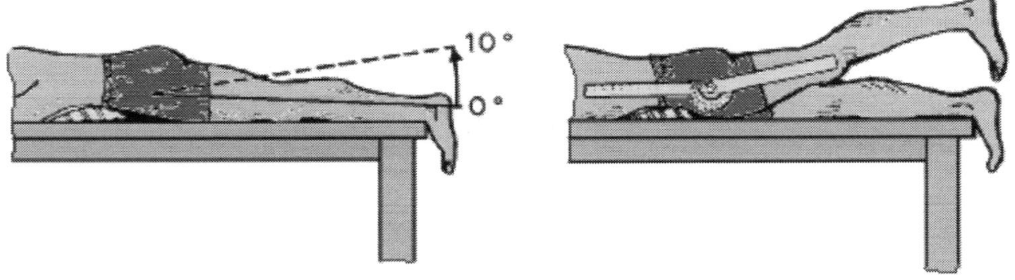

Hip Abduction (0-45 degrees)

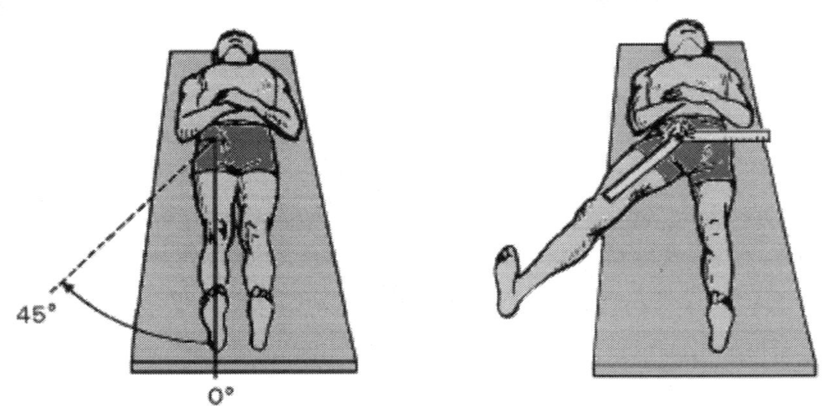

Hip Adduction (0-30 degrees)

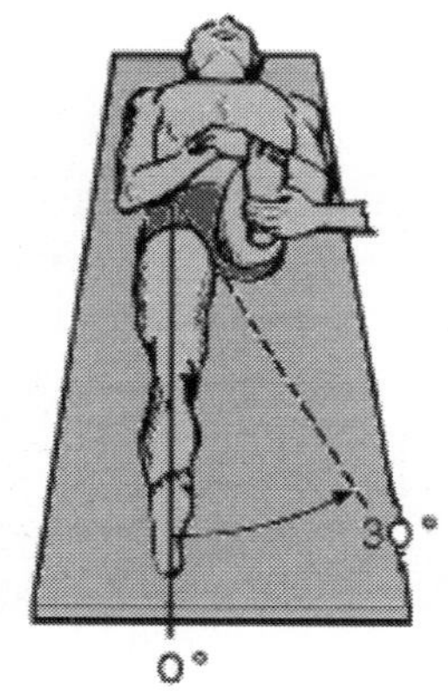

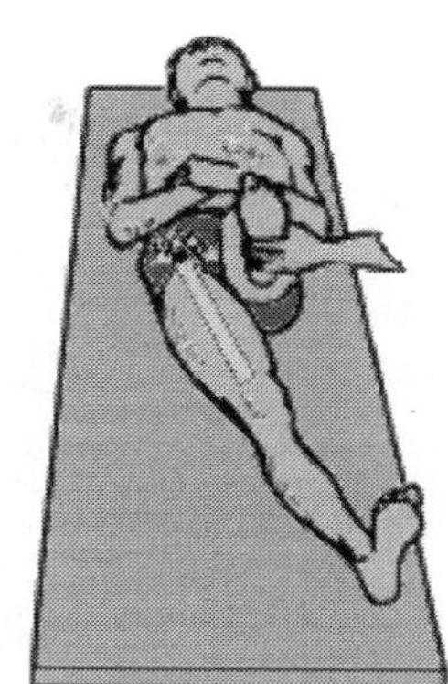

Hip Internal Rotation (0-45 degrees)

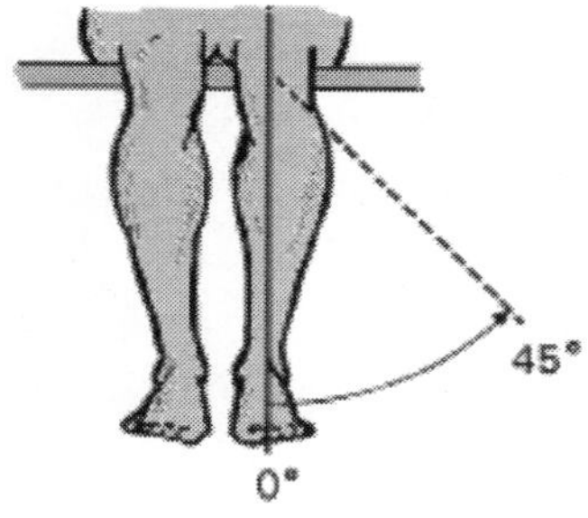

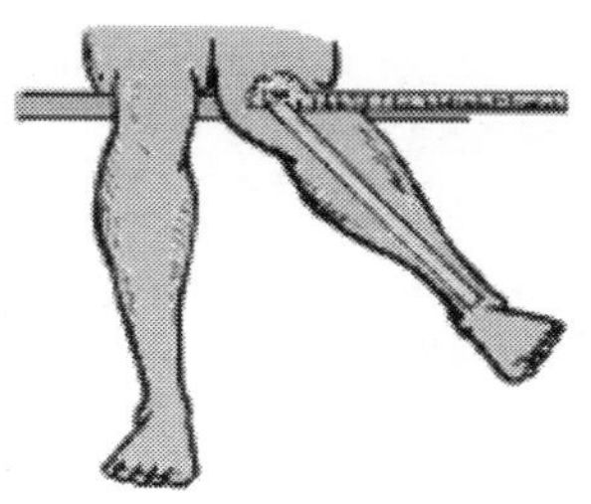

Hip External Rotation (0-45 degrees)

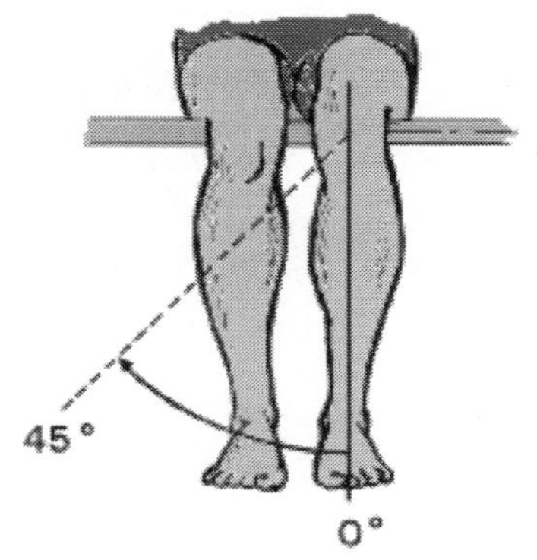

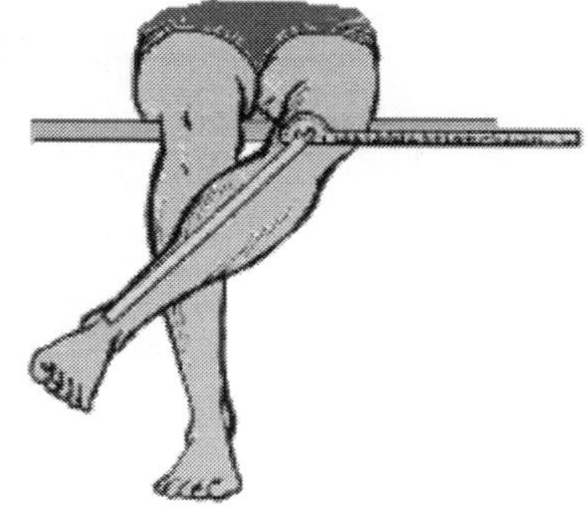

KNEE

Bones -
- Patella
- Femur
- Tibia
- Fibula

Joints -
- Tibial – Femoral Jt. – modified hinge
- Patello – Femoral Jt. – gliding

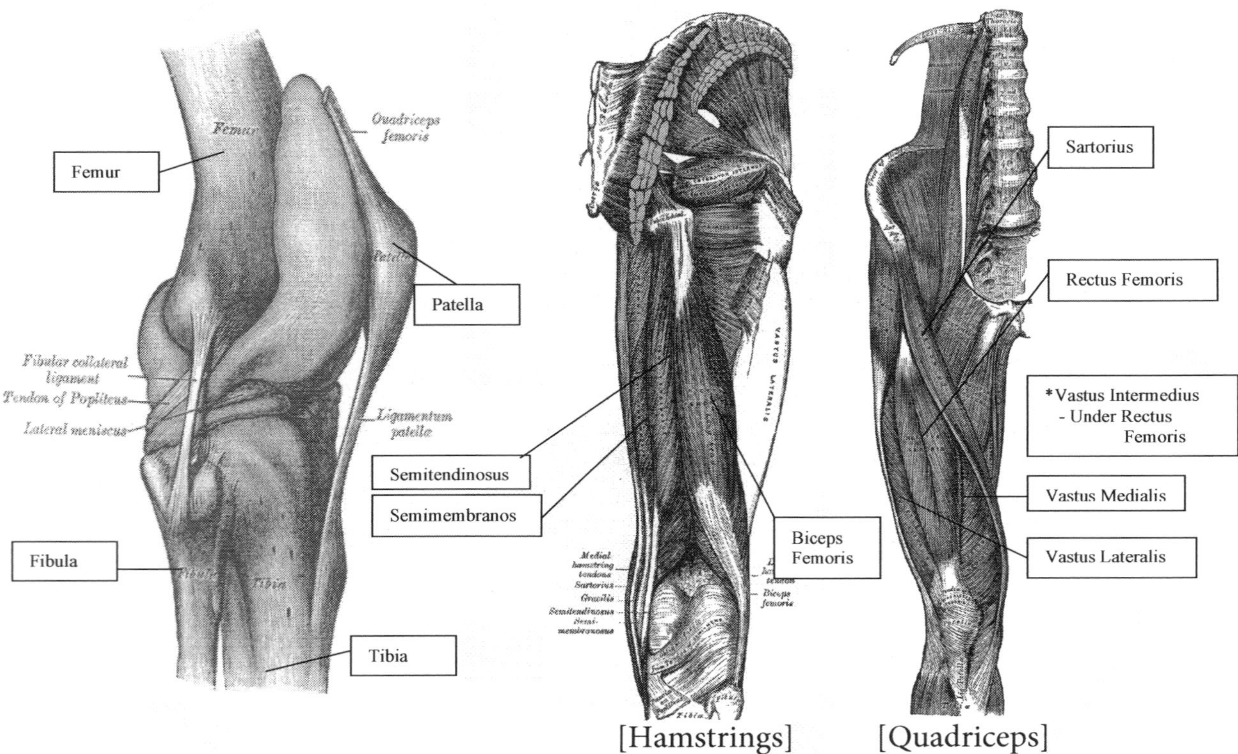

[Hamstrings] [Quadriceps]

Muscles -
- **Flexion** – Hamstrings:
  1. Biceps Femoris
  2. Semitendinosus
  3. Semimembranosus
- **Extension** – Quadriceps:
  1. Rectus Femoris
  2. Vastus Lateralis
  3. Vastus Medialis
  4. Vastus Intermedius

KNEE
(CONTINUED)

Ligaments – *(enlarged for detail)*

- Patellar Tendon
- Anterior Cruciate Ligament (ACL)
- Posterior Cruciate Ligament (PCL)
- Medial Collateral Ligament (MCL)*
- Lateral Collateral Ligament (LCL)^

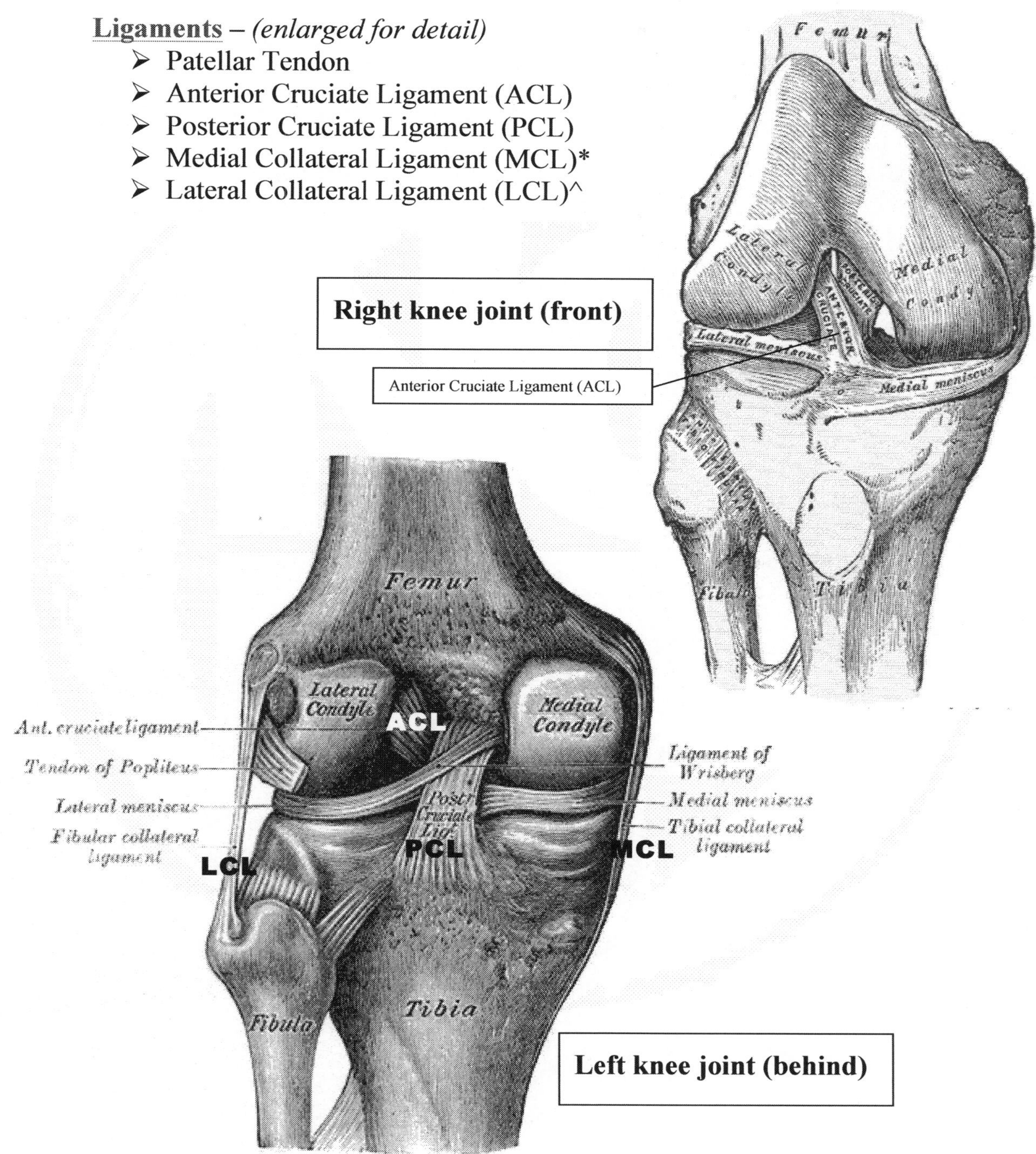

*The Medial Collateral Ligament (MCL) is also referred to as the Tibial Collateral Ligament
^ The Lateral Collateral Ligament (LCL) is also referred to as the Fibular Collateral Ligament

Knee Flexion (0-135 degrees)

(Knee Extension is merely returning to Neutral, 0 degrees, from a flexed position)

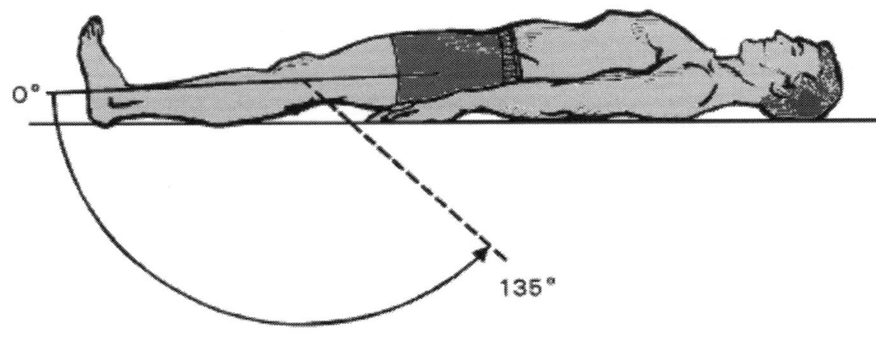

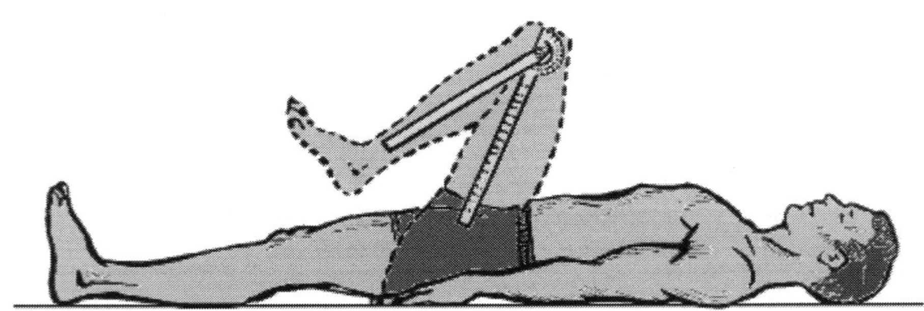

FOOT AND ANKLE

Bones -

- Tibia
- Fibula
- Talus
- Calcaneus

Muscles -

- **Plantar ~~Extension~~** – Gastrocnemius, Soleus
- **Dorsi Flexion** – Anterior Tibialis

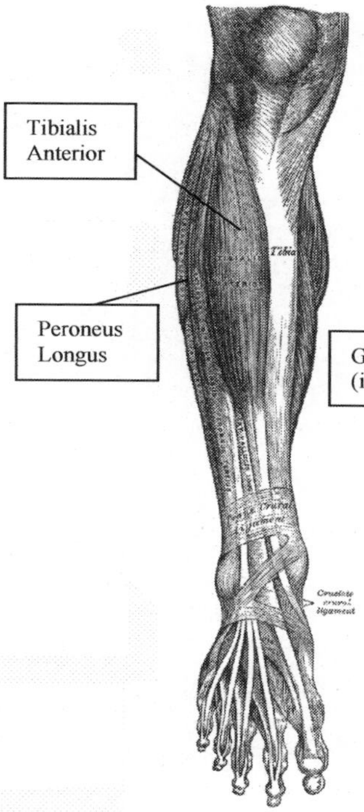

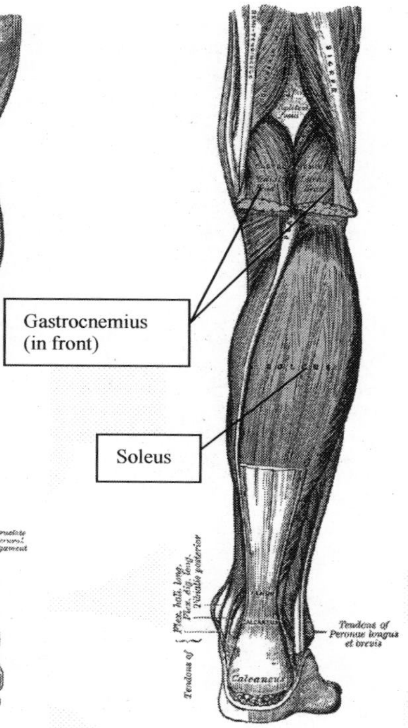

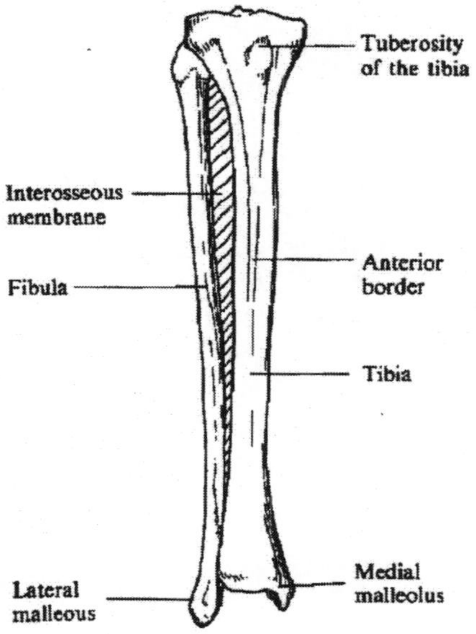

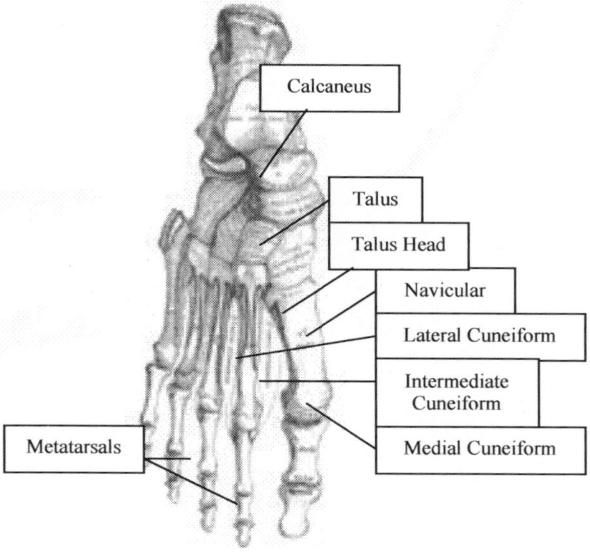

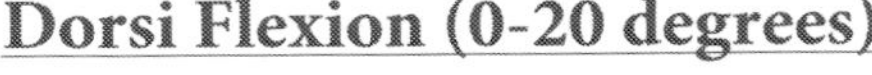

Dorsi Flexion (0-20 degrees)

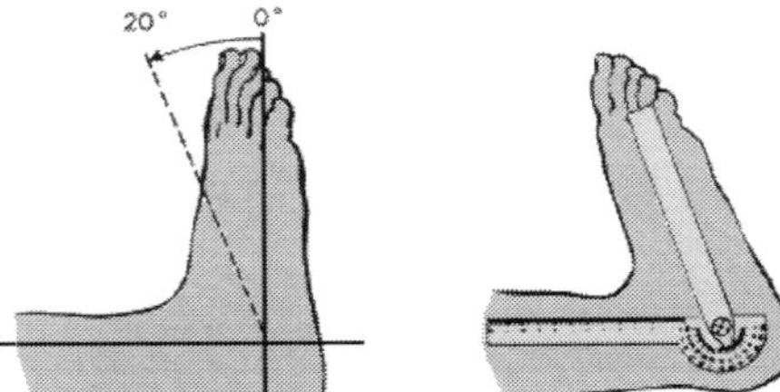

Plantar Flexion (0-50 degrees)

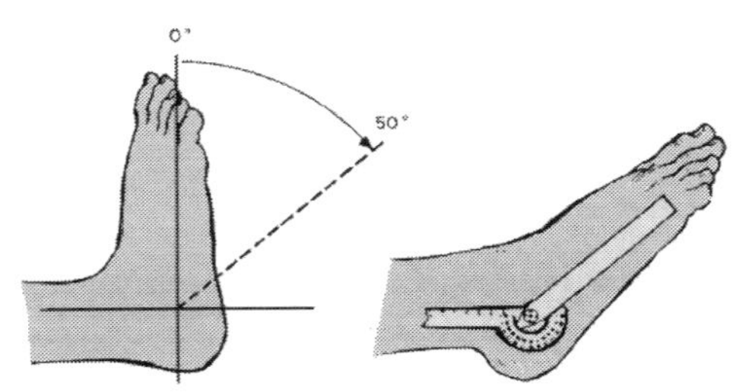

Inversion (0-5 degrees) Right Foot

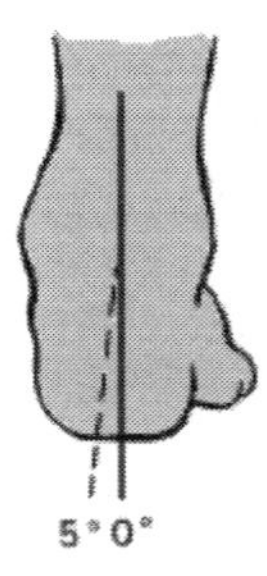

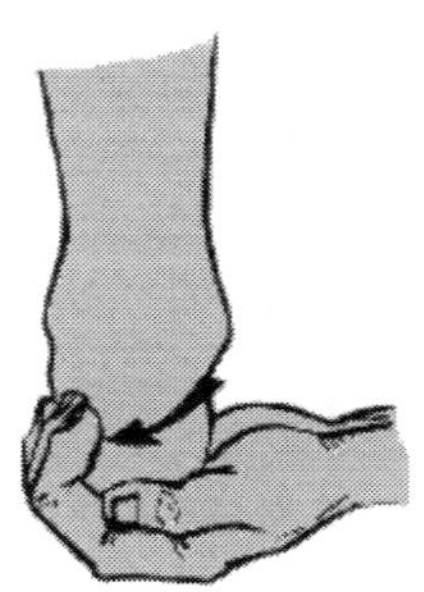

Eversion (0-5 degrees) Right Foot

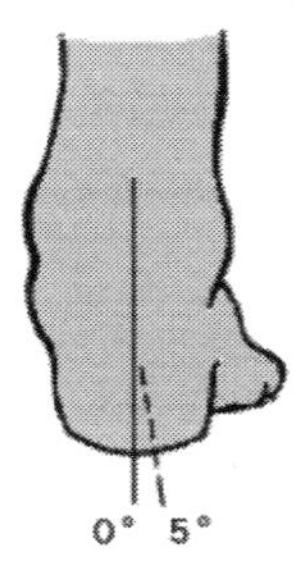

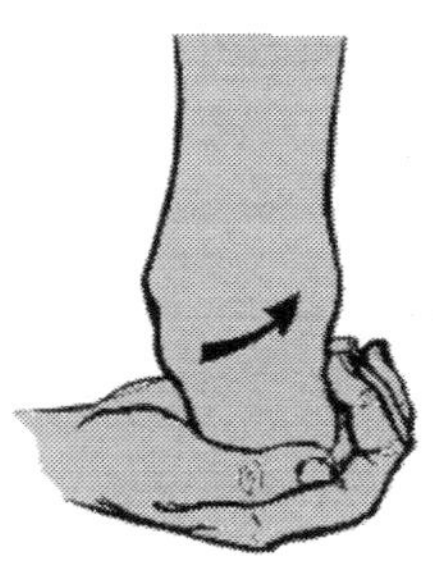

Supination (0-35 degrees) Adduction (0-40 degrees)

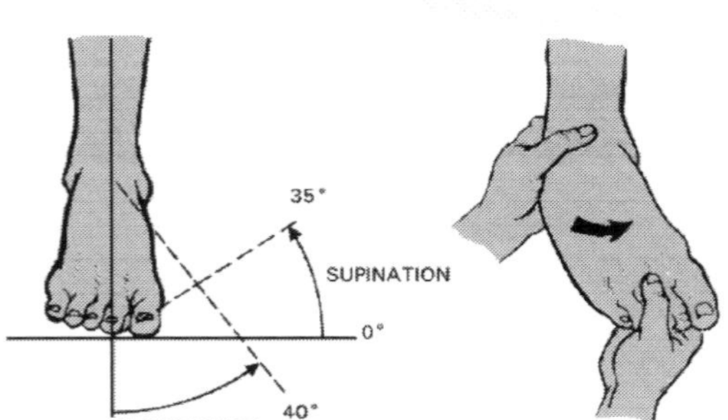

Pronation (0-15 degrees) Abduction (0-30 degrees)

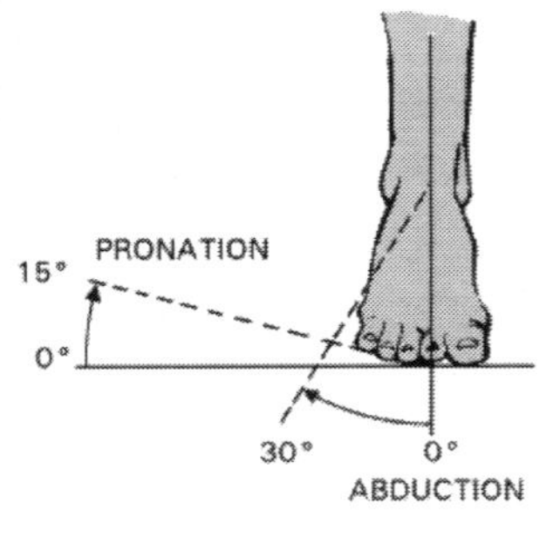

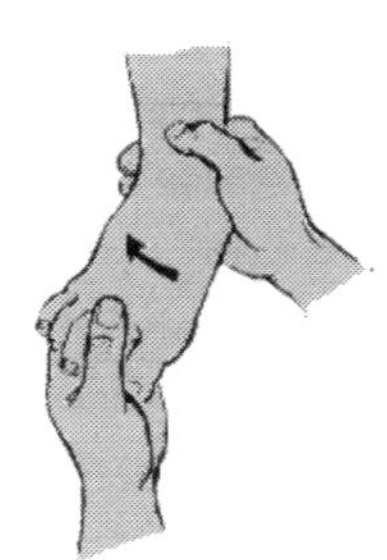

CHAPTER THIRTEEN

Functional Anatomy

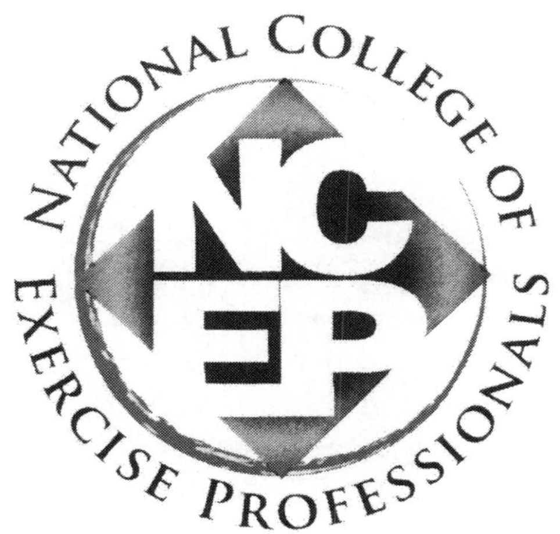

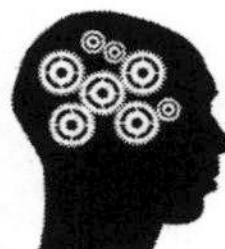

FUNCTIONAL ANATOMY

Why Functional Anatomy?

When most students learn anatomy for the first time they are introduced to what is called "Gross Anatomy." Gross anatomy was invented by a doctor who used cadavers to find out the muscle function and also to learn where they attached inside your body. Gross Anatomy is a very good name for it. If you are not into the forensic sciences, it is really gross to work on a cadaver. Unfortunately, there are some glaring problems with trying to determine the function of a muscle on a dead person. First, most of the clients you will work with as a personal trainer are not dead. (Yes, that was our attempt at humor.) Let's list some of the biggest problems and go over each one by one:

1. ***Position of the body, only looking at "open chain" movements***
2. ***Only measures the concentric contraction***
3. ***Brain is not working***

First, the position of the body can really be a big factor—and a big issue. To understand how a muscle worked, the scientist would cut the muscle closest to one of the attachments (usually the origin) and pull on it. Whichever direction the limb or part of the body moved, they would label that movement as the muscle's function. If we look at someone lying down, it means their feet are not in contact with the ground, or an "open kinetic chain." When an individual is standing, the foot is in contact with the ground and thus, when a muscle contracts it is a completely different outcome. Let's look at the upper body as an example. In an open chain (i.e., "Lat pull down"), the pulling movement would bring an object towards the body. In a closed chain (i.e., "pull up") the pulling would bring the body up to the stationary bar. It doesn't sound like there is a big difference, but the body recognizes it as a night and day difference. That is why some non-functional people can pull down amazing amounts of weight but cannot even complete one single pull up.

Second, when a scientist pulls on one end of the muscle it is creating a shortening of the muscle, also known as a concentric contraction. We know from our physiology chapter that there are three types of contractions: concentric, eccentric and isometric. Throw in to the equation that there are three planes of motion as well: saggital, frontal and transverse, and now we need to know the function of the muscle for at least nine different possibilities. Unfortunately, gross anatomy is limiting: it typically only tells us one function of the muscle in one plane of movement. Often times the one function gross anatomy tells you is not even the one that is used most often. For example, the gross anatomy function of the gluteus medius is to concentrically abduct the hip. The most dominant function of the gluteus medius is to isometrically stabilize the hip and to eccentrically decelerate femoral internal rotation during heel strike in the gait cycle.

Third, the last and possibly most definitive problem with Gross Anatomy is that the brain has stopped functioning or sending signals to the muscles. There is no muscle in the human body that works in isolation. In other words, when the brain sends a signal for movement to occur, it alerts all the muscles in the entire body that the movement will be occurring and every muscle prepares for the movement either by assisting in the actual movement or by stabilizing a part of the body so it does not move. As you know, the mind and body work together, and studying cadavers—and not considering how muscles work in unison with each other in living, active people—does not make much sense.

Overall, we just wanted to give you a brief synopsis of why Gross Anatomy is just not sufficient for exercise professionals. The following chapter will give you a glimpse of Functional Anatomy and how it used in training. If you want to learn more about how to incorporate mopre of this knowledge in to your workouts we offer a full weekend class of Functional Anatomy.

SECTION 1: SPINAL MUSCULATURE

RECTUS ABDOMINUS

EXTERNAL OBLIQUE

INTERNAL OBLIQUE

TRANSVERSE ABDOMINUS

ERECTOR SPINAE

QUADRATUS LUMBORUM

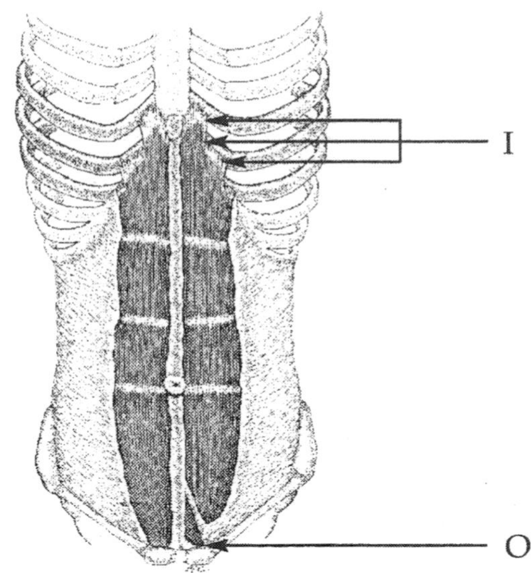

RECTUS ABDOMINUS
(REC-TUS AB-DOM-I-NUS)

Origin:
Pubic Crest

Insertion:
Cartilage of fifth, sixth and seventh ribs, xyphoid process

True Function:

- *Concentric acceleration of spinal flexion*
- *Assists in concentric acceleration of posterior pelvic rotation*
- *Assists in eccentric deceleration of spinal extension, lateral flexion, and rotation*
- *Assists in eccentric deceleration of anterior pelvic rotation*
- *Assists in dynamic stabilization of the lumbo-pelvic hip complex*

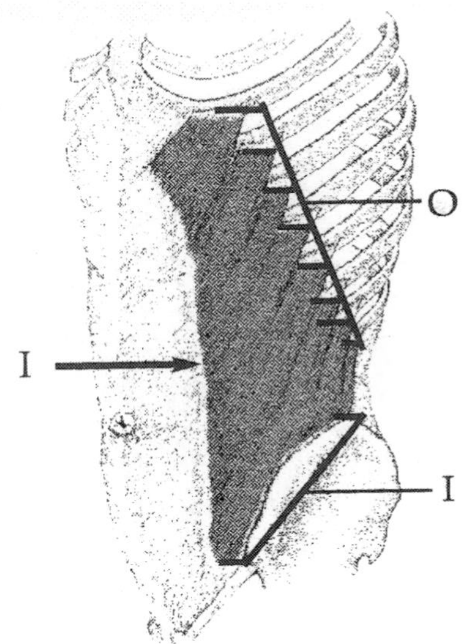

EXTERNAL OBLIQUE
(O-BLEEK)

Origin:
External surfaces of lower eight ribs

Insertion:
Fibers insert into the abdominal aponeurosis and the anterior portion of the iliac crest

True Function:

- *Assists in concentric acceleration of spinal flexion*
- *Assists in concentric acceleration of contralateral rotation of the spine*
- *Assists in concentric acceleration of posterior pelvic rotation*
- *Assists in eccentric deceleration of spinal extension*
- *Assists in eccentric deceleration of spinal rotation*
- *Assists in eccentric deceleration of anterior pelvic rotation*
- *Assists in dynamic stabilization of the lumbo-pelvic hip complex*

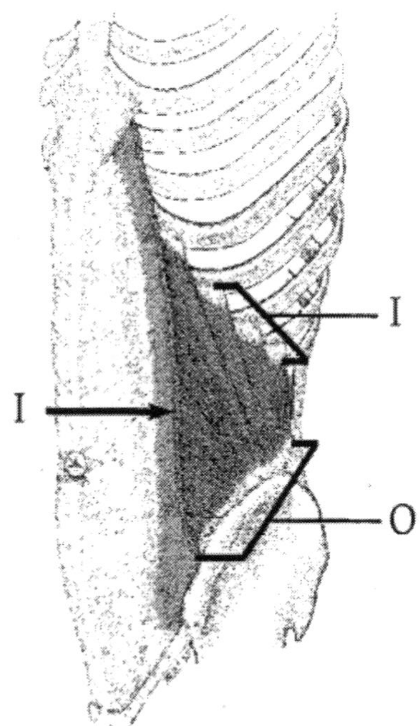

INTERNAL OBLIQUE
(O-BLEEK)

Origin:
Iliac Crest, inguinal ligament and the thoracolumbar fascia

Insertion:
Linea alba, pubic crest, last three ribs

True Function:
- *Assists in concentric acceleration of flexion of the spine*
- *Assists in concentric acceleration of the ipsilateral rotation*
- *Assists in eccentric deceleration of spinal extension*
- *Assists in eccentric deceleration of contralateral rotation*
- *Assists synergistically with the transversus abdominis, deep erector spinae and multifidi to create a posterior shear force at L5-S1*
- *Assists synergistically with the transversus abdominis to provide rotational and translational stability to the lumbar spine secondary to its attachment to the thoracolumbar fascia*

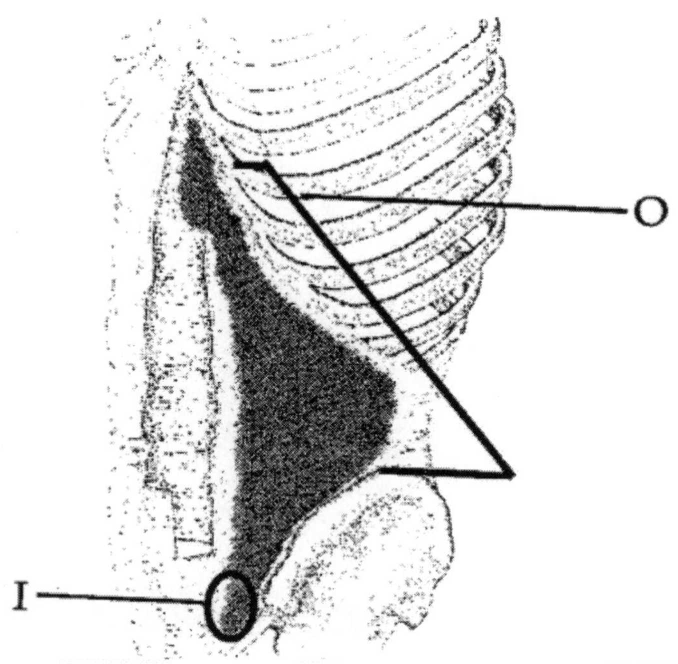

TRANSVERSUS ABDOMINIS
(TRANZ-VER-SUS AB-DOM-I-NUS)

Origin:
Thoracolumbar fascia, cartilage of the last six ribs; iliac crest

Insertion:
Linea alba, pubic crest

True Function:

- *Increases intra-abdominal pressure*
- *Supports the abdominal viscera*
- *Works synergistically with the internal oblique, multifidus and deep erector spinae to stabilize the lumbo-pelvic-hip- complex*
- *Provides segmental stabilization to the lumbar spine*

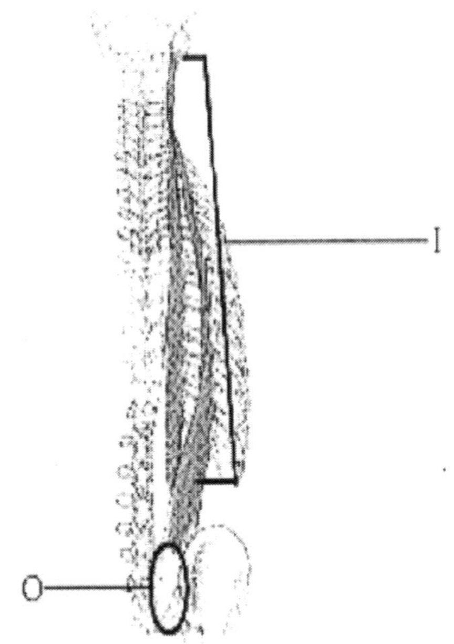

ERECTOR SPINAE
(E-REK-TOR SPY-NEH)

Origin:
1. *SPs of upper lumbar and lower thoracic vertebrae SP of C-7*
2. *TVP of T-1 through T-5*
3. *Posterior surface of ribs 1-12*

Insertion:
1. *SP processes of upper thoracic and cervical vertebrae, except for C-1*
2. *Mastoid process, TVP of thoracic and cervical vertebrae and ribs 4-12*
3. *Ribs 1-12*

True Function:
- *Assists in concentric acceleration of spinal extension, spinal rotation and lateral flexion*
- *Assists in eccentric deceleration of spinal flexion*
- *Assists in eccentric deceleration of spinal rotation*
- *Assists in eccentric deceleration of lateral flexion of lumbar spine*
- *Assists in the dynamic stabilization of the lumbar spine during functional movements*

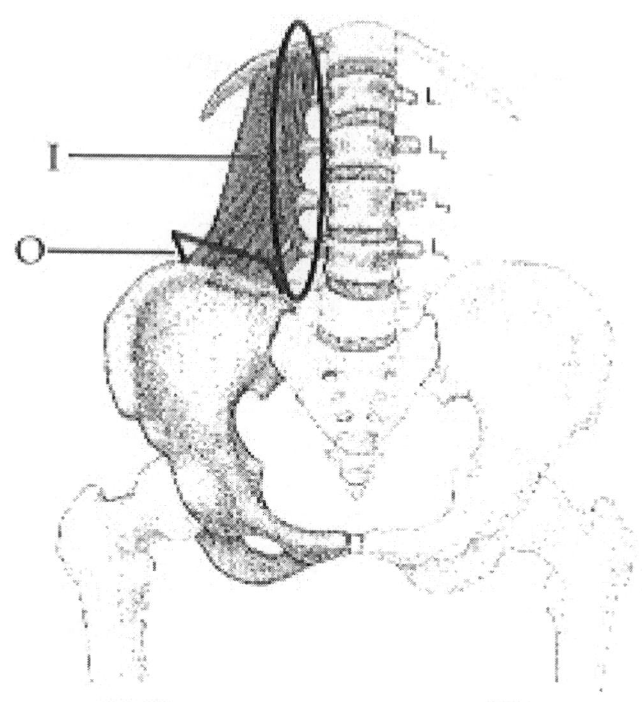

QUADRATUS LUMBORUM
(QUAD-RA-TUS LUM-BORE-UM)

Origin:
Iliac crest and iliolumbar ligament

Insertion:
Transverse processes of L2-L5 and lower margin of 12th rib

True Function:

- *Concentric acceleration of lateral flexion*
- *Assists in eccentric deceleration of lateral flexion*
- *Works synergistically with the gluteus medius, tensor fascia and the adductor complex as the primary frontal plane stabilization mechanism*

SECTION 2: SCAPULAR MUSCULATURE

TRAPEZIUS

RHOMBOIDS MAJOR & MINOR

LEVATOR SCAPULAE

SERRATUS ANTERIOR

PECTORALIS MINOR

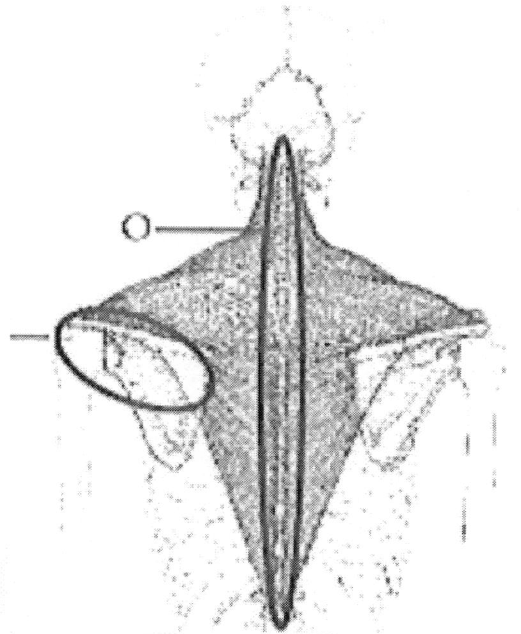

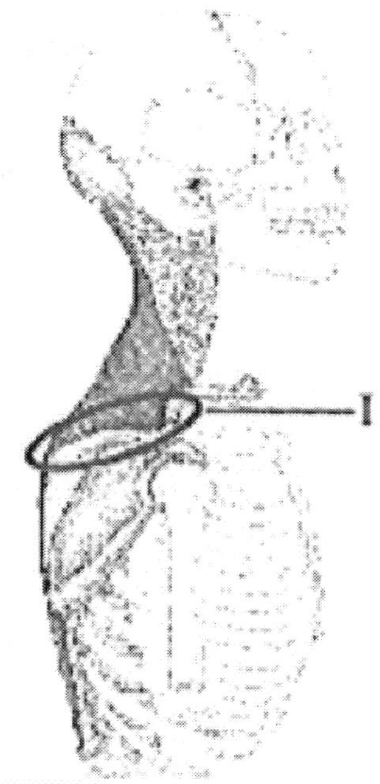

TRAPEZIUS
(TRAH-PEE-ZEE-US)

Origin:
Occipital bone (skull) to the spines of C7 and all the thoracic vertebrae

Insertion:
A continuous insertion along acromion and spine of scapulae and lateral third of clavicle

True Function:

- *Assists in concentric acceleration of scapular elevation, scapular retraction and depression*
- *Upper: functions eccentrically to decelerate cervical flexion, lateral flexion, rotation and assists in providing dynamic stability to the cervical spine and shoulder complex*
- *Middle: eccentrically decelerates scapular protraction and upward rotation, assists in dynamically stabilizing the scapula during functional movements*
- *Lower: eccentrically decelerates scapular elevation, assists in dynamically stabilizing the scapula*

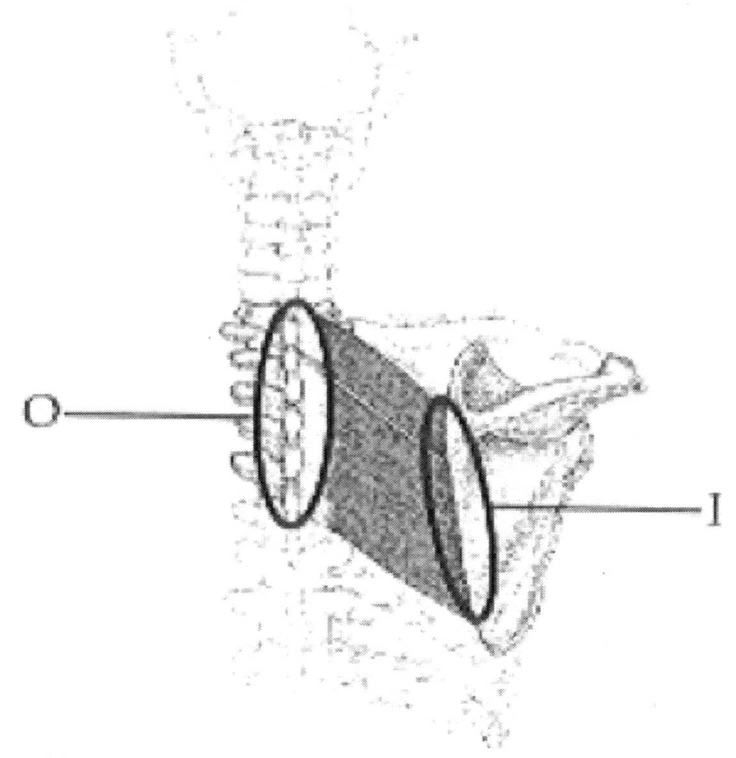

RHOMBOIDS MAJOR AND MINOR
(ROM-BOYDZ)

Origin:
Spinous Processes of C7 and T1 (minor) and spinous processes of T2-T5

Insertion:
Medial Border of scapula

True Function:
- *Assists in concentric acceleration of scapular retraction*
- *Assists in concentric acceleration of downward rotation of the scapula*
- *Assists in eccentric deceleration of upward rotation of the scapula*
- *Assists in dynamic stabilization of the scapula*

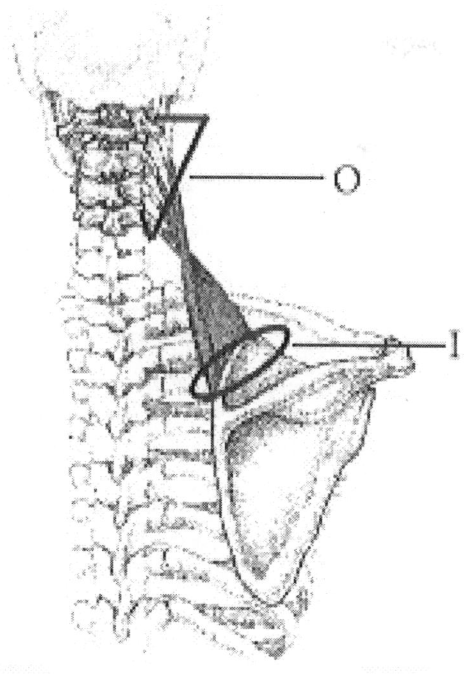

LEVATOR SCAPULAE
(LE-VA-TOR SKAP-YOU-LE)

Origin:
Transverse processes of C1-C4

Insertion:
Superior vertebral border of scapulae

True Function:

- *Assists in concentric acceleration of extension of head and neck bilaterally*
- *Assists in concentric acceleration of elevation and downward rotation of the scapula unilaterally*
- *Assists in concentric acceleration of lateral flexion of the cervical spine unilaterally*
- *Assists in eccentric deceleration of flexion of head and neck bilaterally*
- *Assists in eccentric deceleration of depression and upward rotation of the scapula unilaterally*
- *Assists in eccentric deceleration of later flexion of the cervical spine unilaterally*
- *Assists in dynamic stabilization of the cervical-scapular*

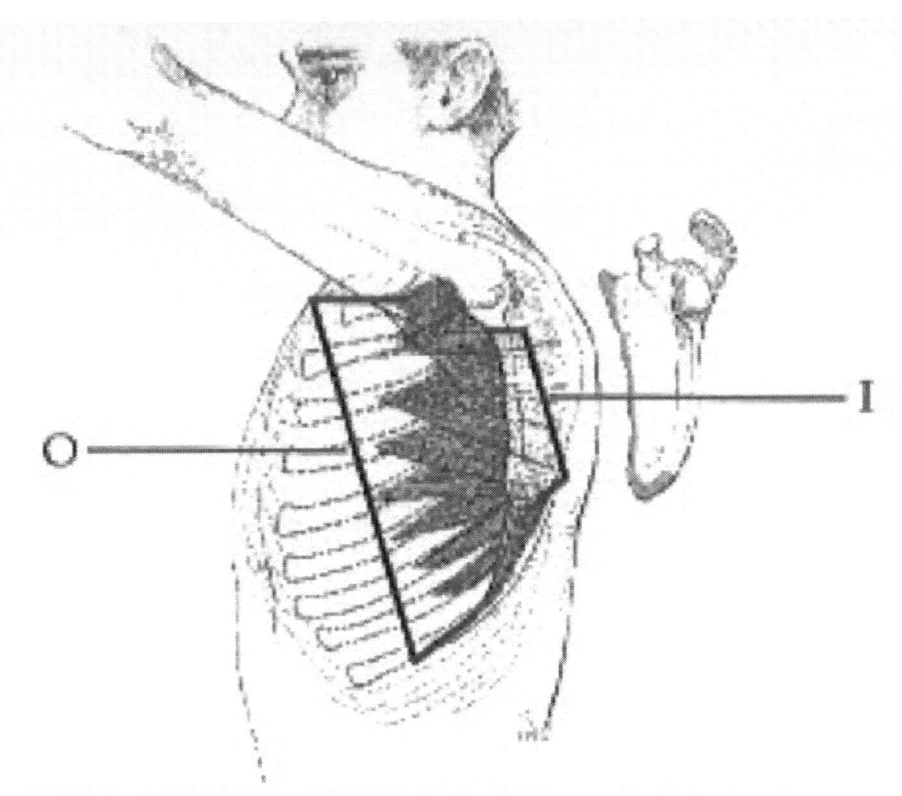

SERRATUS ANTERIOR
(SIR-AH-TUS)

Origin:
Outer surface of upper eight or nine ribs

Insertion:
Entire anterior surface of vertebral (medial) border of scapula

True Function:

- *Assists in concentric acceleration of protraction of the scapula*
- *Assists in eccentric deceleration of retraction of the scapula*
- *Works synergistically with the upper and lower trapezius to provide optimal scapular mobility and stability during shoulder elevation*
- *Assists in dynamic stabilization of the scapula*

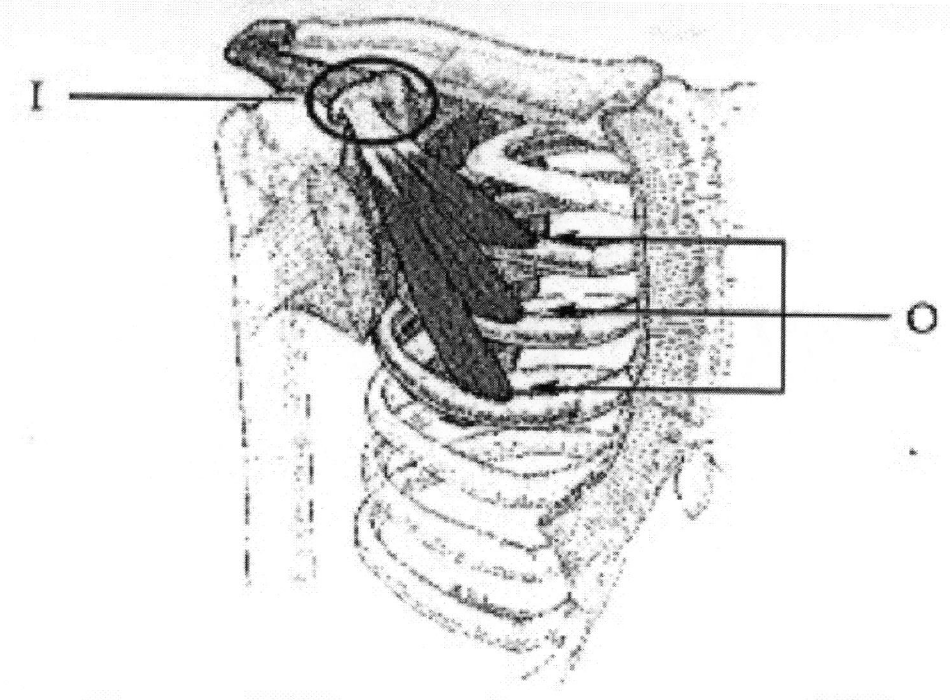

PECTORALIS MINOR
(PECK-TOE-RA-LIS MI-NOR)

Origin:
Anterior surfaces of ribs 3-5

Insertion:
Coracoid process of scapula

True Function:
- *Assists in concentric acceleration of scapular protraction*
- *Assists in eccentric deceleration of scapular retraction*
- *Assists in dynamic stabilization of the scapula during functional movements*

SECTION 3: SHOULDER JOINT MUSCULATURE

SUPRASPINATUS

INFRASPINATUS

TERES MINOR

SUBSCAPULARIS

LATISSIMUS DORSI

TERES MAJOR

PECTORALIS MAJOR

DELTOID

CORACOBRACHIALIS

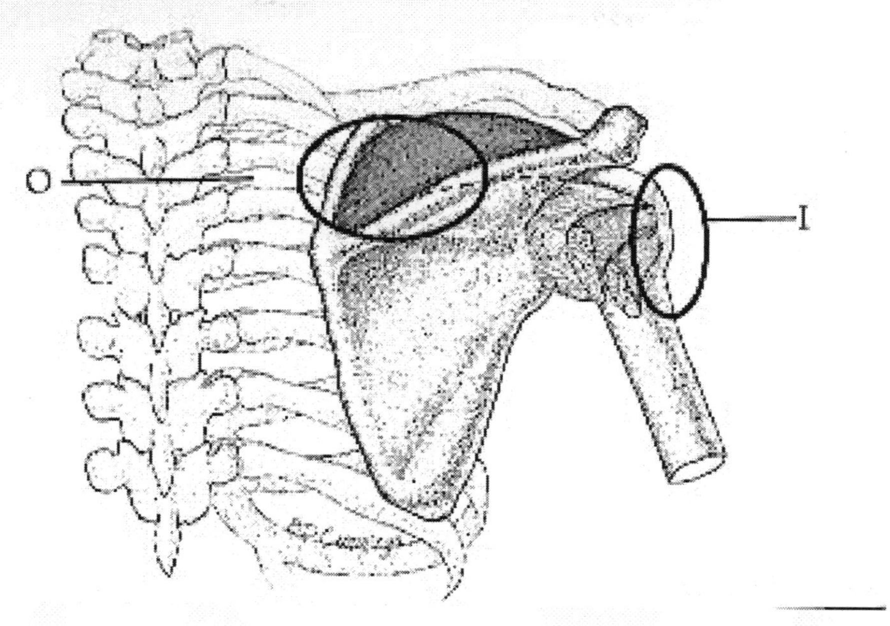

SUPRASPINATUS
(SUE-PRAH-SPY-NAYE-TUS)

Origin:
Supraspinous fossa of the scapula

Insertion:
Superior part of greater tubercle of humerus

True Function:

- *Assist in concentric acceleration of humeral abduction*
- *Assist in eccentric deceleration of humeral adduction*
- *Works synergistically with the other rotator cuff musculature to dynamically stabilize the humeral head in the glenoid fossa*
- *Initiates abduction and dynamic caudal glide while the deltoid acts as the prime mover during shoulder abduction*

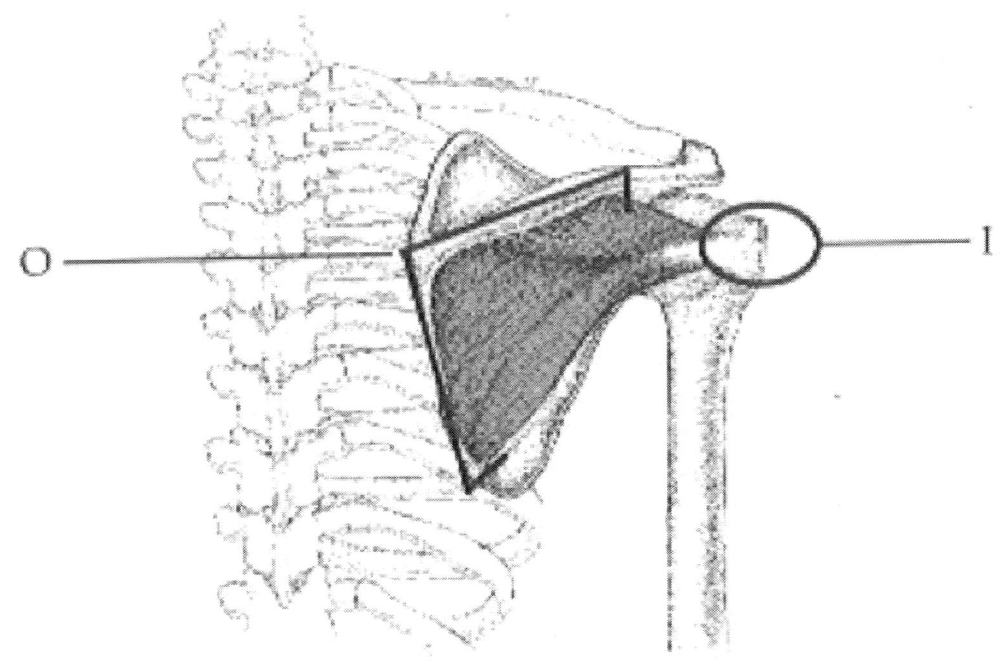

INFRASPINATUS
(IN-FRAH-SPY-NAYE-TUS)

Origin:
Infraspinous fossa of scapula

Insertion:
Greater tubercle of humerus posterior to insertion of supraspinatus

True Function:

- *Assists in eccentric decelerating of internal rotation of the humerus*
- *Works synergistically with the other rotator cuff musculature to dynamically stabilize the humeral head in the glenoid fossa during functional movements*
- *Works synergistically to produce dynamic caudal glide of the humeral head in the glenoid fossa during elevation*
- *Works as an integrated functional unit with the capsule, ligaments, and other cuff musculature to enhance stability and proprioception during functional movements (ligamento-muscular protective reflex)*

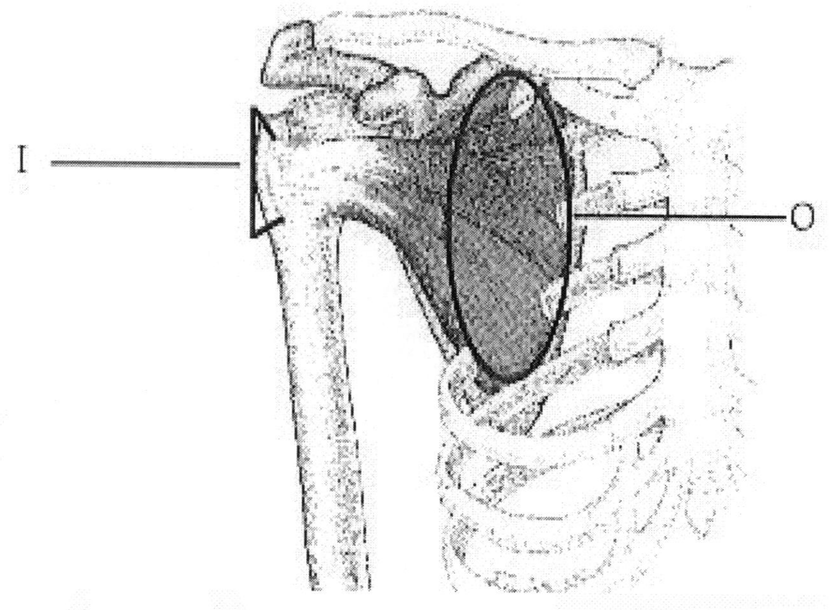

TERES MINOR
(TEH-REZ)

Origin:
Lateral border of scapula, dorsal side

Insertion:
Greater tubercle of humerus inferior to infraspinatus insertion

True Function:

- *Assists in concentric acceleration of external rotation of the humerus*
- *Assists in eccentric deceleration of internal rotation of the humerus*
- *Works synergistically with the other rotator cuff musculature to dynamically stabilize the humeral head in the glenoid fossa during dynamic activity*
- *Works synergistically to produce a dynamic caudal glide of the humeral head in the glenoid fossa during elevation to prevent impingement*
- *Works as an integrated functional unit with the capsule, ligaments, and other cuff musculature to enhance stability and proprioception during functional movements (ligamento-muscular protective reflex)*

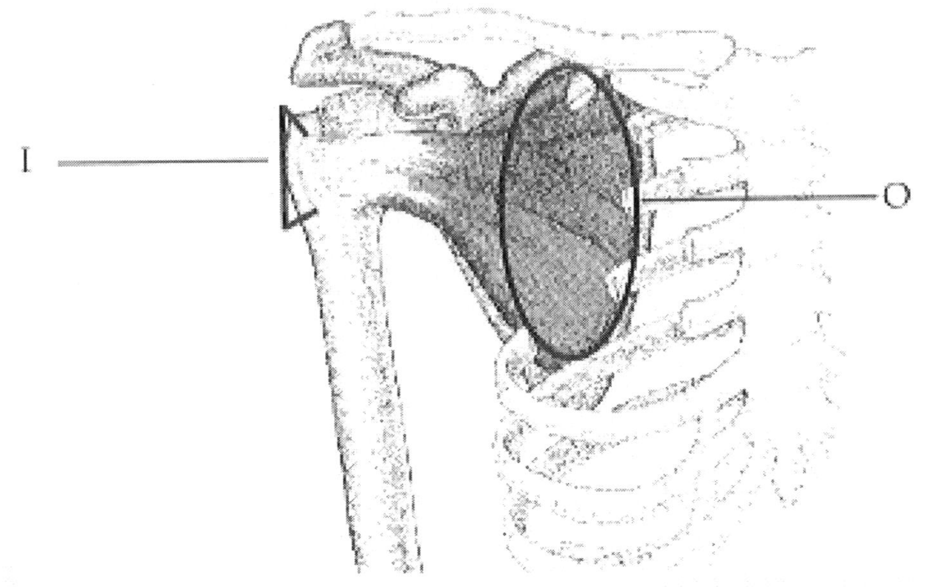

SUBSCAPULARIS
(SUB-SCAP-U-LAHR-US)

Origin:
Subscapular fossa of scapula

Insertion:
Lesser tubercle of humerus

True Function:
- *Assists in concentric acceleration of internal rotation of the humerus*
- *Assists in eccentric deceleration of external rotation of the humerus*
- *Works synergistically with the other rotator cuff musculature to stabilize the humeral head in the glenoid fossa during functional activities*

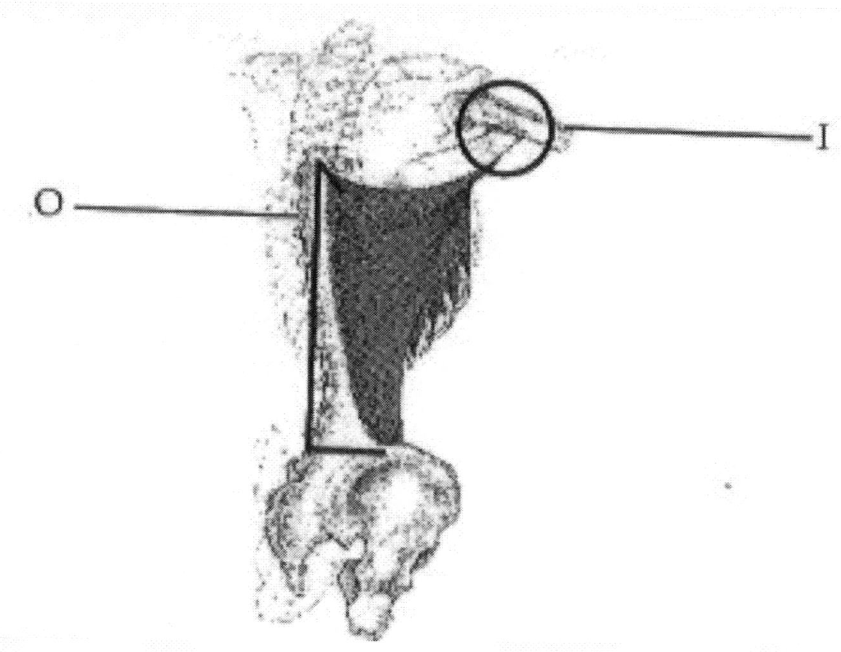

LATISSIMUS DORSI
(LAH-TISS-I-MUS DOR-SEYE)

Origin:
Indirect attachment via thoracolumbar fascia into spines of the lower six thoracic vertebrae, lumbar vertebrae, lower three to four ribs and iliac crest, also from scapula's inferior angle

Insertion:
Spirals around teres major to insert on the anterior humerus

True Function:

- *Assists in concentric acceleration of adduction of the humerus*
- *Assists in concentric acceleration of extension of the humerus*
- *Assists in concentric acceleration of internal rotation of the humerus*
- *Assists in eccentric deceleration of flexion of the humerus*
- *Assists in eccentric deceleration of external rotation of the humerus*
- *Assists in dynamic stabilization of the lumbo-pelvic hip complex through the thoracolumbar fascia mechanism (Posterior Oblique System)*

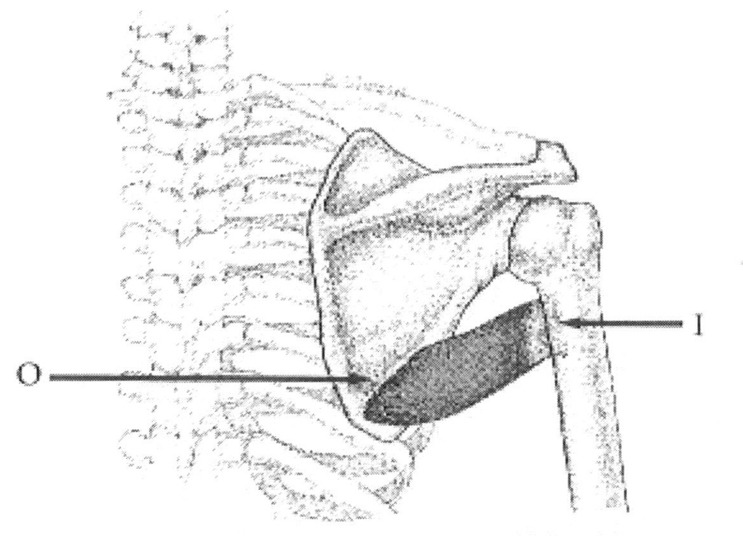

TERES MAJOR
(TEH-REZ)

Origin:
Posterior surface of scapula at inferior angle

Insertion:
Lesser tubercle on anterior humerus; insertion tendon fused with that of the latissimus dorsi

True Function:
- *Assists in concentric acceleration of adduction of the humerus*
- *Assists in concentric acceleration of internal rotation of the humerus*
- *Assists in concentric acceleration of extension of the shoulder*
- *Assists in eccentric deceleration of abduction of the humerus*
- *Assists in eccentric deceleration of external rotation of the humerus*
- *Assists in eccentric deceleration of the flexion of the shoulder*
- *Assists in dynamic stabilization of the glenohumeral joint*

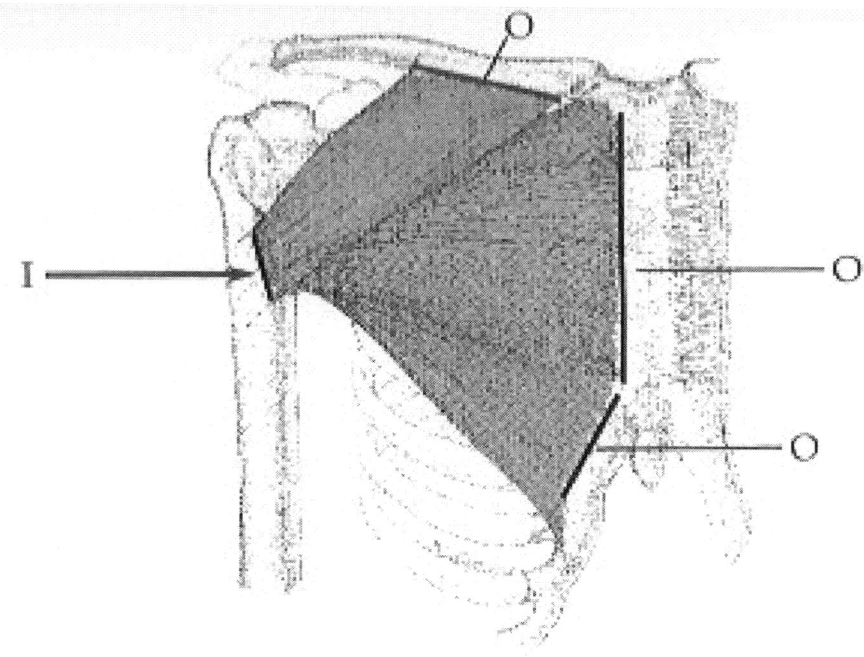

PECTORALIS MAJOR
(PECK-TOE-RA-LIS)

Origin:
Anterior Surfaces of ribs 3-5

Insertion:
Coracoid process of scapula

True Function:
- *Assists in concentric acceleration of scapular protraction*
- *Assists in eccentric deceleration of scapular retraction*
- *Assists in dynamic stabilization of the scapula during functional movements*

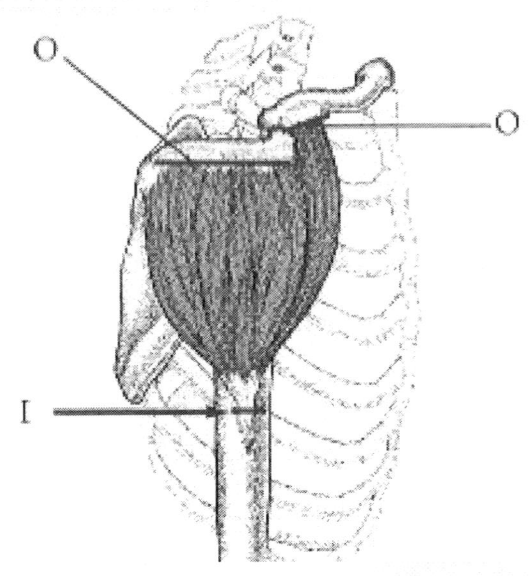

DELTOID
(DELL-TOYD)

Origin:
Embraces insertion of the trapezius, lateral third of clavicle, acromion, and spine of scapula

Insertion:
Deltoid tuberosity of humerus

True Function:
- *Assists in concentric acceleration of shoulder flexion and extension*
- *Assists in concentric acceleration of shoulder abduction and horizontal adduction*
- *Assists in concentric acceleration of internal and external rotation of the shoulder*
- *ALL: assists in dynamic stabilization of the glenohumeral joint during functional movements*
- *ANTERIOR DELTOID: Assists in eccentric deceleration of shoulder extension and external rotation, works as a neutralizer during shoulder abduction*
- *MIDDLE DELTOID: Assists in eccentric deceleration of shoulder adduction*
- *POSTERIOR DELTOID: Assists in eccentric deceleration of shoulder flexion, internal rotation and horizontal adduction, works as a neutralizer during shoulder abduction*

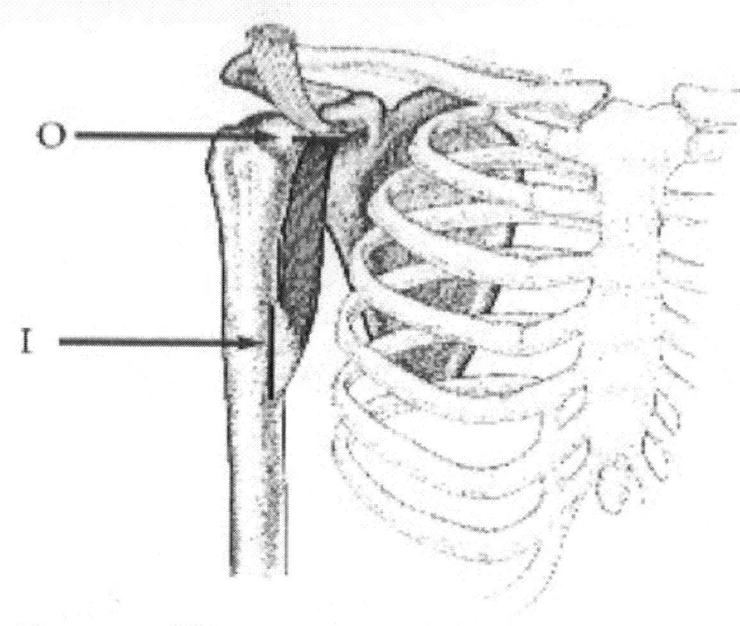

CORACOBRACHIALIS
(CORE-AH-KO-BRAY-KEE-AL-US)

Origin:
Coracoid process of scapula

Insertion:
Medial surface of humerus shaft

True Function:
- *Assists in concentric acceleration of shoulder flexion*
- *Assists in concentric acceleration of shoulder adduction*
- *Assists in eccentric deceleration of shoulder extension*
- *Assists in eccentric deceleration of shoulder abduction*
- *Assists in dynamic stabilization of the shoulder complex*

SECTION 4: ELBOW JOINT MUSCULATURE

BICEPS BRACHII

BRACHIALIS

BRACHIORADIALIS

TRICEPS BRACHII

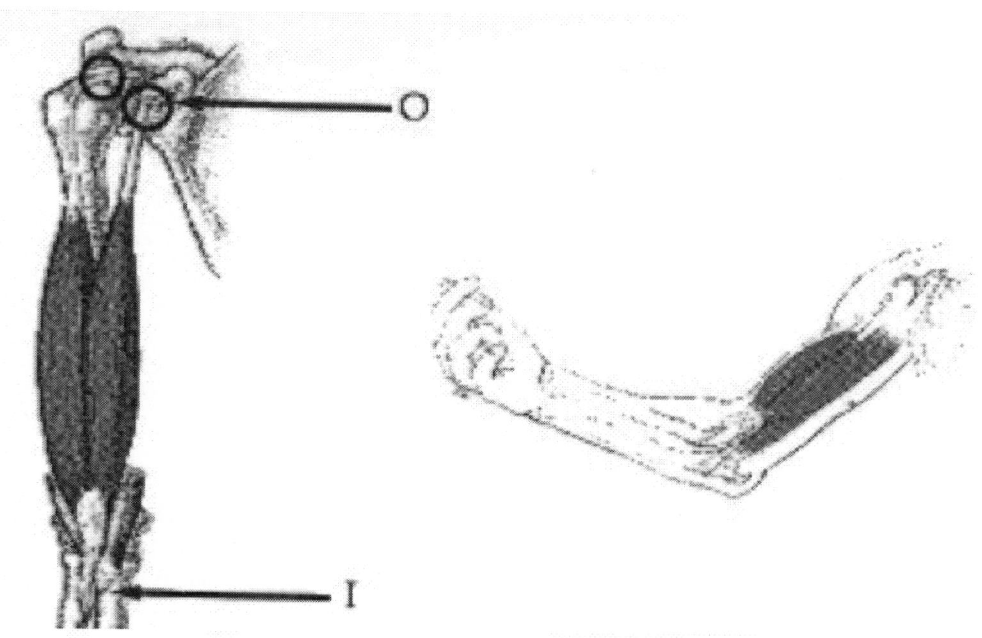

BICEPS BRACHII
(BI-SEPS BRAY-KEE-EYE)

Origin:
Short Head: coracoid process
Long Head: tubercle above glenoid cavity and lip of glenoid

Insertion:
By tendon into the radial tuberosity

True Function:

- *Assists in concentric acceleration of elbow flexion*
- *Assists in concentric acceleration of supination of the radio-ulnar joint*
- *Assist in concentric acceleration of shoulder flexion*
- *Assists in eccentric deceleration of elbow extension*
- *Assists in eccentric decelerates pronation of the radioulnar joint*
- *Assists in eccentric deceleration of shoulder extension*
- *Assists in dynamic stabilization of the humeral head during functional movements*

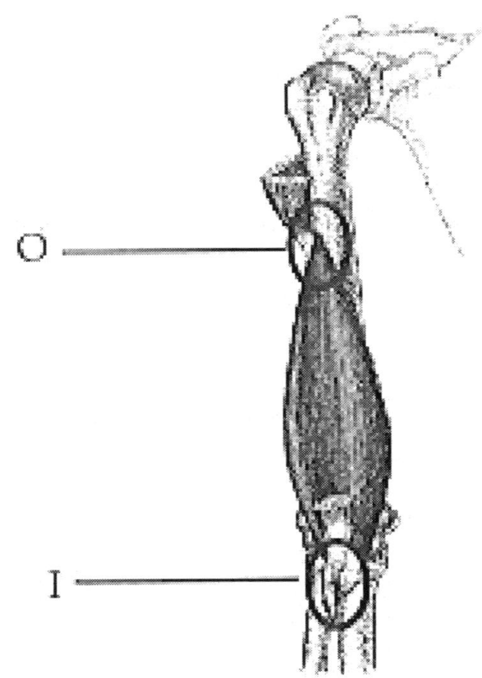

BRACHIALIS
(BRAY-KEE-AL-US)

Origin:
Anterior Aspect of distal half of humerus

Insertion:
Coronoid process of ulna and capsule of elbow joint

True Function:
- *Assists in concentric acceleration of elbow flexion*
- *Assists in eccentric deceleration of elbow extension*
- *Assists in dynamic stabilization of the elbow complex*

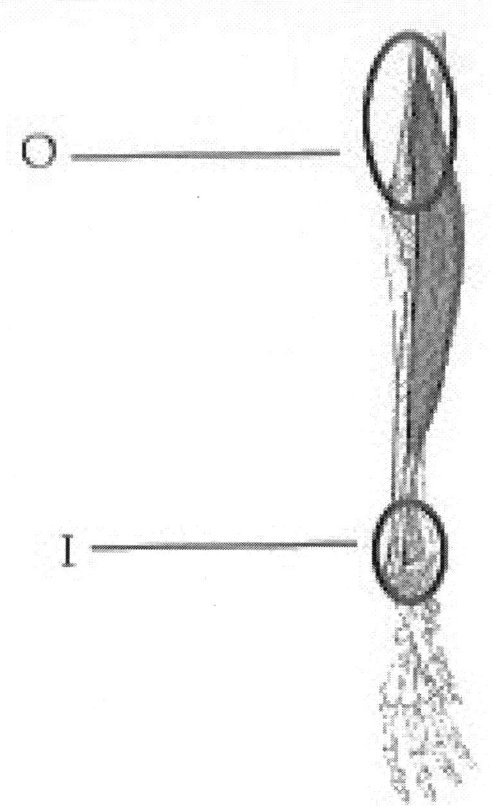

BRACHIORADIALIS
(BRAY-KEE-O-RAY-DEE-AL-US)

Origin:
Distal 1/3 of humerus

Insertion:
Distal 1/3 of radius

True Function:

- *Assist in concentric acceleration of elbow flexion*
- *Assists in eccentric deceleration of elbow extension*
- *Assists in dynamic stabilization of the elbow complex*

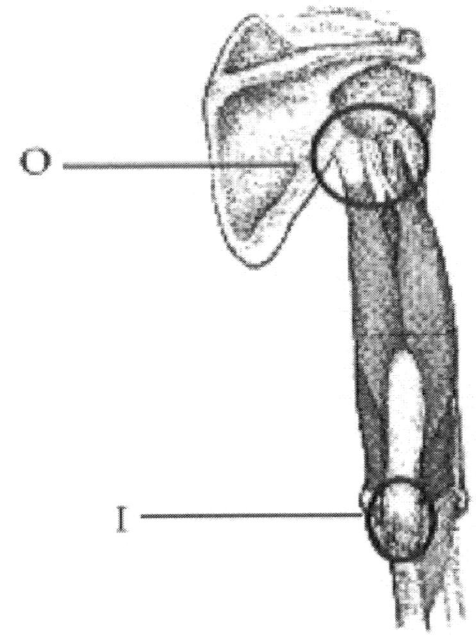

TRICEPS BRACHII
(TRY-SEPS BRAY-KEE-EYE)

Origin:
Long Head: infraglenoid tubercle of scapula
Lateral Head: posterior humerus
Medial Head: posterior humerus

Insertion:
By tendon into olecranon process of ulna

True Function:

- Assists in concentric acceleration of elbow extension
- Assists in concentric acceleration of shoulder extension
- Assists in eccentric deceleration of elbow flexion
- Assists in eccentric deceleration of shoulder flexion
- Assists in dynamic stabilization of the glenohumeral joint

SECTION 5: HIP JOINT MUSCULATURE

GLUTEUS MAXIMUS
GLUTEUS MEDIUS
GLUTEUS MINIMUS
ADDUCTORS
GRACILIS
SARTORIUS
PIRIFORMIS
PECTINEUS
PSOAS MAJOR
ILIACUS
TENSOR FASCIAE LATAE

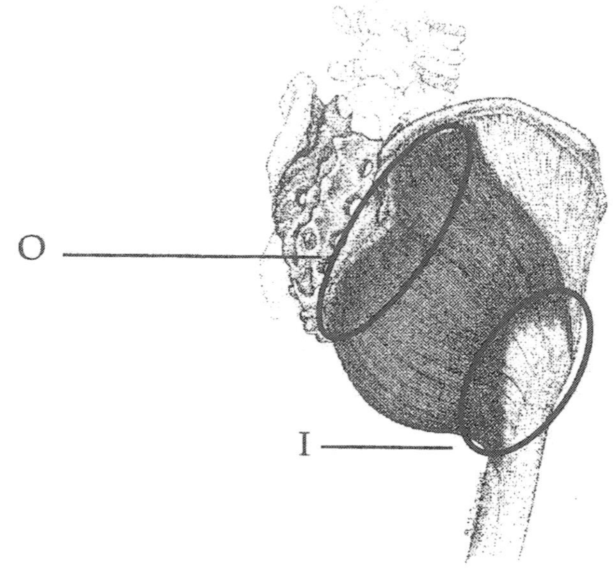

GLUTEUS MAXIMUS
(GLOO-TEE-US MAX-UH-MUS)

Origin:
Iliac crest, sacrum, coccyx and the sacrotuberus and sacroiliac ligaments

Insertion:
Iliotibial tract of fascia lata and gluteal tuberosity of femur

True Function:
- *Concentric acceleration of hip extension*
- *Assists in concentric acceleration of hip external rotation*
- *Eccentric deceleration of hip flexion, hip adduction, and hip internal rotation during the stance phase*
- *Assists in dynamic stabilization of the sacroiliac joint via the sacrotuberus ligament and the lateral knee via the iliotibial band*

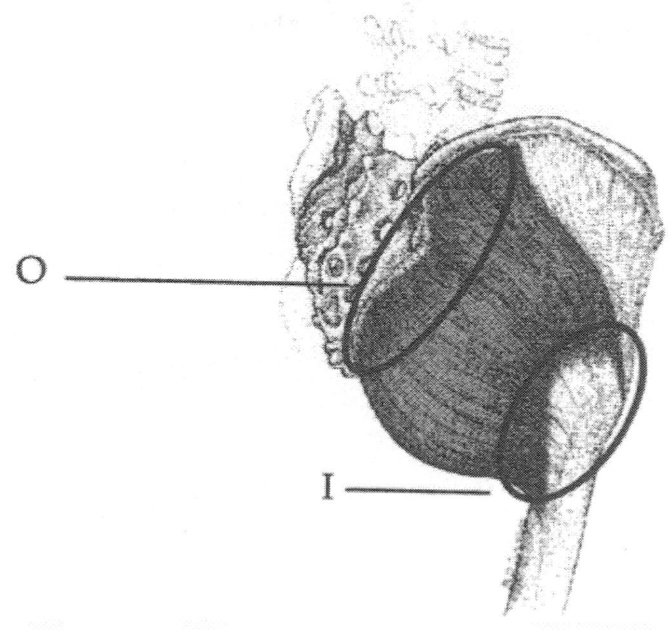

GLUTEUS MEDIUS
(GLUE-TEE-US MEE-DEE-US)

Origin:
The ilium, between the PSIS and iliac crest

Insertion:
Greater trochanter of femur

True Function:

- *Assist in concentric acceleration of femur abduction*
- *Assist in eccentric deceleration of hip adduction and*
- *Assists in dynamic stabilization of the lumbo-pelvic-hip complex in the frontal plane*
- *Anterior Fibers:*
    - *Assist in concentric acceleration of hip internal rotation*
    - *Assist in eccentric deceleration of hip external rotation*
- *Posterior Fibers:*
    - *Assist in concentric acceleration of hip external rotation*
    - *Assist in eccentric deceleration*

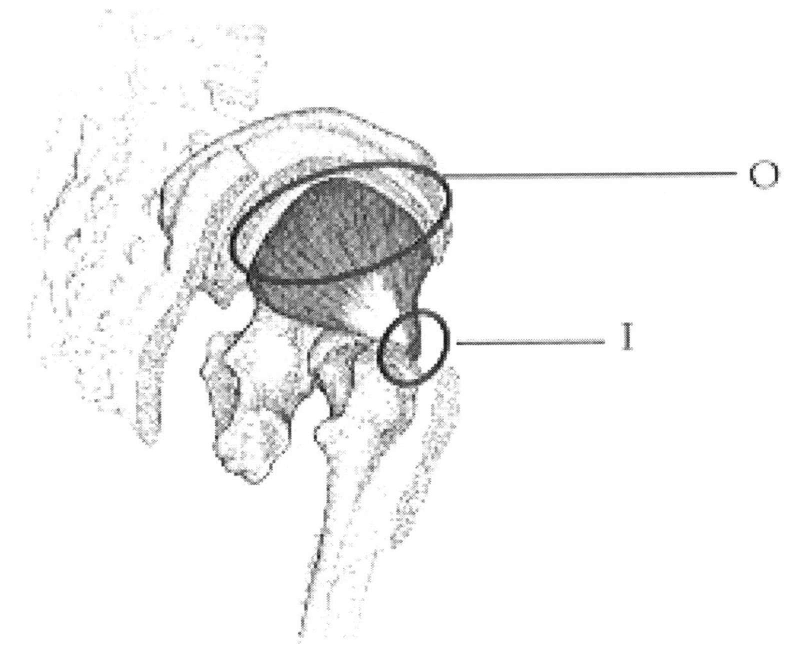

GLUTEUS MINIMUS
(GLUE-TEE-US MIH-NUH-MUS)

Origin:
Ilium, deep to the gluteus medius

Insertion:
Greater trochanter of femur

True Function:
- *Assists in concentric acceleration of hip abduction*
- *Assists in concentric acceleration of hip internal rotation*
- *Assists in eccentric deceleration of hip adduction*
- *Assists in eccentric deceleration of hip external rotation*
- *Assists in dynamic stabilization of the lumbo-pelvic hip complex*

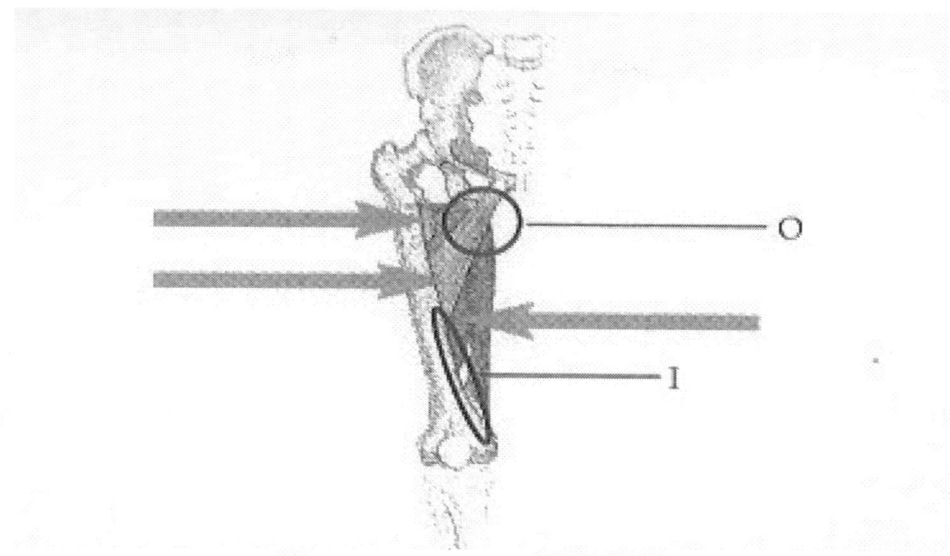

ADDUCTOR COMPLEX
(AH-DUK-TORES LON-GUS, BREH-VIS, MAG-NUS)

1. Adductor Longus 2. Adductor Brevis 3. Adductor Magnus

Origin:
1. *Pubic tubercle*
2. *Inferior ramus of pubis*
3. *Inferior ramus of pubis, ramus of ischium and ischial tuberosity*

Insertion:
1. *Medial lip of the linea aspera*
2. *Pectineal line and medial lip of linea aspera*
3. *The adductor tubercle and lateral lip of linea aspera*

True Function:
- *Assists in concentric acceleration of femoral adduction, flexion, and internal rotation*
- *The adductor magnus assists in concentric acceleration of hip extension*
- *Assists in dynamic stabilization of the LPHC during functional movements*
- *Assists in eccentric deceleration of femoral abduction, extension, and external rotation*
- *The Adductor Magnus assists in eccentric deceleration of hip flexion*

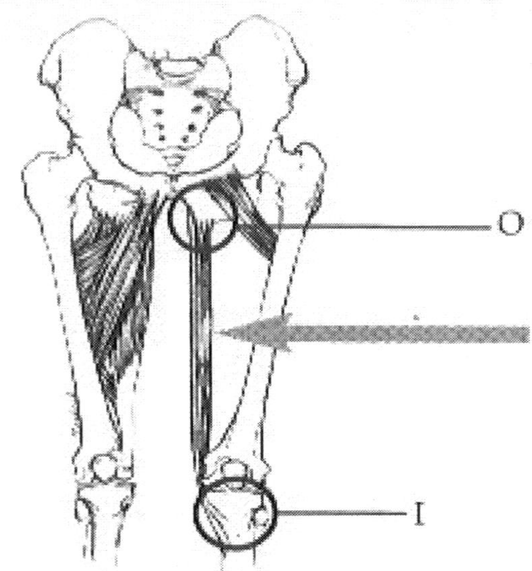

GRACILIS
(GRASS-ILL-US)

Origin:
Pubic symphysis and pubic ramus

Insertion:
Proximal, medial surface of tibia, joining at the Pes Anserinus tendon

True Function:

- *Assists in concentric acceleration of adduction of the femur*
- *Assists in concentric acceleration of internal rotation of the femur*
- *Assists in eccentric deceleration of knee extension prior to heel strike*
- *Assists in eccentric deceleration of hip abduction*
- *Assists in dynamic stabilization of the hip in the frontal plane and the knee in transverse plane*

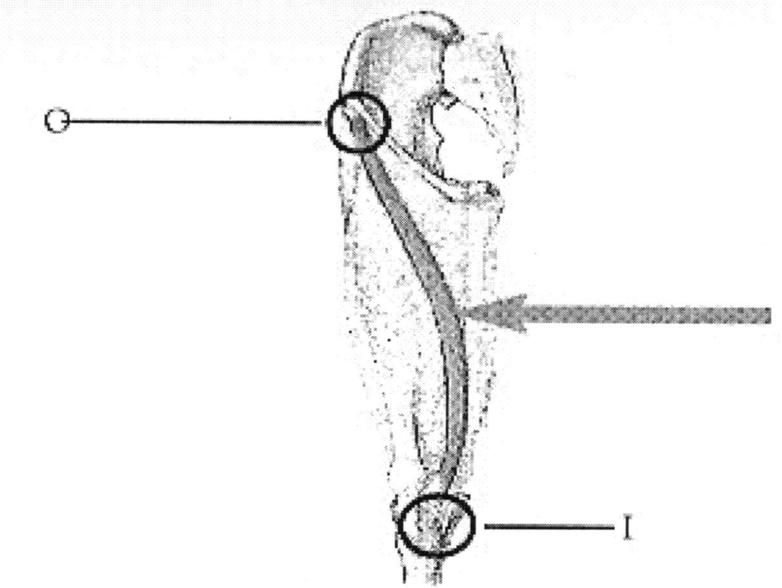

SARTORIUS
(SAR-TOR-EE-US)

Origin:
Anterior superior iliac spine (ASIS)

Insertion:
Proximal, medial surface of tibia, joining at the Pes Anserinus tendon

True Function:

- *Assists in concentric acceleration of internal rotation of the tibia*
- *Assists in concentric acceleration of abduction of the tibia*
- *Assists in concentric acceleration of knee flexion*
- *Assists in concentric acceleration of hip flexion and hip external rotation*
- *Assists in eccentric deceleration of external rotation of the tibia*
- *Assists in eccentric deceleration of adduction of the tibia*
- *Assists in eccentric deceleration of knee extension*
- *Assists in eccentric deceleration of hip extension and hip internal rotation*
- *Assists in dynamic stabilization of the lumbo-pelvic-hip complex, ilio-femoral joint and the tibio-femoral joint*

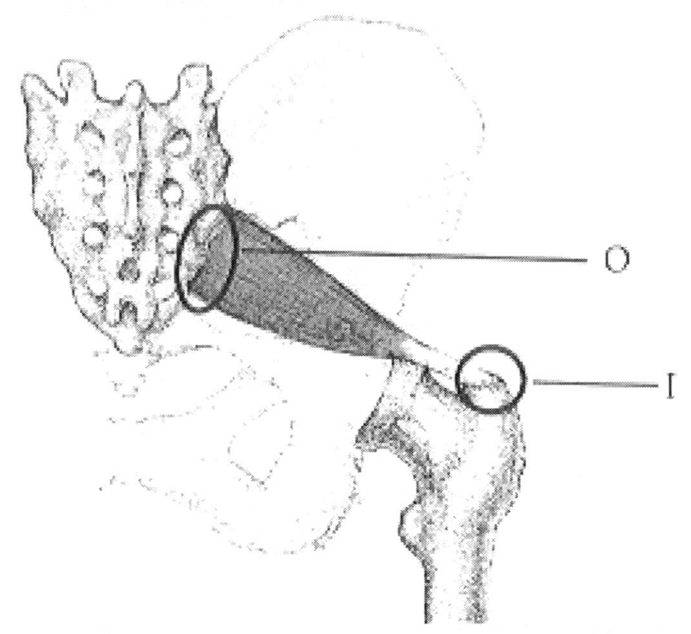

PIRIFORMUS
(PER-IH-FORM-US)

Origin:
Anterior aspect of the sacrum

Insertion:
Superior border of the greater trochanter of the femur

True Function:

- *Concentric acceleration of external rotation of the hip*
- *Assists in concentric acceleration of hip extension*
- *Assists in concentric acceleration of hip abduction when the hip is flexed*
- *Assists in eccentric deceleration of internal rotation of the hip*
- *Assists in eccentric deceleration of hip flexion*
- *Assists in eccentric deceleration of hip adduction when the hip is flexed*
- *Assists in dynamic stabilization of the lumbo-pelvic hip complex*
- *Assists in providing pelvo-femoral dynamic stabilization during function movements*

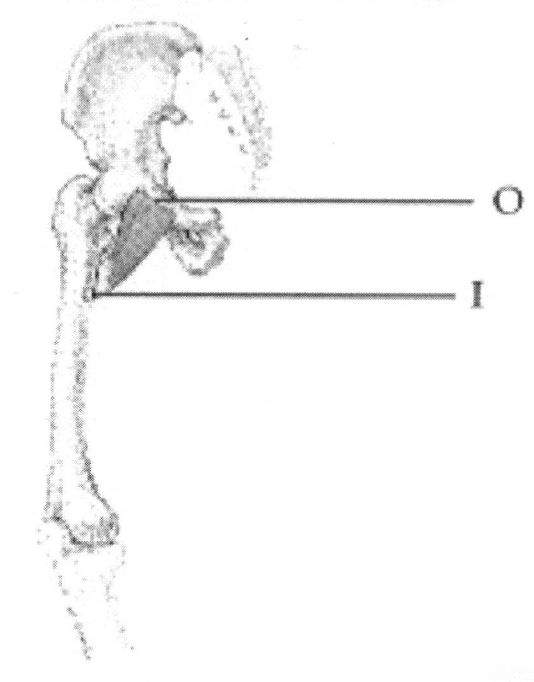

PECTINEUS
(PECK-TIN-EE-US)

Origin:
Superior Ramus of pubis

Insertion:
Pectineal line of femur, between lesser trochanter and linea aspera

True Function:
- *Assists in concentric acceleration of femur adduction*
- *Assists in concentric acceleration of internal rotation of the hip*
- *Asssits in eccentric deceleration of abduction of the femur*
- *Assists in eccentric deceleration of external rotation of the hip*
- *Assists in dynamic stabilization of the lumbo-pelvic-hip complex*

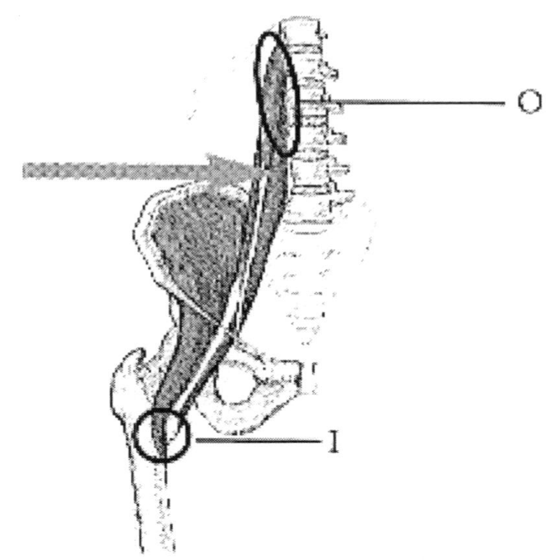

PSOAS MAJOR
(SO-US)

Origin:
Transverse processes and bodies of lumbar vertebrae

Insertion:
Lesser trochanter of femur

True Function:

- *Assists in concentric acceleration of hip flexion*
- *Assist in concentric acceleration of hip external rotation*
- *Assists in eccentric deceleration of hip extension*
- *Assists in eccentric deceleration of femoral internal rotation at heel strike*
- *Assists in dynamic stabilization of the lumbo-pelvic-hip complex during functional movements*

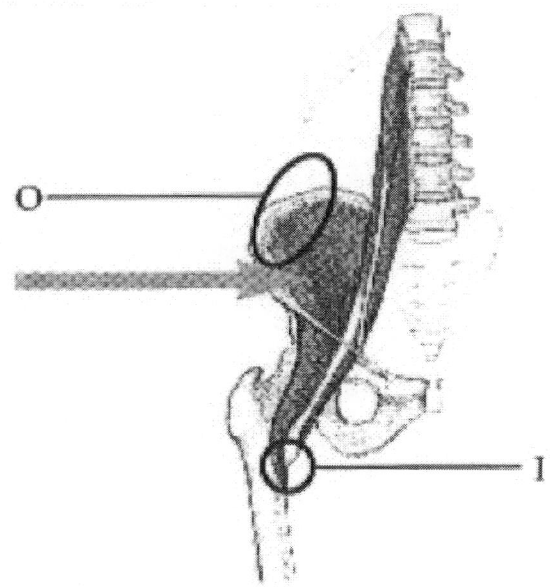

ILIACUS
(ILL-EE-AK-US)

Origin:
Illiac fossa

Insertion:
The lesser trochanter of the femur

True Function:
- *Assists in concentric acceleration of the flexion of the hip*
- *Assists in concentric acceleration of hip external rotation*
- *Assists in eccentric deceleration of hip extension*
- *Assists in eccentric deceleration of femoral internal rotation at heel strike*
- *Assists in dynamic stabilization of the lumbar spine during functional movements*

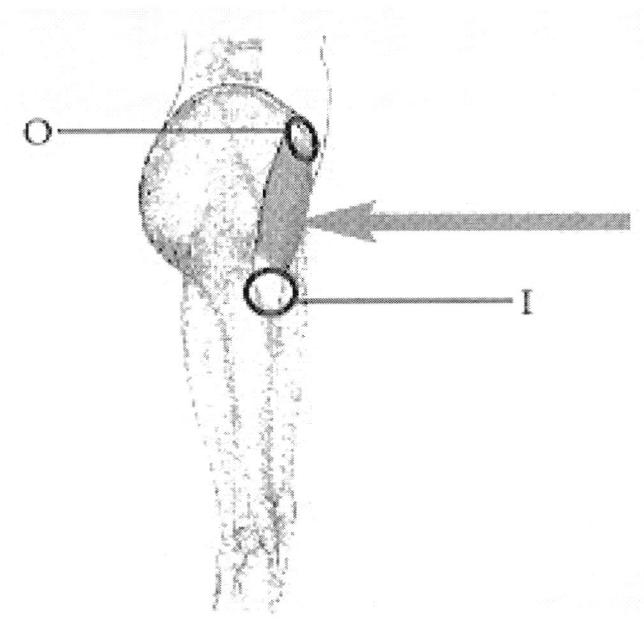

TENSOR FASCIAE LATAE
(TEN-SOR FA-SHEE-UH LA-TAH)

Origin:
Iliac crest, posterior to the ASIS

Insertion:
Tibia by way of the iliotibial tract

True Function:
- *Assists in concentric acceleration of hip flexion*
- *Assists in concentric acceleration of hip abduction*
- *Assists in concentric acceleration of internal rotation of the hip*
- *Assists in eccentric deceleration of hip extension*
- *Assists in eccentric deceleration of hip adduction*
- *Assists in eccentric deceleration of external rotation of the hip*
- *Assists in dynamic stabilization of the lumbo-pelvic-hip complex and the tibio-femoral joint*

SECTION 6:
KNEE JOINT MUSCULATURE

RECTUS FEMORIS
VASTUS INTERMEDIUS
VASTUS LATERALIS
VASTUS MEDIALIS
VASTUS FEMORIS
SEMIMEMBRANOSUS
SEMITENDINOSUS

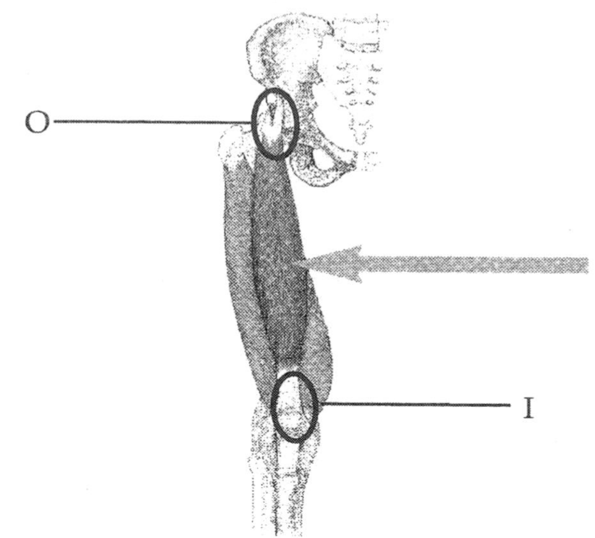

RECTUS FEMORIS
(REK-TUS)

Origin:
Anterior inferior iliac spine (AIIS)

Insertion:
Tibial tuberosity by way of patellar tendon

True Function:

- *Assists in concentric acceleration of knee extension*
- *Assists in concentric acceleration of hip flexion*
- *Assists in eccentric deceleration of knee flexion, adduction, and internal rotation during heel strike*
- *Assists in dynamic stabilization of the knee during functional movement patterns*
- *Assists in deceleration of hip extension and knee flexion during functional movement patterns*
- *Assists in dynamic stabilization of the ilio-femoral joint*

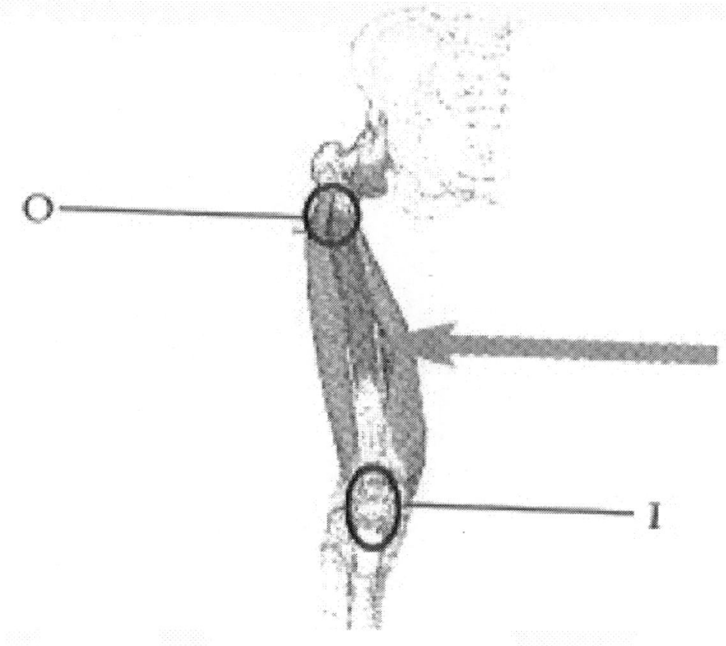

VASTUS INTERMEDIUS
(VAS-TUS IN-TER-MEE-DEE-US)

Origin:
Anterior and lateral surfaces of body of the femur

Insertion:
Tibial tuberosity through the patellar tendon

True Function:
- *Assists in concentric acceleration of knee extension*
- *Assists in eccentric deceleration of knee flexion, adduction and internal rotation during heel strike*
- *Assists in dynamic stabilization of the knee during functional movement patterns*

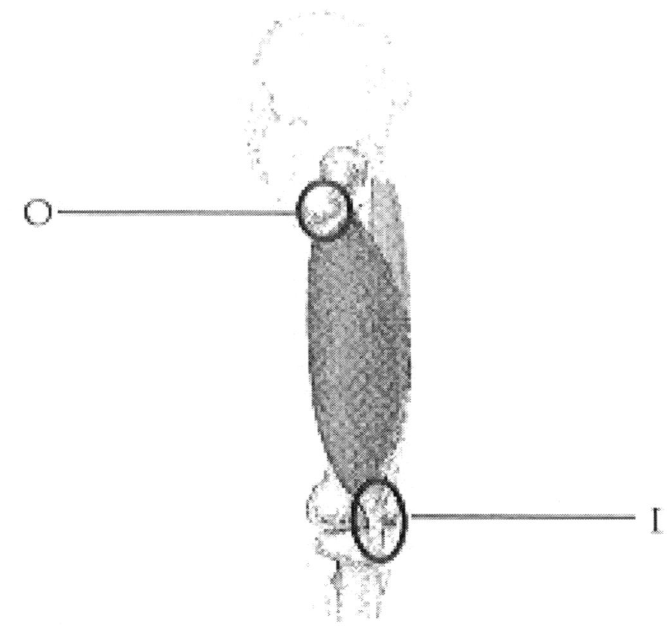

VASTUS LATERALIS
(VAS-TUS LAT-ER-AH-LUS)

Origin:
Greater trochanter and linea aspera of the femur

Insertion:
Tibial tuberosity through the patellar tendon

True Function:
- *Assists in concentric acceleration of knee extension*
- *Assists in eccentric deceleration of knee flexion, adduction and internal rotation during heel strike*
- *Assists in dynamic stabilization of the knee during functional movement patterns*

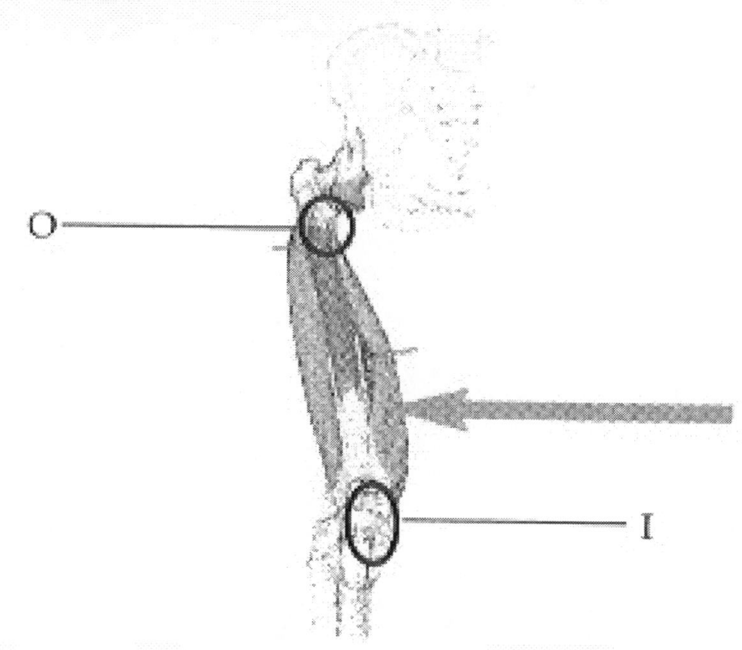

VASTUS MEDIALIS
(VAS-TUS MEE-DEE-AH-LUS)

Origin:
Linea aspera of the femur

Insertion:
Tibial tuberosity through the patellar tendon

True Function:

- *Assists in concentric acceleration of knee extension*
- *Assists in eccentric deceleration of knee flexion, adduction and internal rotation during heel strike*
- *Assists in dynamic stabilization of the knee during functional movement*
- *patterns*
- *Assists in dynamic stabilization of the patella-femoral joint*

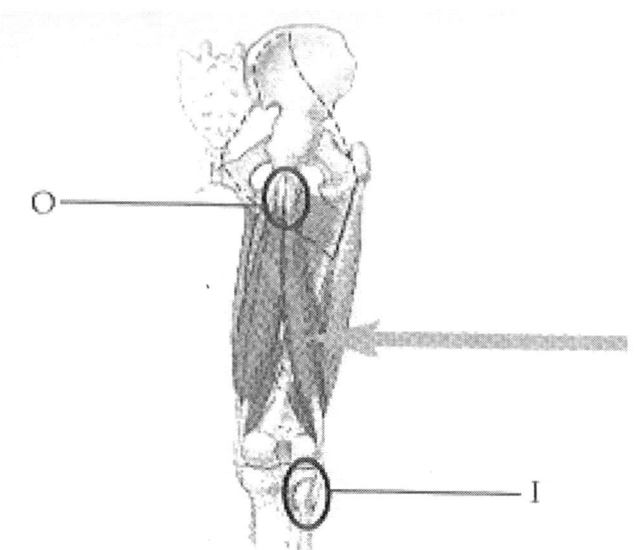

BICEPS FEMORIS
(BI-SEPS FEM-O-RIS)

1. ***Short head of bicep femoris***

Origin:
1. Linea aspera of the femur

Insertion:
1. Head of fibula and lateral condyle of tibia

2. ***Long head of bicep femoris***

Origin:
2. Ischial tuberosity

Insertion:
2. Head of fibula and lateral condyle of tibia

True Function:

- *Assists in concentric acceleration of knee flexion, hip extension and external tibial rotation*
- *Assists in eccentric deceleration of knee extension, hip flexion, and internal rotation at heel strike*
- *Assists in eccentric deceleration of iliosacral anterior rotation during functional movements*
- *Assists in dynamic stabilization of the lumbo-pelvic-hip complex during functional movement patterns*
- *Assists in dynamic stabilization of the proximal tibio-fibular joint*

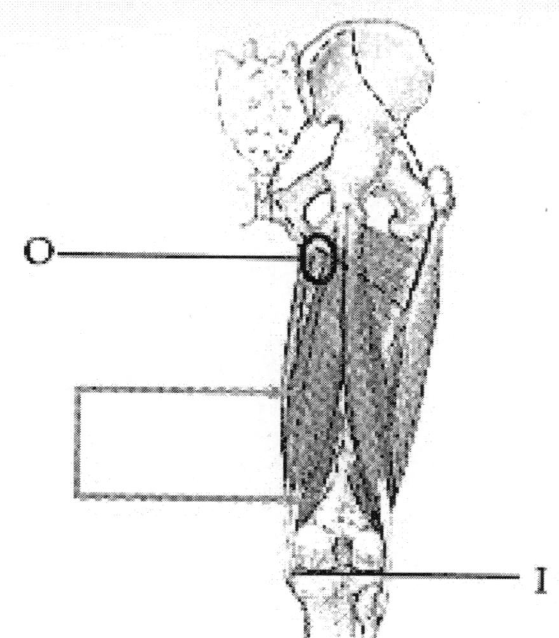

SEMIMEMBRANOSUS
(SEM-EE-MEM-BRAH-NO-SUS)

Origin:
Ischial tuberosity

Insertion:
Medial condyle of the tibia

True Function:
- *Assists in concentric acceleration of knee flexion*
- *Assists in concentric acceleration of hip extension*
- *Assists in concentric acceleration of internal rotation of the tibia*
- *Assists in eccentric deceleration of knee extension prior to heel strike and eccentric deceleration of hip flexion at heel strike*
- *Assists in eccentric deceleration of iliosacral anterior rotation during functional movements*
- *Assists in dynamic stabilization of the lumbo-pelvic-hip complex during functional movement patterns*
- *Assists in dynamic stabilization of the tibio-femoral joint*

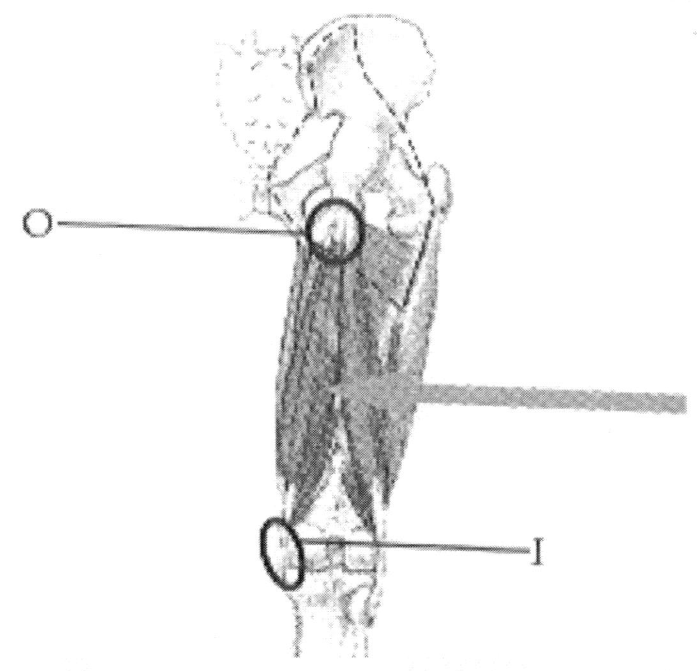

SEMITENDINOSUS
(SEM-EE-TEN-DEH-NO-SUS)

Origin:
Ischial tuberosity

Insertion:
Proximal part of the medial surface of the body of the tibia

True Function:
- *Assists in concentric acceleration of knee flexion*
- *Assists in concentric acceleration of hip extension*
- *Assists in concentric acceleration of tibia internal rotation*
- *Assists in eccentric deceleration of knee extension during swing phase and eccentric deceleration of hip flexion at heel strike*
- *Assists in eccentric deceleration of iliosacral anterior rotation during functional movements*
- *Assists in dynamic stabilization of the lumbo-pelvic-hip complex during functional movement patterns*
- *Assists in dynamic stabilization of the tibio-femoral joint*

SECTION 7: ANKLE JOINT MUSCULATURE

GASTROCNEMIUS
SOLEUS
TIBIALIS ANTERIOR
PERONEALS

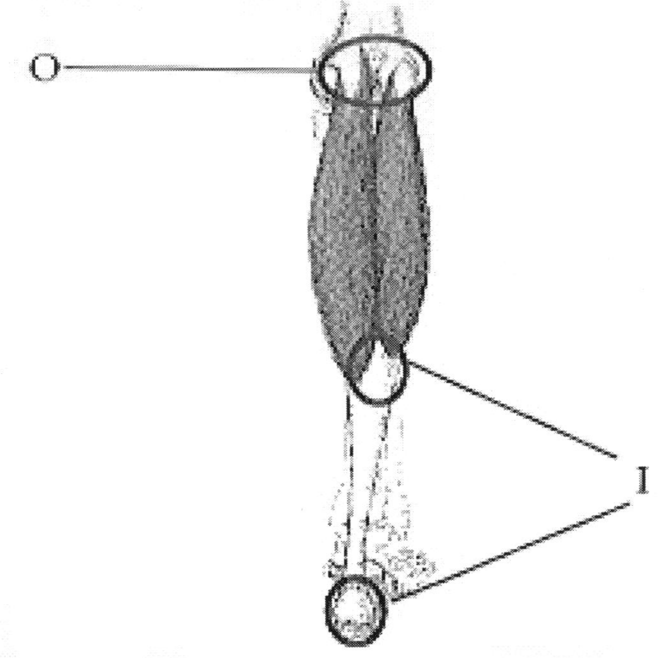

GASTROCNEMIUS
(GAS-TROCK-NEE-MEE-US)

Origin:
Lateral and medial condyles of femur and capsule of knee

Insertion:
Calcaneus by way of the Achilles tendon

True Function:

- *Assists in concentric acceleration of ankle plantar flexion*
- *Assists in concentric acceleration of knee flexion*
- *Assists in eccentric deceleration of femoral internal rotation and deceleration of subtalar joint pronation*
- *Assists in dynamic stabilization of the subtalar joint and tibio-femoral joint during transitional movements*
- *Accelerates subtalar joint supination at the end of mid-stance and is the prime mover during propulsion*
- *Assists in concentric acceleration of external rotation of the knee during propulsion*

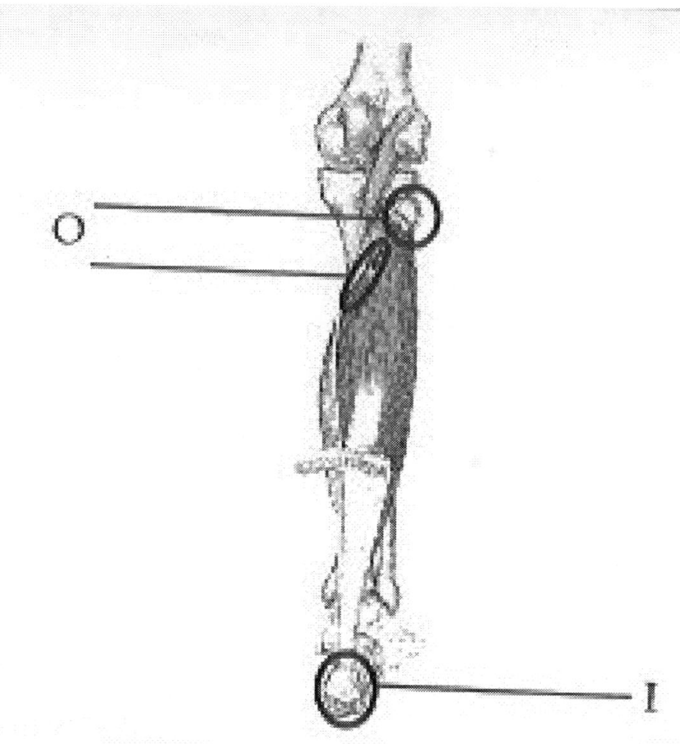

SOLEUS
(SO-LEE-US)

Origin:
Head of fibula and medial border of the tibia

Insertion:
Calcaneus by way of the Achilles tendon

True Function:

- *Assists in concentric acceleration of plantar flexion*
- *Assists in concentric acceleration of STJ supination*
- *Assists in eccentric deceleration of subtalar joint pronation and internal rotation of lower leg at heel strike*
- *Assists in dynamic stabilization of the subtalar joint during transitional movements*
- *Assists in extension of the knee during gait*

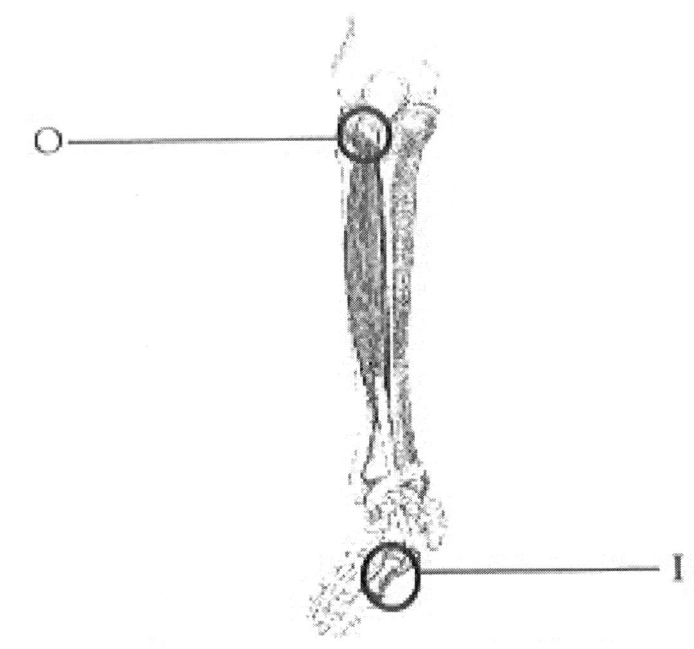

TIBIALIS ANTERIOR
(TIB-EE-AH-LUS)

Origin:
Lateral condyle and the body of the tibia

Insertion:
First metatarsal and first cuneiform

True Function:
- *Assists in concentric acceleration of ankle dorsiflexion at heel strike*
- *Assists in eccentric deceleration of everseion of the mid-foot during mid stance*
- *Assists in dynamic stabilization of the midtarsal joint during functional movements*
- *Assists in concentric acceleration of supination of the foot prior to heel strike*

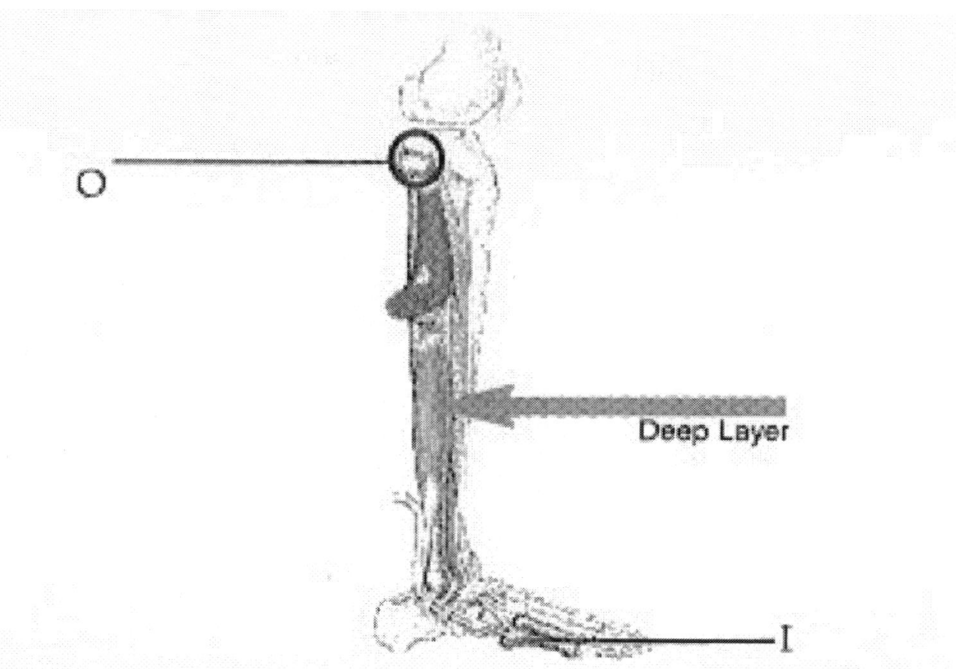

PERONEALS
(PER-O-NEE-ILLS)

1. ***Peroneus Brevis***

Origin:
1. Distal 2/3 of lateral fibula

Insertion:
2. Tuberosity of 5th metatarsal

2. ***Peroneus Longus***

Origin:
2. Proximal 2/3 of lateral fibula

Insertion:
2. Base of the 1st metatarsal and medial cuneiform

True Function:

- *Assists in concentric acceleration of eversion of the ankle*
- *Assists in concentric acceleration of ankle plantar flexion*
- *Assists eccentric deceleration of inversion of the subtalar joint during propulsion*
- *Assists in eccentric deceleration of ankle dorsiflexion*
- *Assists in dynamic stabilization of the first ray in the transverse plane allowing proper foot function*

CHAPTER FOURTEEN

Mechanics of Common Movements

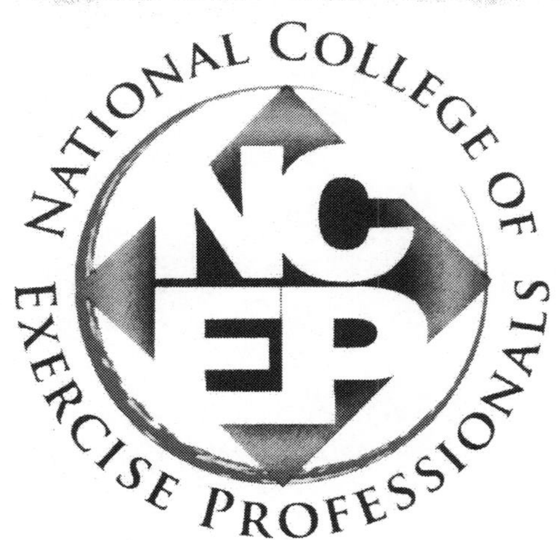

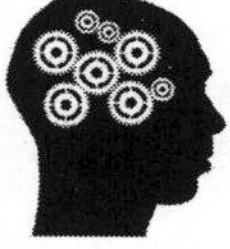

EXERCISE PROGRESSION

"Stability Before Mobility"

This short chapters offers tips for helping improve your clients' posture via a step-by-step progression. As discussed throughout this manual, proper posture is critical to your clients' quality of life, and knowing how to cue them for good posture is a useful tool.

Basic Progression to Strengthen Client's Postural Endurance

1. Find clients ideal alignment (neutral)
2. Teach awareness
3. Challenge ideal alignment

NOTE: *Sometimes, the ability to stabilize will depend on skill more than strength*

This chapter also has anatomy charts for the seven primary movements to study. *It is important to know the appropriate joints, actions, and muscles that are happening in each movement (i.e., correct form) before advancing your client to more difficult movements (including adding resistance).*

Seated Posture Trainer

Goal: To teach proper body alignment and increase postural control and strength.

Level 1: Stable platform (bench, chair)

1. Seated with arms crossed for comfort and to nullify temptation to push with the hands
2. Thighs parallel to ground (may have to manipulate to maintain neutral); note that thighs being too high encourages slouched posture
3. Extend the chest up
4. Head up over shoulders. Optimal: cheekbone bisecting with collarbone
5. Position pelvis in neutral (teach pelvic "rock" awareness)
6. Feet flat with a wide base of support
   -Determine the difficulty of this position by asking how the client "feels"
   -Depending on imbalances, this may be very challenging
   -Progress when seated for 1-3 minutes is not a challenge

Unstable Exercise Progressions

Different levels will depend on the client's level of control. Can your client maintain optimal alignment of their joints? If client deviates, you must correct! Progress slowly!

Examples:

- Smaller base of support
- Lift one leg up – switch
- Manual resistance
- No feet
- Close one eye – switch – both
- Unstable object under foot, progress to two unstable objects

EXERCISE AND JOINT ACTIONS
(CONCENTRIC PORTION)

SQUAT

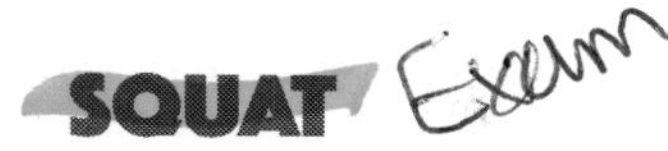

BONES	JOINTS	ACTION	MUSCLES
pelvis, femur	hip	hip extension	glutes, hamstrings
femur, tibia	knee	knee extension	quadriceps
tibia, talus, calcaneus	ankle	ankle plantar flexion	gastrocnemeous, soleus

PUSH

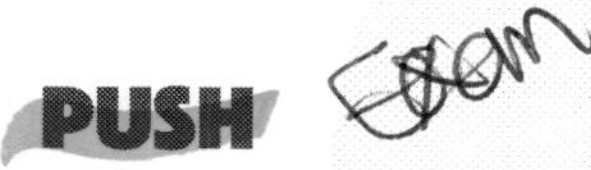

BONES	JOINTS	ACTION	MUSCLEs
humerus, radius, ulna	elbow	elbow extension	triceps
humerus, scapula, clavicle	GH shoulder	shoulder flexion or horizontal adduction	pectoralis, anterior deltoids
scapulae, thoracic vertebrae	ST Scapulo-thoracic	scapular abduction	serratus anterior

PULL

BONES	JOINTS	ACTION	MUSCLES
humerus, radius, ulna	elbow	elbow flexion	biceps
humerus, scapula, clavicle	GH shoulder	shoulder extension or adduction	latissimus dorsi, posterior deltoids
scapulae, thoracic vertebrae	ST Scapulo-thoracic	scapular adduction	rhomboids

BEND

BONES	JOINTS	ACTION	MUSCLES
vertebrae	spine	spinal flexion	rectus abdominus

TWIST

BONES	JOINTS	ACTION	MUSCLES
vertebrae	spine	spinal flexion and rotation	rectus abdominus, TVA, external obliques

LUNGE

BONES	JOINTS	ACTION	MUSCLES
pelvis, femur	hip	hip extension	glutes, hamstrings
femur, tibia	knee	knee extension	quadriceps
tibia, talus, calcaneus	ankle	ankle plantar flexion	gastrocnemius, soleus

GAIT
(SEE ADVANCED CURRICULUM)

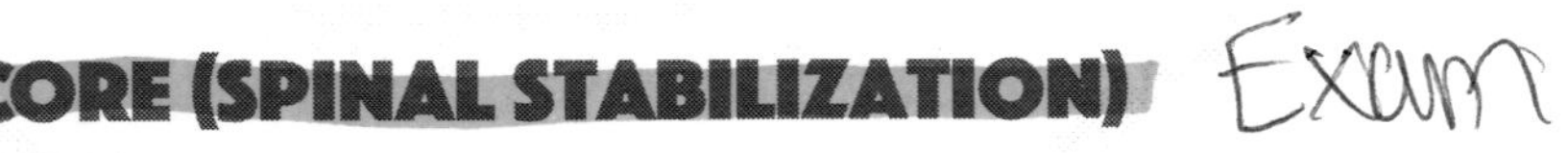

CORE (SPINAL STABILIZATION)

BONES	JOINTS	ACTION	MUSCLES
vertebrae	spine	stabilization	TVA (transverse abdominals)

CHAPTER FIFTEEN

Postural Dysfunctions

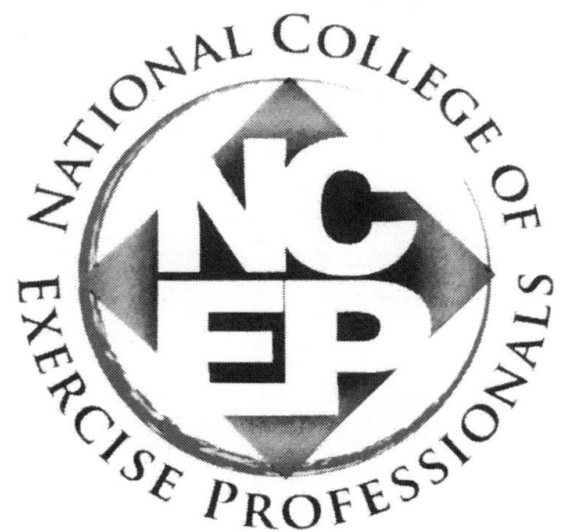

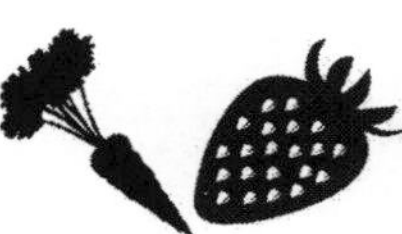

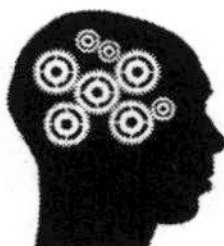

COMMON DYSFUNCTIONS

As an exercise professional and discussed throughout this manual, identifying your clients' posture is key to designing an excellent, individualized exericse program. This chapter explains, in detail, three of the most common postural dysfunctions that you will see.

ROUNDED SHOULDER PATTERN

HEALTH HISTORY ORTHOPEDIC AND LIFESTYLE INFORMATION	• Office job, sits large part of the day • Experiences some low back pain • Possible sore muscles: Levator scapulae, upper traps, SCM, rectus capitus, and scalenes • Mild pain or soreness between scapulae • Common injuries: rotator cuff, general shoulder problems, lateral epicondylitis, and eventually thoracic outlet syndrome • Headaches are common especially after being at the computer • Resistance training routines with too much pushing versus pulling especially heavy bench presses
POSTURAL ASSESSMENT EVALUATION	• Forward head • Rounded shoulders • No neck • Increased thoracic curve • Winging and/or tipping scapula
DYNAMIC ASSESSMENT EVALUATION	• Chin juts out during curl up assessment • Scapula wings during push-up assessment • Early/excessive scapula elevation during shoulder abduction
FLEXIBILITY	• Tight muscles: 1) pectoralis major/minor 2) levator scapulae 3) upper trapezius 4) latissimismus dorsi 5) subscapularis 6) SCM/rectus capitus/scalenes
CORE ASSESSMENT	• Weak lower abdominals • Inability to control TVA; drawing in maneuver • Over developed upper abdominals

NOTE: We do not diagnose or treat conditions. We are merely assessing and matching appropriate exercises.

ROUNDED SHOULDER PATTERN

FLEXIBILITY

STRETCH	SETS	REPS	TIME	NOTES
1. foam roll - *lats and upper back*	1	Only one to start	30 seconds to 2 minutes (what is tolerable)	May be tender, be very careful
2. neck - *stretch to all sides*	1	3-5 each side	About 10 seconds	DO NOT FORCE; ease into motion
3. chest - *passive and active*	1	3-5 each side	20-30 seconds each side	Ease into movement
4. lats - *up on a ball or table*	1	3-5 each side	20-30 seconds each side	Keep humerus externally rotated

RESISTANCE EXERCISES

BODY PART	EXERCISE	REPS	SETS	REST	NOTES
PULL (upper body stabilization)	*PRONE COBRA*	15 with 10 seconds on/off	1-3	1-2 minutes	Keep head parallel to ground, very challenging
PUSH	*4 POINT PUSH UP HOLDS*	30 sec – 3 min holds	1-3	30-90 seconds (active)	Keep TVA contracted, and spine in neutral
PULL	*PULL UPS*	Till fatigue	1-3	30-90 seconds (active)	May have to use assistance if client do at least 5 reps
BEND	*BENT OVER ROW*	15-25	1-3	30-90 seconds (active)	Keep scapula-humerus rhythm until end range
LUNGE	*MULTI PLANAR LUNGE*	15-25 total lunges	1-3	30-90 seconds (active)	Keep scapula retracted/ depressed

ROUNDED SHOULDER PATTERN

POSTURAL DEVIATIONS

Head - *forward and neck hyper-extended*

Scapulae - *more than 2 inches from the spine, medial borders not parallel-winged, inferior angle not articulating with ribs*

Humerus - *internally rotated, palms facing backwards*

Thoracic - *increased kyphotic curve*

POSSIBLE WEAK MUSCLES

Rhomboids

Mid/Lower Trapezius

Serratus Anterior

Teres Minor / Infraspinatus

Posterior Deltoids

Longus Coli / Capitus

POSSIBLE TIGHT MUSCLES

Pectoralis Major/Minor

Levator Scapulae

Upper Trapezius

Latissimus Dorsi

Subscapularis

Sternocleidomastoid

PELVIC TILT PATTERN

HEALTH HISTORY ORTHOPEDIC AND LIFESTYLE INFORMATION	• Office job, sits large part of the day • Experiences some low back pain • SI joint instability, pre-post natal • Possible sore muscles: adductors, rectus femoris, superficial erector spinae and psoas • Common injuries: hamstrings, adductor strains and ankle sprains • Client wears high-heeled shoes often • Tightness in hips and low back • Over training of cycle sports
POSTURAL ASSESSMENT EVALUATION	• Lumbar hyperextension • Anterior pelvic tilt • Noticeable abdomen distension • Does not distribute weight evenly on both legs
DYNAMIC ASSESSMENT EVALUATION	• Increased hyperextension of lumbar region during push-up assessment • Unable to control TVA during leg lowering assessment • Unable to extend hip beyond neutral w/out pelvic compensation • Increased lateral sway on single leg stance and squat
FLEXIBILITY	• Tight muscles: 1) iliopsoas 2) superficial erector spinae 3) rectus femoris 4) adductors 5) upper rectus abdominus
CORE ASSESSMENT	• Weak lower abdominals • Inability to control TVA and drawing in maneuver • Over developed upper abdominals

NOTE: We do not diagnose or treat conditions. We are merely assessing and matching appropriate exercises.

PELVIC TILT PATTERN

FLEXIBILITY

STRETCH	SETS	REPS	TIME	NOTES
1. foam roll - *quads, adductors, piriformis*	1	Only one to start	30 seconds to 2 minutes (what is tolerable)	May be tender, be very careful
2. iliopsoas - *stand-ing, staggered stance*	1	3-5 each side	20-30 seconds	DO NOT FORCE (ease into motion)
3. hip flexors - *from the knees*	1	3-5 each side	20-30 seconds each side	Squeeze glutes and post. tilt pelvis
4. gastrocnemius and soleus - *against a wall, bent and straight back leg*	1	3-5 each side	20-30 seconds each side	Keep femur internally rotated
5. adductor - *standing, staggered stance*	1	3-5 each side	20-30 seconds each side	Keep TVA tight and pelvis posteriorly tilted

RESISTANCE EXERCISES

BODY PART	EXERCISE	REPS	SETS	REST	NOTES
BEND (lower body stabilization)	*SUPINE BRIDGE ON BALL*	30 seconds to 3 minutes	1-3	30-90 seconds (active)	Keep head on ball, glutes tight
PUSH	*STABILITY BALL HOLD (in push up position)*	15-25 (iso first-30 seconds)	1-3	30-90 seconds (active)	Keep TVA contracted, and spine in neutral
PULL	*BALL BACK EXTENSION*	15-25	1-3	30-90 seconds (active)	Vary arm position to change effects
TWIST	STANDING ROTATIONS (MED BALL?)	15-25	1-3	30-90 seconds (active)	Keep hips still while rotating spine
SQUAT	STRAIGHT ALIGNMENT SQUAT W/ HOLD	30 sec to 3 min holds	1-3	2-5 minutes	Everything in perfect alignment

PELVIC TILT PATTERN

POSTURAL DEVIATIONS

Lumbar - *hyper-extended*

Pelvis - *anterior tilt*

Lower Abdominals - *distended*

Feet - *pointing outward*

FUNCTIONALLY WEAK MUSCLES

Transverse Abdominus

Lower Rectus Abdominus

External Oblique

Multifidus

Gluteus Maximus

Biceps Femoris

FUNCTIONALLY TIGHT MUSCLES

Psoas

Iliacus

Superficial Erector Spinae

Upper Rectus Abdominus

Rectus Femoris

Hip Adductors

PRONATION DISTORTION PATTERN

HEALTH HISTORY ORTHOPEDIC AND LIFESTYLE INFORMATION	• Weak glutes and lower abdominals • Low back pain • Possible soreness in calves • Common injuries: sesmoiditis, plantar fascitis, posterior tibialis tendonitis, and ITB tendonitis • Wears high heeled shoes often • Often times in runners
POSTURAL ASSESSMENT EVALUATION	• Weakened or flattened arch of foot • Lower part of femur rotated medially • Knock knees (genu valgum) • Excessive Q-angle • Lower abdomen distension
DYNAMIC ASSESSMENT EVALUATION	• Poor balance standing on one foot • Feet cave in medially when on one foot • Knees go inward when doing one legged squat • Inability to extend hip beyond neutral w/out pelvic compensation
FLEXIBILITY	• Tight muscles: 1) gastrocnemieus/soleus 2) peroneals 3) TFL/ITB 4) hamstrings (biceps femoris, if LBP) 5) psoas 6) adductors
CORE ASSESSMENT	• Weak lower abdominals • Inability to control TVA and drawing in maneuver

NOTE: We do not diagnose or treat conditions. We are merely assessing and matching appropriate exercises.

PRONATION DISTORTION PATTERN

FLEXIBILITY

STRETCH	SETS	REPS	TIME	NOTES
1. foam roll - *ITB, quads, adductors, piriformis*	1	Only 1 to start	30 seconds to 2 minutes (what is tolerable)	May be tender, be very careful
2. iliopsoas - *standing, staggered stance*	1	3-5 each side	20-30 seconds	DO NOT FORCE; ease into motion
3. hamstrings - *supine, active and passive*	1	3-5 each side (bent leg and straight leg)	20-30 seconds each side	Have client use a towel or strap to help assist
4. gastrocnemius & soleus - *against a wall, bent and straight back leg*	1	3-5 each side	20-30 seconds each side	Keep femur internally rotated
5. adductor - *standing, staggered stance*	1	3-5 each side	20-30 seconds each side	Keep TVA tight and pel-vis posteriorly tilted

RESISTANCE EXERCISES

BODY PART	EXERCISE	REPS	SETS	REST	NOTES
BEND (lower body stabilization)	*4- POINT OPPOSITE ARM, LEG HOLD*	30 seconds to 2 minutes	1-3	30-90 seconds (active)	Ankle neutral, knee track over 2nd toe
PUSH	*SINGLE LEG ALT. ARM PRESS (CABLE)*	15-25	1-3	30-90 seconds (active)	Keep TVA contracted, and ankle in neutral
PULL	*SINGLE LEG ONE ARM ROW W/ TWIST*	15-25	1-3	30-90 seconds (active)	Tight TVA & control eccen-tric twist
TWIST	SINGLE LEG WOOD CHOPS	15-25	1-3	30-90 seconds (active)	Tight TVA and ankle in neutral
SQUAT	SINGLE LEG SQUAT AND REACH	15-25	1-3	30-90 seconds (active)	Ankle neutral, knee track over toe

PRONATION DISTORTION PATTERN

POSTURAL DEVIATIONS

Foot - *weakened or dropped arches*

Knees - *pointing inward*

Hip - *excessive "Q" angle at the hip*

FUNCTIONALLY WEAK MUSCLES

Posterior Tibialis

Flexor Digitorum Longus

Flexor Hallucis Longus

Anterior Tibialis

Vastus Medialis

Biceps Femoris

Hip External Rotators / Piriformis

Gluteus Medius

FUNCTIONALLY TIGHT MUSCLES

Peroneals

Gastrocnemius / Soleus

Pes Anserine group

Tensor Fascia Latae / IT Band

Psoas

CHAPTER SIXTEEN

Case Study

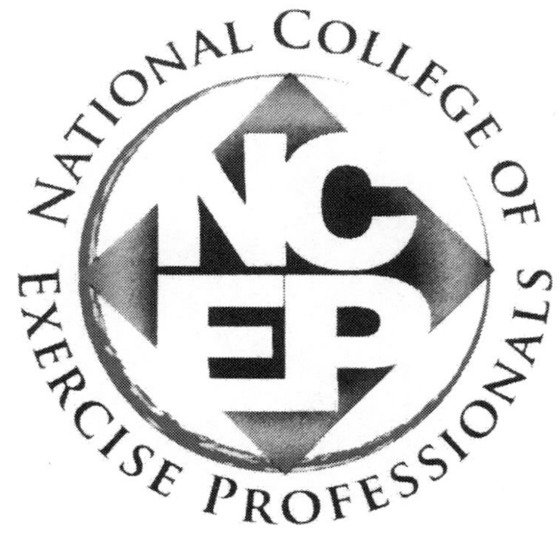

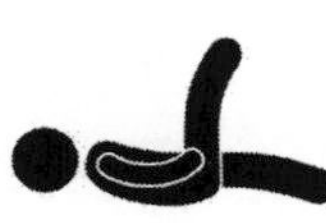
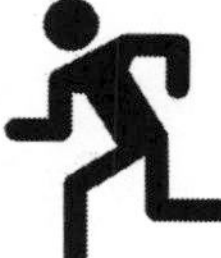

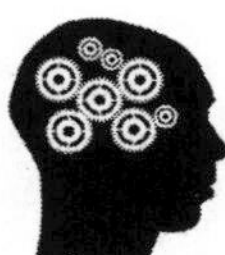

CASE STUDY

Julie Johnson is 36 years old and a mother of two. Her cholesterol level is 192. Her blood pressure is 126/87. She is 15 pounds over weight. She has off/on low back pain that her doctor says she just has to live with. She tries to get to the gym at least 2 or 3 times per week to do an aerobics class. Someone told her she should hire a personal trainer to help her, so here she is. She is willing to commit about 1 hour a day on the days she does not go to group classes.

GOAL: *to lose the 15 extra pounds and be able to play with her kids better without having to worry about her back*

1. According to the ACSM, what Risk Stratification is she?
A: *Apparently Healthy - AH*

2. What risk Cardiovascular Risk Factors does she have?
A: *NONE (although she is close on many)*

3. What Signs or Symptoms does she have for Cardiovascular Disease?
A: *NONE*

4. Based on the information provided, does she need a nutritionist referral?
A: *NO, but you may want to provide her some advice*

5. Assessments:
Flexibility - *during the overhead squat she could not go very far down, her knees went in, her feet rolled out and her butt stuck way out*
Strength -
Core: *breathes out of chest, poor TVA contraction*
Relative: *body drops during push-up test*

Balance - *wobbles on one foot and her knee starts to come in*
Vertical Jump - *maybe 6 inches*
Coordination - *poor side to side and with rotation during multi-planar step and hold*

6. Movements:
Push - *lost form with 4 point push up*
Pull - *lost form during pull up*
Bend - *bent less than 75 degrees*
Twist - *much better to the right then left*
Squat - *poor ROM and poor form*
Lunge - *poor stability both left and right*

7. Evaluation of the assessments:
It seems Julie has a need for stabilization training. She is very unstable throughout her core, and has poor ROM and needs to build a bit of strength along the way. Based on the way she moved, I will create a *CORE-based resistance program* that also incorporates flexibility for the Pelvic Tilt and Pronation Distortion Patterns.

NAME: Julie Johnson **DATE:_____** **SESSION: 1**

EXERCISE	REPS	SETS	COMMENTS
Belly breathing w/ BP cuff	15-25 breaths if possible	1-2	Do not let pressure change
Foam roll: calves, inner leg, outer leg, front of leg, side of butt	1-2 minutes each	1-2	Stay on the part that you feel discomfort
Balance on one leg - use a toe from the other foot if needed	Hold as long as you can up to 2 minutes	1-2	Keep your TVA tight, squeeze your toes into the ground
4 point hold - work up to lifting one hand (iso-push)	Hold as long as you can up to 2 minutes	1-2	Keep shoulder blades squeezed together
Form squats with med ball rotations (iso-squat, twist)	Go down slowly, Hold bottom position 10 rotations each way	1-2	Go down as far as you can in perfect form, TVA tight, chest up, knees over toes
Lunge and hold with cable pulls (iso-lunge, pull)	Hold lunge as long as you can and try to do 15-25 reps	1-2	Keep feet pointing straight, body straight up, TVA tight
Multi-planar step and hold	3-5 reps in each direction	1-2	Hold each position until your leg is not wobbling; drag other toe if needed

WARM UP: dynamic warm up done after foam rolling
TOTAL TIME: between 50-60 minutes 3-5 days/week for 2 to 4 weeks

CHAPTER SEVENTEEN

Becoming an Exercise Professional

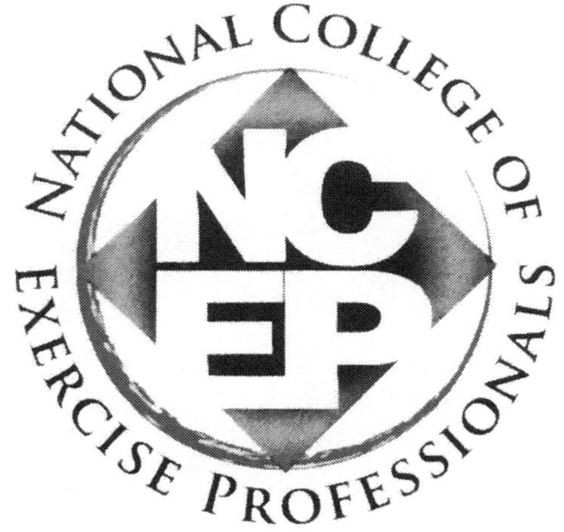

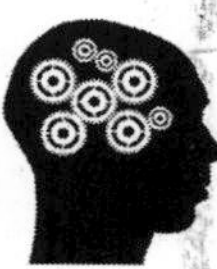

EXERCISE PROFESSIONAL

You will often hear this common refrain as your enter the fitness industry: results are the most important thing for the client. Yet, the same is true for you in your career as a trainer. In order to stay in the industry and be successful, you must achieve professional success. Learning how to become, as we iterated throughout this manual, an "exercise professional" is vital—and it is the "professional" part that has its own separate skillset that must be learned and internalized. Being knowledgeable about health and fitness, and even being a brilliant trainer on the floor with a client, does not necessarily mean that you are well-versed in professionalism. After all, it does not matter how great you may be as a trainer if you are not able to convince clients to train with you!

To be fair, most personal trainers prefer to only instruct fitness, often declaring that they do not like to "sell." However, in reality, once you position yourself as a trainer and employee, you are constantly "selling" yourself and your services. However, the great thing about working in the health and fitness industry is that we are selling something that we all strongly believe in: health and fitness as a lifestyle. Truly believing in fitness—not to mention being knowledgeable about it—makes it easy for us to sell personal training and fitness programs. The key is knowing how to effectively present the sale opportunity and effectively closing the sale. This chapter outlines a few of our strategies for becoming an exercise professional and tips for your sales approach.

"Sales Through Service" Approach

We at the National College of Exercise Professionals advocate the "Sales Through Service" approach, which was originally developed by the Sports Club Company (see our history). This philosophy is simple: when you provide great service, you are also *selling* your services. While you do not want to completely give your service away, it is important to give potential clients a "sample" of what you can offer. For example, in the restaurant industry, a chef will occasionally give a small sample so that people will become intrigued and want to have more. As for you, a great exercise professional will provide the service of posture tips, exercise suggestions and encouragement for helping a person change his/her lifestyle. This creates a connection and a entry level of trust that will naturally lead to the opportunity to present your services in full.

In the fitness industry, some people discourage offering a "free first workout" because if you give your product or service away, it has no perceived value. For example, doctors do not give away a free first visit and lawyers rarely give away their time. However, due to the prevalence of the free first session in our industry, at the very least, we suggest that a trainer provide a *complimentary consultation/assessment*. For those that do chose to offer a free first workout, it may be advantageous to perform two sessions as part of the introductory program; remember, the first workout is not really a workout, usually entailing a client's health history, goal setting, and assessments (and then maybe a few exercises). In doing this, you should always explain to the potential client that you will be designing an exercise program based on his/her health history, goals, and assessments. Then, he/she will be able to truly experience your workout design and personal training services.

NCEP CONSULTATION

1. Health History - *Fill out for the prospective client to build trust and respect; ask "why" to find his/her deeper motivations; use Stability Balls if available to introduce core stabilization and balance principles*

2. Risk Stratification (AH, IR, KD) - *If IR or KD, physician's clearance form needed; must stop until form is completed and may have to reschedule*

3. Discuss the 5 Components of Fitness - *Nutritional Strategy, ROM/Flexibility Training, Cardiovascular Training, Resistance Training, and Attitude Training; also discuss core/balance/stability training, power/speed, and Athletic Performance Enhancement Training*

4. SMFR – *Foam Rolling (demonstrate and discuss to show knowledge)*

5. Core - *4 Point Assessment; TVA breathing; core training introduction using mat exercises and Stability Ball*

6. Flexibility - *Active/Dynamic stretching introduction*

7. Assessments - *Overhead Squat Assessment, then Gait Assessment*

   ------ (if time) ------

8. Cardiovascular Training - *Level 1: Testing Phase (Talk Test, Leveling Test, and Recovery Test)*

Save at least 5-10 minutes for presentation of personal training services and/or schedule next appointment.

NOTE: During the consultation, remember to drop "seeds" throughout each of these activities, making sure to communicate to your potential client your vast array of fitness knowledge. So, when you sit down with this individual for the final 5-10 minutes, it is not the first time you are expressing why he/she should train with you.

Another tip during your consultation hour is that when you ask questions/communicate with your client, ask "closed-ended" (i.e., yes/no) questions, such as: "are you having a good time?" and "can you see yourself doing this on a continual basis?" This helps limit the intimidation factor.

Understanding Sales and the "Menu"

As you see above in our sample consultation, it is vital to save at least a few minutes at the end of the consultation or complimentary session(s) to present the personal training packages and explain the costs and process of signing up. To accomplish this, it is essential to have a professional price sheet. If you are working at a health club or gym, they will undoubtedly have their own club price sheet for personal training services. Conversely, if you are working independently or starting your own program, you will want to create a sharp looking price sheet with your name, company name and/or logo at the top. How much you charge will depend on several factors including your level of expertise, the facility, and the going rate in your community (i.e., the cost of services differs in various parts of the country). For example, some trainers charge hundreds of dollars per session and some offer their service for a much lower rate. It is important to be honest and realistic with your pricing—while you do not want to undersell your services, you also want to avoid a price that may appear overpriced when all these factors are considered. Regardless of the cost for one session, it is common in our industry (and many other retail sales environments) to lower the unit price for a larger package. Here is an example of the price sheet breakdown:

Personal Training Packages

AMOUNT	COST PER SESSION	TOTAL	SAVINGS
1 session	$75	$75	--
3 sessions	$70	$210	6% off per session
5 sessions	$65	$325	13% off per session
10 sessions	$55	$550	17% off per session
20 sessions	$50	$1000	23% off per session

While you will develop your own strategies as you gain experience, we have a specific four step strategy that you can follow once you place a price sheet—or what we like to think of as a "menu"—in front of your potential client. (We will refer to the one above for this example.)

STEP ONE: *While you hold the price sheet, discuss that a session regularly costs $75. Note that we think this should be the only time you mention a dollar value (unless he/she asks, of course).*

STEP TWO: *Then, show client that the best value is the 20 session package because of the 23% savings. Again, we recommend that you do not mention dollar amount because he/she can already see it.*

STEP THREE: *Next, while still holding the price sheet, point to one of the middle packages and say: "This one is the best one for you" or "this is one of our most popular packages," or a similar refrain. What you pick out depends on the individual; for a person who seems adamant about hiring a trainer, you might recommend the 10 session package whereas you might recommended the 3 session package for a person who seems more hesitant or unsure.*

STEP FOUR: *Finally, gently hand the "menu" to the individual and politely ask: "which one do you like?," or a similar refrain. This final step is key, and we recommend that you do not say anything more—give the potential client the opportunity to think, and we do not recommend applying pressure or "hardselling."*

To be sure, there are many people in the fitness industry who practice hard selling techniques and attempt to make people feel guilty about their health and fitness. These trainers also use psychological techniques to coerce people into signing up for a package. However, these are the same people who seldom follow up with quality service and true commitment to changing someone's life, and often give our industry a bad reputation. While there may be times to provide a gentle nudge and encourage a person to take the first step, it is important that you let them make the decision and be professional at all times. We advocate using a polite, professional, service-oriented sales approach and we believe that this approach will lead to long-term sales and business success.

A quick note about the logistics of personal training packages: it is also important to have an expiration date on the package, that you clearly state a twenty-four hour cancellation policy (or he/she will be charged for the session), and that the sessions are non-refundable and non-transferable. That being said, we also believe that it is good business to operate by a philosophy of "Do the Right Thing" and not just sticking to your policies. There may be situations where you will refund a client (for example because of a family emergency), and where you will excuse a late cancellation or no show. Yet, you also must avoid allowing people to take advantage of your good nature and you should always explain your policy clearly when you are making an exception and let them know that it is a special situation.

The Importance of Personality and Professionalism

Another component of building trust and establishing a business relationship with clients revolves around your personality. In fact, most successful trainers are very gregarious and positive—they are the "host of the party" type of people. Fitness can be a very fun experience and, like we discussed back in the first chapter, people like trainers who help them feel happy and motivated. However, there is also a place for trainers who are stoic and stern, as some people prefer a trainer who acts like a drill sergeant. Just remember that people naturally gravitate towards others who are like them, so be true to yourself and your personality, and you will find your niche.

Finally, understand that professional etiquette is also critical to your success and top trainers always conduct themselves with class and integrity. It is extremely important to be polite, punctual, well-mannered, dignified, humble, and honest. Also note that the fitness industry is a physical environment and people are often wearing clothing that can be revealing. Sexual comments and innuendo are completely inappropriate and we also caution entering into a romantic relationship with clients or with co-workers. As for attire, the best approach is Casual Professional. The fitness industry obviously involves movement and therefore the clothing should be comfortable fitting and either light or warm depending on the exact temperature of the training environment. However, your outfit should always look sharp, and be clean and neat. The same goes for hygiene and overall appearance. In fact, the "Casual Professional" approach is also excellent for your general attitude. You should feel relaxed and comfortable when talking to clients, but always maintain a sense of polite professionalism. While each of these tips seem like common sense, you would be surprised how many trainers—potentially great ones—whose failure to abide by these simple guidelines hinder their success.

One of the keys to great success is education and we believe that it is important that you keep an attitude of always learning and always growing. Be proud of the education that you have and continue to add more knowledge and more credentials. Also, be sure to proudly include your education on your resume, marketing materials, and website.

A Note About Your Options in the Fitness Industry

We would be remiss if we did not acknowledge that there is always an initial (and ongoing) consideration for the exercise professional: to work in a corporate or company gym, or become an independent trainer. There are pros and cons to both, and we generally recommend that for a first-time trainer, working in a gym/health club is the best option. The advantage of working as a trainer for a club company is that they will usually take care of insurance, marketing, purchasing equipment, billing, and collections. They will often also handle sales, difficult customers, and other liability issues. In addition, if they are a quality company, they provide leadership, mentoring, and the opportunity to advance. On the other hand, if you work independently, you will keep all of the gross income for yourself or your own company. While you will have the expenses of insurance and the added responsibilities of finding a location, buying and maintaining equipment, etc., you will have the opportunity to build and shape your own business and company to your liking.

Overall, the great thing about our industry is that there are many amazing opportunities for success. You can become a top trainer, move into management with a club company, start your own fitness company, become a fitness blogger, create new programs, make videos/media, become an educator, etc. Whatever you choose to do, you can go on to change the world—and many individuals' lives—through teaching about fitness. Your success is up to you and there are truly no limits to what you can achieve.

ABOUT NCEP

The Origins: A Need for Holistic Personal Training

The National College of Exercise Professionals (NCEP) has a unique history, one that is organic in growth and has evolved over time. NCEP was born out of the original Sports Club Company in Los Angeles in the late 1990s where Michael DeMora, the Founder and President of NCEP, was a Fitness Manager for the Sports Club Company. Eventually, Mike became the Director of Education for the prestigious Spectrum Clubs, a new (at the time) gym chain that branched out of the Sports Club Company.

In this position of Director of Education, Mike came in contact with hundreds of clients who appreciated his holistic approach to health and fitness, and the type of functional training that became a staple of the gym chains he managed. Out of these experiences, combined with his elite education with two masters degrees, Mike realized that there was a need—a need for a "better" way to educate people about health and fitness that went beyond the confines of a gym and encompassed wholesale lifestyle changes. Thus, operating out of a local office in Southern California, Mike created NCEP as an alternative personal training certification, along with other courses, that focused on functional training through a holistic approach. Throughout the 2000s, NCEP has taught over thousands of trainers, or more accurately, what we like to call "exercise professionals," who have gone on to great success in the field. Since these early days, he has worked to build NCEP from the grassroots—focusing on people, relationships, and cutting-edge research in ways that make NCEP different among its competitors.

NCEP in the Present: Re-imagining Personal Training Certification

Remaining faithful to Mike's founding, today, NCEP is a rapidly growing company seeking to offer would-be personal trainers a more hands-on way to seek certification through our acclaimed Standard Certification course, among other courses we offer. NCEP is now national in scope, teaching courses in cities all over the United States with a team of instructors and exercise professionals committed to "teaching it forward" in a personalized way.

While we are a smaller company than some of the certification mills in our industry, we are growing in our reputation and recognition. As we like to say in our courses, "we're small but we're mighty" or as Shakespeare wrote, "though she be but little, she is fierce." We continue to work harder and smarter than our competition, and offer a lower price with a much better value—and pride ourselves on doing things the "right way" no matter what.

The NCEP Difference: A Unique Focus on Functional Training

There are many significant difference between the National College of Exercise Professionals and other organizations, and those who take our courses know why. For starters, we are a fitness education industry group dedicated to the most cutting-edge exercise science, primarily in the form of "functional training." The best gym club companies in the fitness industry are embracing the functional training approach—and we truly believe that our methods take this approach to an even higher level while still being the foundation of our Standard Certification course. We also offer a variety of other proprietary courses and continuing education workshops related to functional training, such as what we refer to as Athletic Performance Enhancement (APE) and a focus on bio-mechanics and advanced body assessments. The fact that we also include these various philosophies as part of our introductory course illustrates our commitment to functional training and focus on human movement.

NCEP is accredited by the National Exercise Therapy Association National Board of Certification, and we work with many high end health club companies around the country. We are a preferred certification and education provider for the Sports Club Company (owners and operators of the Sports Club/LA clubs across the country), the Oregon Athletic Clubs (an elite club chain in the Portland area), the Honolulu Club (the finest club in the state of Hawaii), and others. We have also worked closely with many other top national club companies including the Spectrum Clubs, Lifetime Fitness, Golds Gym, Fitness 19, Retro Fitness, in addition to being an accepted certification at large gym chains such as Equinox Sports Clubs and 24-Hour Fitness.

Putting the "Personal" in Personal Training Certifications

Finalyl, another major difference in our approach is our personalized model of education. While many—if not most—other certification companies require online exams at a testing center, we strongly believe in teaching our classes live and in person. We believe that people learn best with visual interaction and demonstration because, after all, personal fitness itself is based on personal interactions and demonstrations between trainer and client. Online tests, we feel, are antithetical to our industry despite its widespread prevalence and convenience for the certification companies. Instead, all of our courses are taught in-person, and we maintain a low student to faculty ratio often generally under 15 students per class to offer a more conducive atmosphere to learn. We believe firmly in "getting out" into communities and teaching our classes at the club level. Most of all, what makes our courses special is our staff dedicated to teaching students the most up to date information in an easily digestible manner. Our courses offer a holistic approach to fitness, and always include information about sales and professional etiquette—we seek to make sure individuals who take our course are not just ready to become personal trainers, but true "exercise professionals" in the field.

For more information, please visit ncepfitness.com.

JOIN THE MOVEMENT

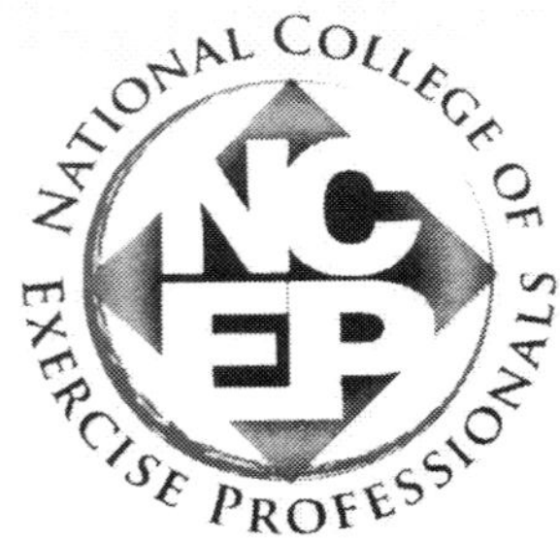

NOTES

Made in the USA
San Bernardino, CA
25 January 2018